Intraoperative Neurophysiological Monitoring

Second Edition

Intraoperative Neurophysiological Monitoring

Second Edition

Aage R. Møller, PhD

University of Texas at Dallas
Dallas, TX

HUMANA PRESS ✳ TOTOWA, NEW JERSEY

Production Editor: Jennifer Hackworth

Cover design by Patricia F. Cleary

For additional copies, pricing for bulk purchases, and/or information about other Humana titles, contact Humana at the above address or at any of the following numbers: Tel.: 973-256-1699; Fax: 973-256-8341; E-mail: orders@humanapr.com; or visit our www.humanapress.com

eISBN: 978-1-59745-018-8

Printed in the United States of America. 10 9 8 7 6 5 4 3

Library of Congress Cataloging-in-Publication Data

Møller, Aage R.
  Intraoperative neurophysiological monitoring / Aage R. Møller. -- 2nd ed.
    p. cm.
  Includes bibliographical references and index.
  ISBN 978-1-58829-703-7 (alk. paper)
   1. Neurophysiologic monitoring. 2. Evoked potentials (Electrophysiology) I. Title.

  RD52.N48M65 2006
  617.4'8--dc22

                                        2005050259

Preface

This book is based on two earlier works: Aage R. Møller: *Evoked Potentials in Intraoperative Monitoring* published in 1988 by Williams and Wilkens; and more directly by Aage R Møller: *Intraoperative Neurophysiologic Monitoring* published in 1995 by Gordon and Breach under the imprint of Harwood academic publishers. The present book represents an expansion and extensive rewriting of the 1995 book. In particular, new chapters related to monitoring of the spinal motor system and deep brain stimulation (DBS) have been added. The anatomical and physiological basis for these techniques are described in detail as are the practical aspects of such monitoring. Chapters on monitoring of sensory systems and monitoring in skull base surgery have been rewritten as has the chapter on monitoring of peripheral nerves.

The general principles of intraoperative monitoring are discussed in Section I where Chapter 2 describes the basis for intraoperative monitoring and Chapter 3 discusses the various forms of electrical activity that can be recorded from nerve fibers and nerve cells; near-field activity from nerves, nuclei, and muscles recorded with monopolar and bipolar electrodes. This chapter also discusses far-field potentials and the responses from injured nerves and nuclei. Chapter 4 discusses practical aspects of recording evoked potentials from nerves, nuclei, and muscles including a discussion of various stimulus techniques.

Section II covers sensory systems. Chapter 5 covers the anatomy and physiology of the auditory, somatosensory and visual systems. Monitoring of the auditory system is covered in Chapter 6; Chapter 7 covers monitoring the somatosensory system and Chapter 8, monitoring the visual system.

Section III discusses motor systems. The anatomy and physiology that is of interest for intraoperative monitoring is discussed in Chapter 9 and practical aspects of the spinal motor and brainstem motor systems are covered in Chapters 10 and 11, respectively.

Section IV is devoted to peripheral nerves, and Chapter 12 covers the anatomy and physiology, whereas Chapter 13 discusses practical aspects of monitoring peripheral nerves.

Section V discusses different ways that intraoperative electrophysiological recordings can guide the surgeon in an operation. Chapter 14 discusses methods to identify motor and sensory nerves and map the spinal cord and the floor of the fourth ventricle. Chapter 15 describes methods that can guide the surgeon in an operation, such as microvascular decompression operations for hemifacial spasm and placement of electrodes for DBS and for making lesions in the thalamus and basal ganglia.

Section VI discusses practical aspects of intraoperative monitoring. Chapter 16 covers the role of anesthesia in monitoring and Chapter 17 discusses general matters regarding monitoring such as how to reduce the risk of mistakes and how to reduce the effect of electrical interference of recorded neuroelectrical potentials. Chapter 18 discusses equipment and data analysis related to intraoperative monitoring. This chapter also discusses electrical stimulation of nervous tissue. The final chapter, Chapter 19 discusses the importance of evaluation of the benefits of intraoperative neurophysiological monitoring, to the patient, the surgeon, and the field of surgery in general.

Aage R. Møller

Acknowledgments

I have had valuable help from many individuals in writing this book. Mark Steckert, MD, PhD, provided important comments on several aspects of this second edition.

I want to thank Hilda Dorsett for preparing much of the new artwork and for revising some of the illustrations from the first edition of the book. I thank Renee Workings for help with editing the manuscript and Karen Riddle for transcribing many of the revisions of the manuscript.

I also want to thank Richard Lansing and Jennifer Hackworth, production editor, of Humana Press for their excellent work on the book.

I would not have been able to write this book without the support from the School of Behavioral and Brain Sciences at the University of Texas at Dallas.

Last but not least I want to thank my wife, Margareta B. Møller, MD, PhD, for her support during writing of this book and for her valuable comments on earlier versions of the book manuscript.

Aage R. Møller

Contents

SECTION VI: PRACTICAL ASPECTS OF ELECTROPHYSIOLOGICAL RECORDING IN THE OPERATING ROOM

1

Introduction

Surgery can generally be regarded as a risk-filled method for treating diseases, and it has a potential for causing injury to the nervous system. Because such injuries might not be detected by visual inspection of the operative field by the surgeon, they could occur and progress without the surgeon's knowledge. Intraoperative neurophysiological monitoring involves the use of neurophysiological recordings for detecting changes in the function of the nervous system that are caused by surgically induced insults.

Intraoperative recording of neuroelectric potentials makes it possible to assess function nearly continuously throughout an operation. Although evoked potentials are important in making clinical diagnoses, there are often alternative methods available to obtain the required information in the clinical setting, such as imaging modalities (computed axial tomography [CAT] and magnetic resonance imaging [MRI]), which have made evoked potentials and other electrophysiological studies less important for clinical diagnosis of neurological disorders. However, although the CAT scan is available in a few operating rooms (mainly for stereotaxic surgery and biopsy), it is not practical for monitoring neural injuries, at least not yet. Imaging methods mainly detect changes in structures, whereas neurophysiological methods assess changes in function, therefore providing obvious advantages for intraoperative monitoring.

Appropriate use of intraoperative recording of various types of neuroelectric potential makes it possible to assess the function of specific parts of the nervous system continuously during an operation and detect changes in neural function with little delay. Early detection of such functional changes can reduce the risk of postoperative deficits caused by iatrogenic injuries to the nervous system. These methods makes it possible to identify which specific surgical step has

caused a problem so that the surgeon can reverse the step that caused the injuries before they become severe enough to result in permanent neurological deficits.

The benefits to the patient and to the surgeon of using appropriate neurophysiological monitoring methods during operations in which neural tissue is at risk of being injured are well recognized, and intraoperative neurophysiological monitoring is now widely practiced in many hospitals in connection with such operations. Individuals on the neurophysiological monitoring team are now accepted as members of the operating room team. Although monitoring of patients' vital signs in the operating room has been done for many years, monitoring the function of the nervous system is a relatively new addition to the operating room and it has a wider range of applications than just the monitoring function.

During the late 1970s and early 1980s, the application of electrophysiological methods in the operating room was primarily focused within university centers and a few large hospitals. It soon became evident that standard laboratory techniques transplanted to the operating room could reduce the risk of inadvertently injuring neural tissue and thereby reduce the risk of permanent neurological deficits. This new use of standard laboratory techniques became known as intraoperative neurophysiological monitoring.

Routine use of intraoperative neurophysiological monitoring developed during the 1980s, and during that time, intraoperative neurophysiological monitoring got its own society in the United States (the American Society for Neurophysiological Monitoring [ASNM]).

Although it is assumed that the era of intraoperative neurophysiological monitoring started in the late 1970s, electrophysiological methods were used in the operating room for the purpose of reducing the risk of permanent neurological deficits even before that time. In the early 1960s, monitoring of the facial nerve

From: *Intraoperative Neurophysiological Monitoring: Second Edition*
By A. R. Møller
© Humana Press Inc., Totowa, NJ.

was mainly done to reduce the risks of facial paresis or palsy after operations for vestibular schwannoma *(1,2)*.

Leonid Malis, a neurosurgeon, used recordings of evoked potentials from the sensory cortex in his neurosurgical operations. Malis, however, fascinated by the development of microneurosurgery, stated later that microneurosurgery had made intraoperative monitoring unnecessary *(3)* although others expressed the opposite opinion in support of the usefulness of intraoperative monitoring *(4)*.

Orthopedic surgery was one of the first specialties to make systematic use of intraoperative neurophysiological monitoring, particularly in operations involving the spine. In the 1970s, work by Dr. Richard Brown, a neurophysiologist, reduced the risk of damage to the spinal cord during scoliosis operations by using recordings of somatosensory evoked potentials *(5,6)*, and intraoperative neurophysiological monitoring has been used for several decades for many additional types of neurosurgical operations *(5)*.

Monitoring of auditory brainstem evoked responses (ABRs) was also one of the earliest applications of intraoperative neurophysiological monitoring and was used in microvascular decompression (MVD) operations for hemifacial spasm (HFS) and trigeminal neuralgia pioneered by Grundy *(7)* and Raudzens *(8)* in the early 1980s and others *(9,10)* thereafter. Direct recordings from the exposed intracranial structures such as the eighth cranial nerve and the cochlear nucleus decreased the time to get an interpretable record *(11,12)*. Such recordings had been used earlier for research purposes *(13)*.

In the 1980s, intraoperative neurophysiological monitoring was introduced in operations for large skull base tumors *(14,15)* and later by other investigators *(16)*. Intraoperative neurophysiological monitoring for such operations could involve monitoring of cranial motor nerves, including CN III, IV, and VI, especially for tumors involving the cavernous sinus, and the motor portion of CN V (portio minor).

Later, intraoperative monitoring of the function of the ear and the auditory nerve came into general use by neurosurgeons and its use

spread to other surgical specialties, such as otoneurological surgery and to plastic surgery, where it serves mainly to preserve the function of peripheral nerves.

The spread of the use of intraoperative neurophysiological monitoring to other types of hospital came in the beginning of the 1990s when also certification processes were established by the American Board for Neurophysiological Monitoring, (ABNM) that certifies Diplomats of the American Board for Neurophysiological Monitoring (DABNM). Certification in Neurophysiological Intraoperative Neurophysiological Monitoring (CNIM) is available through the American Board of Registration of Electroencephalographic and Evoked Potential Technologists (ABRET).

While the techniques that were used in the beginning of the era of intraoperative neurophysiological monitoring were transplanted from the animal laboratories, the increased use of intraoperative neurophysiological monitoring promoted the development of specialized techniques to become commercially available by several companies.

Methods for monitoring of spinal motor systems advanced during the 1990s with the development of techniques using magnetic *(17)* and electrical stimulation *(18)* of the motor cortex and stimulation of the spinal cord *(19)*. Methods that provided satisfactory anesthesia and also permitted activation of motor system by stimulation of the motor cortex were developed *(20,21)*.

Intraoperative neurophysiological monitoring is an inexpensive and effective method for reducing the risk of permanent postoperative deficits in many different operations where nervous tissue is being manipulated. It provides real-time monitoring of function to an extent that makes it superior to imaging methods that provide information about structure and that are impractical for use in the operating room. Intraoperative neurophysiological monitoring relates to the spirit of the Hippocratic oath: namely "Do no harm." We might not be able to relieve suffering from illness, but we should at least not harm the patient in our attempts to relieve the patient from illness. Intraoperative neurophysiological monitoring provides an example in medicine and surgery of improvements accomplished specifically by reducing failures and, thus, improving performance by reducing failures, a principle that is now regarded with great importance in the design of complex applications, such as in military procedures and space exploration.

Although the greatest benefit of intraoperative neurophysiological monitoring is that it provides the possibility to reduce the risk of postoperative neurological deficits, it can also be of great value to the surgeon by providing other information about the effects of the surgeon's manipulations that is not otherwise available. Intraoperative recordings of neuroelectric potentials can help the surgeon identify specific neural structures, making it possible to determine the location of neural blockage on a nerve. Intraoperative neurophysiological recordings can often help the surgeon carry out the operation and, in some cases, to determine when the therapeutic goal of the operation has been achieved. Intraoperative neurophysiological monitoring can often give the surgeon a justified increased feeling of security.

We are now seeing the beginning of an era of treatment of certain movement disorders and severe pain that moves away from the use of medications and toward the use of complex procedures such as deep brain stimulation (DBS) and other forms of functional intervention, some of which involve prompting the expression of neural plasticity.

Using neurophysiological methods is critical for treatments using DBS and selective lesioning of brain tissue for treating movement disorders and severe pain. The obvious advantage of such procedures as DBS and selective lesions is that the treatment is directed specifically to structures that are involved in producing the symptoms, whereas other general medical (pharmaceutical) treatment, even when applied in accordance with the best known experience, is much less specific and often has severe side effects and limited beneficial effect. Although any licensed physician can prescribe any drug, even such drugs that have complex actions and known and unknown side effects, procedures such as DBS can only be done, at

least adequately, by teams of experts that include members with a thorough understanding of neuroscience and the pathophysiology of the disorders that are to be treated.

There is little doubt that the use of procedures such as DBS will expand to include disorders that are currently treated with medication alone. The implementation of stimulation treatments will be broadened, consequently increasing the demands on neurosurgeons who perform these procedures, as well as neurophysiologists who are providing the neurophysiological guidance for proper placement of such stimulating electrodes.

Neurophysiology in the operating room also provides an opportunity for research and study of the normal function of the human nervous system as well as the function of the diseased nervous system. In fact, use of neurophysiology in the operating room for research was practiced before it came into general use for intraoperative monitoring. For the neurophysiologist, the operating room offers possibilities for research that are otherwise not available. Performing studies on patients undergoing neurosurgical operations often makes it possible to do intracranial recordings in a unique way to examine the normal functions of parts of the nervous system that are not affected by the disorder for which the patient is undergoing the operation. Electrophysiological recording during operations also offers unique possibilities to study the pathophysiology of disease processes, because it is possible to record electrical activity directly from the parts of the nervous system that are affected by the disease.

There are two kinds of research that can be done in the operating room. The first is basic research, the purpose of which is to gain new knowledge but no direct benefit to patients is expected. However, experience has taught us that even basic research can provide (unexpected) immediate as well as long-term benefit to patient treatment. The other kind of research, applied research, has as its aim to provide immediate improvement of treatment, including reduction of postoperative deficits. This means that both types of research can be beneficial to the patients either in providing better therapeutic achievements or by reducing the risk of postoperative permanent neurological deficits.

There are several advantages of doing research in the operating room. Humans are different from animals and the results are directly applicable to humans. Second, but not least, it is easier to study the physiology of diseased systems in humans than trying to make animal models of diseases. Humans can respond and tell you how they feel, which is an advantage when evaluating results of, for instance, efforts to reduce postoperative deficits.

Research in the operating room has a longer history that intraoperative neurophysiological monitoring. One of the first surgeons-scientists who understood the value of research in the neurosurgical operating room was Wilder Penfield (1891–1976), who founded the Montreal Neurological Institute in 1934. Penfield was a neurosurgeon who had a solid background in neurophysiology, inspired by Sherrington during a Rhodes Scholarship to Oxford. He stated that, "Brain surgery is a terrible profession. If I did not feel it will become different in my lifetime, I should hate it," (1921). Penfield might be regarded as the founder of intraoperative neurophysiological research and he did ground-breaking work in many areas of neuroscience. His work on the somatosensory system is especially known (22,23). In the 1950s, he used electrical stimulation to find epileptic foci, and in connection with these operations, he did extensive studies of the temporal lobe, especially with regard to memory.

Other neurosurgeons have followed Penfield's tradition, such as George A. Ojemann, who has contributed much to understanding pathologies related to the temporal lobe as well as to provide basic research regarding memory and, in particular, regarding the large individual variations of the brain. Like Penfield, he operated on many patients for epilepsy, and during these operations, he mapped the temporal lobe and studied the centers for memory and speech using electrical current to inactivate specific regions of the brain in patients who were awake and therefore were able to respond and perform memory tasks.

Ojemann, working with Otto Creutzfeldt from Germany, developed methods for microelectrode recordings from the brain of awake patients. They studied neuronal activity during face recognition, but their studies also contributed to the development of the use of microelectrodes in recordings from the human brain.

A neurologist, Gaston Celesia, has expanded our knowledge about the organization of the human cerebral cortex by recordings of evoked responses directly from the surface of the human auditory cortex (24,25). Celesia mapped the auditory cortex in humans and studied somatosensory evoked potentials from the thalamus and primary somatosensory cortex (26). Other investigators have studied other structures such as the dorsal column nuclei, the cochlear nucleus, and the inferior colliculus in patients undergoing neurosurgical operations where these structures became exposed (27–30). The methods used to record evoked potentials from the surface of the cochlear nucleus by inserting an electrode into the lateral recess of the fourth ventricle (28,31) became a useful method for monitoring the integrity of the auditory nerve in operations for vestibular schwannoma, where preservation of hearing was attempted (32), as well as in microvascular decompression operations for trigeminal neuralgia, hemifacial spasm, and disabling positional vertigo.

Studies of the neural generators of the ABR have likewise benefited from recordings from structures that became exposed during neurosurgical operations. Recordings from the auditory nerve that were first published in 1981 by two groups, one in Japan (Isao Hashimoto, neurosurgeon) (33) and one in the United States (13) showed that the auditory nerve is the generator of two vertex positive deflections in the auditory brainstem responses, whereas the auditory nerve in small animals such as the rhesus monkey is the generator of only one (major) peak (34–36).

The neurosurgeon Fred Lenz has studied the responses from nerve cells in the thalamus in awake humans using microelectrodes and mapped the thalamus with regard to involvement in painful stimulation as well as in response to innocuous somatosensory stimulation *(37–39)*.

Electrophysiological studies of patients undergoing MVD operations for HFS have supported the hypothesis that the anatomical location of the physiological abnormalities that cause the symptoms of HFS is central to the location of vascular contact with the facial nerve (the facial motonucleus) *(40)* involving mechanisms similar to the kindling phenomenon (described in refs. *41* and *42*), and not primarily caused by ephaptic transmission at the location of the vascular contact that caused the symptoms as another hypothesis had postulated. The findings that a specific sign, the abnormal muscle response (or lateral spread response), disappears when the offending blood vessel is moved off the facial nerve *(43)* is now widely used in such operations as a guide to the surgeon in finding the vessel that is the culprit and in effectively decompressing the facial nerve. It has increased the success rate of the operation, decreased the operating time, and reduced the risk that a reoperation would be necessary. This is again an example of how studies undertaken for pure basic science can result in practical methods that increase the efficacy of an operation, and this case in particular essentially eliminated the need of reoperations, which were not uncommon before that method was introduced.

These examples show clearly that there is no sharp border between basic and applied research. The method used for studies of neural generators for the ABR came into use for monitoring the auditory nerve. Research on speech and language centers in the brain has proven to be important for epilepsy operations. Research on hemifacial spasm provided better outcomes of MVD operations.

Although it has been difficult to use exact scientific methods for assessing the benefits of intraoperative neurophysiological monitoring, it is my opinion based on many years of experience that the skill of the surgeon together with good use of electrophysiology in the operating room can benefit the patient who is being operated on and it can benefit many future patients by the progress in treatment that an effective collaboration between surgeons and neurophysiologists promotes.

REFERENCES

1. Hilger J. Facial nerve stimulator. *Trans. Am. Acad. Ophth. Otolaryngol.* 1964;68:74–76.
2. Kurze T. Microtechniques in neurological surgery. *Clin. Neurosurg.* 1964;11:128–137.
3. Malis LI. Intra-operative monitoring is not essential. *Clin. Neurosurg.* 1995;42:203–213.
4. Sekhar LN, Bejjani G, Nora P, Vera PL. Neurophysiological monitoring during cranial base surgery: is it necessary? *Clin. Neurosurg.* 1995;42:180–202.
5. Nash CL, Lorig RA, Schatzinger LA, Brown RH. Spinal cord monitoring during operative treatment of the spine. *Clin. Orthop.* 1977;126: 100–105.
6. Brown RH, Nash CL. Current status of spinal cord monitoring. *Spine* 1979;4:466–478.
7. Grundy B. Intraoperative monitoring of sensory evoked potentials. *Anesthesiology* 1983;58: 72–87.
8. Raudzens RA. Intraoperative monitoring of evoked potentials. *Ann. NY Acad. Sci.* 1982;388: 308–326.
9. Friedman WA, Kaplan BJ, Gravenstein D, Rhoton AL. Intraoperative brain-stem auditory evoked potentials during posterior fossa microvascular decompression. *J. Neurosurg.* 1985;62:552–557.
10. Linden R, Tator C, Benedict C, Mraz C, Bell I. Electro-physiological monitoring during acoutic neuroma and other posterior fossa surgery. *J. Sci. Neurol.* 1988;15:73–81.
11. Møller AR, Jannetta PJ. Monitoring auditory functions during cranial nerve microvascular decompression operations by direct recording from the eighth nerve. *J. Neurosurg.* 1983;59: 493–499.
12. Silverstein H, Norrell H, Hyman S. Simultaneous use of CO_2 laser with continuous monitoring of eighth cranial nerve action potential during acoustic neuroma surgery. *Otolaryngol. Head Neck Surg.* 1984;92:80–84.
13. Møller AR, Jannetta PJ. Compound action potentials recorded intracranially from the auditory nerve in man. *Exp. Neurol.* 1981;74:862–874.
14. Møller AR. Electrophysiological monitoring of cranial nerves in operations in the skull base.

In: Sekhar LN, Schramm VL, Jr. eds. *Tumors of the Cranial Base: Diagnosis and Treatment.* Mt. Kisco, NY: Futura; 1987:123–132.

15. Sekhar LN, Møller AR. Operative management of tumors involving the cavernous sinus. *J. Neurosurg.* 1986;64:879–889.

16. Yingling C, Gardi J. Intraoperative monitoring of facial and cochlear nerves during acoustic neuroma surgery. *Otolaryngol. Clin. North Am.* 1992;25:413–448.

17. Barker AT, Jalinous R, Freeston IL. Non-invasive magnetic stimulation of the human motor cortex. *Lancet* 1985;1:1106–1107.

18. Marsden CD, Merton PA, Morton HB. Direct electrical stimulation of corticospinal pathways through the intact scalp in human subjects. *Adv. Neurol.* 1983;39:387–391.

19. Deletis V. Intraoperative monitoring of the functional integrety of the motor pathways. In: Devinsky O, Beric A, Dogali M, eds. *Advances in Neurology: Electrical and Magnetic Stimualtion of the Brain.* New York: Raven; 1993:201–214.

20. Sloan TB, Heyer EJ. Anesthesia for intraoperative neurosysiologic monitoring of the spinal cord. *J. Clin. Neurophysiol.* 2002;19:430–443.

21. Sloan T. Anesthesia and motor evoked potential monitoring. In: Deletis V, Shils JL, eds. *Neurophysiology in Neurosurgery.* Amsterdam: Elsevier Science; 2002.

22. Penfield W, Boldrey E. Somatic motor and sensory representation in the cerebral cortex of man as studied by electrical stimulation. *Brain* 1937;60:389–443.

23. Penfield W, Rasmussen T. *The Cerebral Cortex of Man: A Clinical Study of Localization of Function.* New York: Macmillan; 1950.

24. Celesia GG, Broughton RJ, Rasmussen T, Branch C. Auditory evoked responses from the exposed human cortex. *Electroenceph. Clin. Neurophysiol.* 1968;24:458–466.

25. Celesia GG, Puletti F. Auditory cortical areas of man. *Neurology* 1969;19:211–220.

26. Celesia GG. Somatosensory evoked potentials recorded directly from human thalamus and Sm I cortical area. *Arch. Neurol.* 1979;36:399–405.

27. Møller AR, Jannetta PJ, Jho HD. Recordings from human dorsal column nuclei using stimulation of the lower limb. *Neurosurgery* 1990;26:291–299.

28. Møller AR, Jannetta PJ. Auditory evoked potentials recorded from the cochlear nucleus and its vicinity in man. *J. Neurosurg.* 1983;59:1013–1018.

29. Hashimoto I. Auditory evoked potentials from the humans midbrain: slow brain stem responses. *Electroenceph. Clin. Neurophysiol.* 1982;53:652–657.

30. Møller AR, Jannetta PJ. Evoked potentials from the inferior colliculus in man. *Electroenceph. Clin. Neurophysiol.* 1982;53:612–620.

31. Kuroki A, Møller AR. Microsurgical anatomy around the foramen of Luschka with reference to intraoperative recording of auditory evoked potentials from the cochlear nuclei. *J. Neurosurg.* 1995;82:933–939.

32. Møller AR, Jho HD, Jannetta PJ. Preservation of hearing in operations on acoustic tumors: An alternative to recording BAEP. *Neurosurgery* 1994;34:688–693.

33. Hashimoto I, Ishiyama Y, Yoshimoto T, Nemoto S. Brainstem auditory evoked potentials recorded directly from human brain stem and thalamus. *Brain* 1981;104:841–859.

34. Møller AR, Burgess JE. Neural generators of the brain stem auditory evoked potentials (BAEPs) in the rhesus monkey. *Electroenceph. Clin. Neurophysiol.* 1986;65:361–372.

35. Spire JP, Dohrmann GJ, Prieto PS. *Correlation of Brainstem Evoked Response with Direct Acoustic Nerve Potential.* New York: Raven; 1982.

36. Martin WH, Pratt H, Schwegler JW. The origin of the human auditory brainstem response wave II. *Electroenceph. Clin. Neurophysiol.* 1995;96:357–370.

37. Greenspan JD, Lee RR, Lenz FA. Pain sensitivity alterations as a function of lesion localization in the parasylvian cortex. *Pain* 1999;81:273–282.

38. Lenz FA, Dougherty PM. Pain processing in the ventrocaudal nucleus of the human thalamus. In: Bromm B, Desmedt JE, eds. *Pain and the Brain.* New York: Raven; 1995:175–185.

39. Lenz FA, Lee JI, Garonzik IM, Rowland LH, Dougherty PM, Hua SE. Plasticity of pain-related neuronal activity in the human thalamus. *Prog. Brain Res.* 2000;129:253–273.

40. Møller AR, Jannetta PJ. On the origin of synkinesis in hemifacial spasm: results of intracranial recordings. *J. Neurosurg.* 1984;61:569–576.

41. Goddard GV. Amygdaloid stimulation and learning in the rat. *J. Comp. Physiol. Psychol.* 1964;58:23–30.

42. Wada JA. *Kindling 2.* New York: Raven; 1981.

43. Møller AR, Jannetta PJ. Microvascular decompression in hemifacial spasm: intraoperative electrophysiological observations. *Neurosurgery* 1985;16:612–618.

PRINCIPLES OF INTRAOPERATIVE NEUROPHYSIOLOGICAL MONITORING

The basic principles of recording and stimulation of the nervous system used in intraoperative neurophysiological monitoring resemble techniques used in the clinical diagnostic laboratory with some very important differences. The electrical potentials that are recorded from the nervous system in the operating room must be interpreted immediately and are recorded under circumstances of interference of various kinds. This means that the person who does intraoperative neurophysiological monitoring must be knowledgeable about the function of the neurological systems that are monitored, how electrical potentials are generated by the nervous system, and how such potentials change as a result of pathologies that occur because of surgical manipulations. This section provides basic information about the principles of intraoperative neurophysiological monitoring. Chapter 3 describes how electrical activity is generated in the nervous system and how such electrical activity can be recorded and can be used as the basis for detecting injuries to specific parts of the peripheral and central nervous system. Chapter 4 provides some practical information about recording of neuroelectric potentials from the nervous system and how to stimulate the nervous system in anesthetized patients. This chapter also discusses how to record very small electrical potentials in an electrically hostile environment such as the operating room.

2

Basis of Intraoperative Neurophysiological Monitoring

INTRODUCTION

Intraoperative neurophysiological monitoring is often associated with reducing the risk of postoperative neurological deficits in operations where the nervous system is at risk of being permanently injured. Although the main use of electrophysiological methods in the operating room might be for reducing the risk of postoperative neurological deficits, electrophysiological methods are now in increasing use for other purposes. For example, electrophysiological methods are now regarded as necessary for guiding the placement of electrodes for deep brain stimulation or for making lesions in specific structures for treating movement disorders and pain. Intraoperative electrophysiological recordings can also help the surgeon in carrying out other surgical procedures. Finding specific neural tissue such as cranial nerves or specific regions of the cerebral cortex are examples of tasks that are included in the subspecialty of intraoperative neurophysiological monitoring. Neurophysiological methods are in increasing use for diagnostic support in operations such as those involving peripheral nerves. In certain operations, intraoperative electrophysiological recordings

From: *Intraoperative Neurophysiological Monitoring: Second Edition*
By A. R. Møller
© Humana Press Inc., Totowa, NJ.

can increase the likelihood of achieving the therapeutical goal of an operation. Intraoperative neurophysiological recordings have shown to be of help in identifying the offending blood vessel in a cranial nerve disorders (hemifacial spasm).

REDUCING THE RISK OF NEUROLOGICAL DEFICITS

The use of intraoperative neurophysiological monitoring to reduce the risk of loss of function in portions of the nervous system is based on the observation that the function of neural structures usually changes in a measurable way before being permanently damaged. By reversing the surgical manipulation that caused the change within a certain time will result in a recovery to normal or near-normal function, whereas if no intervention had been taken, there would have been a risk that permanent postoperative neurological deficit would have resulted.

Surgical manipulations such as stretching, compressing, or heating from electrocoagulation are insults that can injure neural tissue, as can ischemia caused by impairment of blood supply resulting from surgical manipulations or intentional clamping of arteries, that could also result in permanent (ischemic) injury to neural structures, causing a risk of noticeable postoperative neural deficits.

The effect of such insults represents a continuum; at one end, function decreases for the time of the insult, and at the other end of this continuum, nervous tissue is permanently damaged and normal function never recovers, thus causing permanent postoperative deficits. Between these extremes, there is a large range over which recovery can occur either totally or partially. Thus, up to a certain degree of injury, there can be total recovery, but thereafter, the neural function might be affected for some time. After more severe injury, the recovery of normal function not only takes a longer time but the final recovery would only be partial, with the degree of recovery depending on the nature, degree, and duration of the insult.

Injuries acquired during operations that result in a permanent neurological deficit will most likely reduce the quality of life for the patient for many years to come and maybe for a lifetime. Therefore, it is important that the person responsible for interpreting the results of monitoring is aware that the neurophysiologist has a great degree of responsibility, together with the surgeon and the anesthesiologist, in reducing the risk of injury to the patient during the operation.

Techniques for Reducing Postoperative Neurological Deficits

The general principle of intraoperative neurophysiological monitoring is to apply a stimulus and then to record the electrical response from specific neural structures along the neural pathway that are at risk of being injured. This can be done by recording the near-field evoked potentials by placing a recording electrode on a specific neural structure that becomes exposed during the operation or, as more commonly done, by recording the far-field evoked potentials from, for instance, electrodes placed on the surface of the scalp.

Intraoperative neurophysiological monitoring that is done for the purpose of reducing the risk of postoperative neurological deficits makes use of relatively standard and well-developed methods for stimulation and recordings of electrical activity in the nervous system. Most of the methods that are used in intraoperative neurophysiological monitoring are similar to those that are used in the physiological laboratory and in the clinical testing laboratory for many years.

Sensory System. Intraoperative neurophysiological monitoring of the function of sensory systems has been widely practiced since the middle of the 1980s. The earliest uses of intraoperative neurophysiologic monitoring of sensory systems were modeled after the clinical use of recording sensory evoked potentials for diagnostic purposes.

Sensory systems are monitored by applying an appropriate stimulus and recording the response from the ascending neural pathway, usually by placing recording electrodes on the surface of the scalp to pick up far-field potentials from nerve tracts and nuclei in the brain (far-field responses).

It has been mainly somatosensory evoked potentials (SSEPs) and auditory brainstem responses (ABRs) that have been recorded in the operating room for monitoring the function of these sensory systems for the purpose of reducing the risk of postoperative neurological deficits. Visual evoked potentials (VEPs) are also monitored in some operations. When intraoperative neurophysiological monitoring was introduced, it was first SSEPs that were monitored routinely *(1)*, followed by ABRs *(2–4)*.

Although the technique used for recording sensory evoked potentials in the operating room is similar to that used in the clinical diagnostic laboratory, there are important differences. In the operating room, it is only changes in the recorded potentials that occur during the operation that are of interest, whereas in the clinical testing laboratory, the deviation from normal values (laboratory standard) are important measures. Another important difference is that results obtained in the operating room must be interpreted instantly, which places demands on the personnel who are responsible for intraoperative neurophysiological monitoring that differ from those working in the clinical laboratory. In the operating room, it is sometimes possible to record evoked potentials directly from neural structures of sensory pathways (near-field responses) when such structures become exposed during an operation.

The use of evoked potentials in intraoperative neurophysiological monitoring for the purpose of reducing the risk of postoperative permanent sensory deficits is based on the following:

1. Electrical potentials can be recorded in response to a stimulus.
2. These potentials change in a noticeable way as a result of surgically induced changes in function.
3. Proper surgical intervention, such as reversal of the manipulation that caused the change, will reduce the risk that the observed change in function develops into a permanent neurological deficit or, at least, will reduce the degree of the postoperative deficits.

Motor Systems. Intraoperative neurophysiological monitoring of the facial nerve was probably the first motor system that was monitored systematically. The introduction of skull base surgery in the 1980s *(5)* caused an increased demand for monitoring of other cranial systems, and the use of monitoring for many cranial motor nerves spread rapidly *(6,7)*. Intraoperative neurophysiological monitoring of spinal motor systems was delayed because of technical difficulties, mainly in eliciting recordable evoked motor responses to stimulation of the motor cortex in anesthetized patients. After these technical obstacles in activating descending spinal motor pathways were resolved in the 1990s, intraoperative neurophysiological monitoring of spinal motor systems gained wide use *(8)*. Monitoring of cranial nerve motor systems commonly relies on recordings of electromyographical (EMG) potentials from muscles that are innervated by specific motor nerves, whereas monitoring of spinal motor systems also makes use of recordings directly from the descending motor pathways of the spinal cord. Spinal motor systems are often monitored by recording EMG potentials from specific muscles in response to electrical or magnetic stimulation of the motor cortex (Chap. 10).

Peripheral Nerves. Monitoring of motor nerves is often accomplished by observing the electrical activity that can be recorded from one or more of the muscles that are innervated by the motor nerve or motor system that is to be monitored (evoked EMG potentials). The respective motor nerve might be stimulated electrically or by the electrical current that is induced by a strong magnetic impulse (magnetic stimulation). Recordings of muscle activity that is elicited by mechanical stimulation of a motor nerve or by injury to a motor nerve are important parts of many forms of monitoring of the motor system. Such muscle activity is monitored by continuous recording EMG potentials ("free-running EMG"). When such activity is made audible, it can provide important feedback to the surgeon and the surgeon, can then modify his/her operative technique accordingly.

Monitoring peripheral nerves intraoperatively can be done by electrically stimulating the nerve in question at one point and recording the compound action potentials (CAPs) at a different location. Changes in neural conduction that might occur between these two locations will result in changes in the latency of the CAP and/or in the waveform and amplitude of the CAP. The latency of the CAP is a measure of the (inverse) conduction velocity, and decreased conduction velocity is a typical sign of injury to a nerve. The latency and waveform of the recorded CAP typically increases as a result of many kinds of insult to a nerve.

Interpretation of Neuroelectric Potentials

The success of intraoperative neurophysiological monitoring depends greatly on the correct interpretation of the recorded neuroelectrical potentials. In most situations, the usefulness of intraoperative neurophysiological monitoring depends on the person who watches the display, makes the interpretation, and decides what information should be given to the surgeon. It is, therefore, imperative for success in intraoperative neurophysiological monitoring that the person who is responsible for the monitoring be well trained. It is also important that he/she is familiar with the different steps of the operation and well informed in advance about the patient who is to be monitored.

It is important that information about changes in recorded potentials be presented in a way that contributes specific interpreted detail that the surgeon will find useful and actionable. Surgeons are not neurophysiologists and the knowledge of neurophysiology varies among surgeons. The neurophysiologist who provides results of monitoring to the surgeon must, therefore, present their skilled interpretation of the recorded potentials. The surgeon might not always appreciate data such as latency values because the surgeon might not understand what such data represent. Monitoring is of no value if the surgeon does not take action accordingly. If the surgeon does not understand what the information provided by the neurophysiologist means, then there is little chance that he/she will take appropriate action.

Correct and prompt interpretation of changes in the waveforms of the recorded potentials is essential for such monitoring to be useful. The far-field potentials such as ABR, SSEP, and VEP are often complex and consist of a series of peaks and troughs that represent the electrical activity that is generated by successively activated nerve tracts and nuclei of the ascending neural pathways of the sensory system. Exact interpretation of the changes in such potentials that could occur as a result of various kinds of surgical insult therefore require thorough knowledge of the anatomy and physiology of the systems that are monitored and of how the recorded potentials are generated.

The most reliable indicators of changes in neural function are changes (increases) in the latencies of specific components of sensory evoked potentials, and surgically induced insults to nervous tissue often also cause changes in the amplitude of the sensory evoked potentials.

It must be remembered that the recorded sensory evoked potentials do not measure the function (or changes in function) of the sensory system that is being tested. For example, there is no direct relationship between the change in the ABR and the change in the patient's hearing threshold or change in speech discrimination. This is one reason why it has been difficult to establish guidelines for how much evoked potentials could be allowed to change during an operation without presenting a noticeable risk for postoperative deficits.

Interpretation of sensory evoked potentials is based on knowledge of the anatomical location of the generators of the individual components of SSEP, ABR, and VEP in relation to the structures that are being manipulated in a specific operation. Interpretation of sensory evoked potentials also depends on the processing of the recorded potentials. For example, filtering of various kinds are used and that affects the waveform of the potentials. The amplitude of these sensory evoked potentials is smaller than the background noise (ongoing brain activity [EEG potentials] and electrical noise) and it is, therefore, necessary to use signal averaging to enhance the signal-to-noise ratio of electrical potentials such as sensory evoked potentials. Signal averaging (adding the responses to many stimuli) is based on the assumption that the responses to every stimulus are identical and they always occur at the same time following stimulation. Because the sensory evoked potentials that are recorded in the operating room are likely to change during the time that responses are being averaged, the averaging process might produce unpredictable results. These matters are important to take into consideration when interpreting sensory evoked potentials. (Signal averaging and filtering are discussed in more detail in Chap. 18.)

Different ways to reduce the time necessary to obtain an interpretable recording are discussed and described in Chaps. 4, 6, and 18. The specific techniques that are suitable for intraoperative neurophysiological monitoring of the auditory, somatosensory, and visual systems are dealt with in more detail in Chaps. 4 and 6, respectively.

In some instances, it is possible to record potentials from the structures that actually generate the evoked potentials in question (near-field potentials). Such potentials often have sufficiently large amplitude, allowing observation of the potentials directly without signal averaging. If it is possible to base the intraoperative neurophysiological monitoring on recording of evoked potentials directly from an active neural structure (nerve, nerve tract, or nucleus), little or no signal averaging might be necessary because the amplitudes of such potentials are much larger than those of far-field potentials, such as the ABR and SSEP, and such near-field potentials can often be viewed directly on an computer screen or after only a few responses have been averaged. These matters are also discussed in more detail in the chapters on sensory evoked potentials (Chaps. 4 and 6).

The design of the monitoring system and the way the recorded potentials are processed are important factors in facilitating proper interpretation of the recorded neuroelectric potentials, as is the way the recorded potentials are displayed (*see* Chap. 18). The proper choice of stimulus parameters and the selection of the location along the nervous pathways where the responses are recorded also facilitate prompt interpretation of recorded neuroelectrical potentials.

When recording EMG potentials, it is often advantageous to make the recorded response audible (9,10) so that the neurophysiologist responsible for the monitoring and the surgeon can hear the response and make his/her own interpretation. Still, the possibilities to present the recorded potentials directly to the surgeon are currently few, and it is questionable whether it would be advantageous. Few surgeons are physiologists and most surgeons want the results of monitoring to be presented in an interpreted form rather than raw data.

The importance of being able to detect a change in function as soon as possible cannot be emphasized enough. Prompt interpretation of changes in recorded potentials makes it possible

for the surgeon to accurately identify the step in the operation that caused the change, which is a prerequisite for proper and prompt surgical intervention and, thus, the ability to reduce the risk of postoperative neurological deficits.

Correct identification of the step in an operation that entails a risk of complications might make it possible to modify the way such an operation is carried out in the future and thereby makes it possible to reduce the risk of complications in subsequent operations. In this way, intraoperative neurophysiological monitoring can contribute to the development of safer operating methods by making it possible to identify which steps in an operation might cause neurological deficits, and it thereby naturally also plays an important role in teaching surgical residents and fellows.

When to Inform the Surgeon

It has been debated extensively whether the surgeon should be informed of all changes in the recorded electrical activity that could be regarded to be caused by surgical manipulations or only when such changes reach a level that indicate a noticeable risk for permanent neurological deficits. The question is thus: should the information that is gained be used only as a warning that implies that if no intervention is made, there is a likelihood that the patient will get a permanent postoperative neurological deficit, or should all information about changes in function be conveyed to the surgeon?

If only information that is presumed to indicate a high risk of neurological deficits is given to the surgeon, then it must be known how large a change in the recorded neuroelectrical potentials can be permitted without causing any permanent damage. This question has so far largely remained unanswered. The degree and the nature of the change and the length of time that the adverse effect has lasted are all factors that are likely to affect the outcome, and the effect of these factors on the risk of postoperative neurological deficits are largely unknown. Individual variation in susceptibility to surgical insults to the nervous system and many other factors affect the risk of neurological deficits in mostly unknown ways and degrees. An individual's disposition and homeostatic condition and perhaps the effect of anesthesia are likely to affect the susceptibility to surgically induced injuries.

If the surgeon is given information about any noticeable change in the recorded potentials that may be related to his/her action it is not necessary to know how large a change in recorded potentials can be permitted without a risk of permanent neurologic deficits. The surgeon can use such information in the planning and the decision of how to proceed with the operation, and intraoperative neurophysiological monitoring can thereby effectively help decrease the risk of neurological deficits. This means that it is beneficial to the surgeon to be informed whenever his or her actions have resulted in a noticeable change in the recorded neuroelectrical potentials. In that way, intraoperative neurophysiological monitoring provides information rather than warnings. Changes in the recorded potentials that are larger than the (small) normal variations of the potentials in question should be reported to the surgeon if there is reasonable certainty that these changes are related to surgical manipulations.

If the surgeon is made aware of any change in the recorded potentials that is larger than those normally occurring, it can help the surgeon to carry out the operation in an optimal way with as little risk of adverse affect on neural function as possible. Providing such information gives the surgeon the option of altering his/her course of action in a wide range of time. If the change in the recorded potentials is small, it is likely that the surgeon would be able to reverse the effect by a slight change in the surgical approach or by avoiding further manipulation of the neural tissue affected; alternatively, the surgeon might choose not to alter the technique if the surgical manipulations that caused the changes in the recorded neurophysiological potentials are essential to carrying out the operation in the anticipated way. However, even in such a case, the knowledge that the surgical procedure is affecting neural

function in a measurable way is valuable to the surgeon, and continuous monitoring of the change can keep his/her option to modify the procedure to remain open because monitoring has identified which step in the operation caused the change in function.

If information about a change in the recorded potentials is withheld until the change in the recorded electrical potentials has increased greatly, it would be difficult for the surgeon to determine which step in the surgical procedure caused the adverse effect, and thus it would not be possible for the surgeon to intervene appropriately because it would not be known which step in the procedure caused the change. Also, in such a situation, the surgeon would not have had the freedom of delaying his/her action to reverse the change because it had already reached dangerous levels.

The more knowledge that is gathered about the effect of mechanical manipulation on nerves, the more it seems apparent that even slight changes in measures of electrical activity (such as the CAP) might be signs of permanent injury. However, studies that relate changes in evoked potentials to morphological changes and changes in postoperative function are still rare. Thus, relatively little is known quantitatively about the degree to which a nerve can be stretched, heated, or deprived of oxygen before a permanent injury results, but there is no doubt that different nerves respond in different ways to injury because of mechanical manipulations, heat, or lack of oxygen.

Presenting information about changes in the recorded neuroelectrical potentials as soon as they reach a level where they are detectable also has an educational benefit in that it tells the surgeon precisely which steps in an operation might result in neurological deficit. It is often possible on the basis of such knowledge to modify an operation to avoid similar injuries in future operations.

When conveying information about early changes in the recorded potentials, it is important that it be made clear to the surgeon that such information represents guidance details, as opposed to a warning that the surgical manipulations are likely to result in a high risk of serious consequences if appropriate action is not taken promptly by the surgeon. Warnings are justified, however, if, for instance, there is a sudden large change in the evoked potentials or if the surgeon has disregarded the need to reverse a manipulation that has caused a slow change in the recorded electrical potentials.

The surgeon should be informed of the possibility of a surgically induced injury even in cases in which the change (or total disappearance of the recorded potentials) could be caused by equipment or electrode malfunction. Thus, only after assuming that the problem is biological in nature can equipment failure be considered as a possible cause.

False Alarms

The question of false-positive and false-negative responses in intraoperative neurophysiological monitoring has been extensively debated. In some of these discussions, a false-positive response meant that the surgeon was alerted of a situation that would not have led to any noticeable risk of neurological deficits if no action had been taken.

Before discussing false-positive and false-negative responses in intraoperative neurophysiological monitoring, the meaning of false-positive and false-negative responses should be clarified. A typical example of a false-positive result of a test for a specific disease occurs when the test showed the presence of a disease when there was, in fact, no disease present. Using the same analogy, a false-negative test would mean that the test failed to show that a certain individual in fact had the specific disease. In the clinic or in screening of individuals without symptoms, false-negative results are more serious than false-positive results: false-positive results might lead to an incorrect diagnosis or unnecessary treatment, whereas false-negative results might have the dire consequence of no treatment being given for an existing disease.

These definitions cannot be transposed directly to the field of intraoperative neurophysiological monitoring. One reason is that the purpose of intraoperative neurophysiological

monitoring is not to detect when a certain surgical manipulation will cause a permanent neurological deficit. Instead, the purpose is to provide information about when there is a (noticeable) risk that a permanent neurological deficit might occur. In fact, in most cases when intraoperative neurophysiological monitoring shows changes in function that indicates a risk of causing neurological deficits, no permanent deficits occur. There is no serious consequences associated with this kind of false-positive responses in intraoperative neurophysiological monitoring. A situation in which the surgeon was mistakenly alerted of a change in the recorded potentials that was afterward shown to be a result of a technical fault or a harmless change in the nervous system rather than being caused by surgical manipulations might be regarded as a true false-positive response.

The occurrences of false-negative results, which mean that a serious risk has occurred without being noticed, indicate a failure in reaching the goal of intraoperative neurophysiological monitoring and it might have serious consequences.

Therefore, the conventional definition of false-positive and false-negative results cannot be applied to intraoperative neurophysiological monitoring because the purpose of monitoring is not to identify an individual with a neurological deficit but to identify signs that have a certain risk of leading to such deficits if no action is taken.

Nonsurgical Causes of Changes in Recorded Potentials

Alerting the surgeon as soon as a change occurs naturally always implies a faint possibility that a change in evoked potentials might be caused by technical problems that affected some part of the equipment that is used or by a loss of contact of one or more of the electrodes. The characteristics of changes caused by technical problems are usually so different from those of changes caused by injury from surgical manipulations that these two phenomena can easily be distinguished by an experienced neurophysiologist. It is possible that a total loss of recorded potentials can be caused by a technical failure, but it could also be caused by a major failure in the part of the nervous system that is being monitored. However, if such an event should occur, it is much better to first assume that the cause is biological and to promptly alert the surgeon accordingly and then do trouble-shooting of the equipment. In general, when something unusual happens, it is advisable to alert the surgeon promptly that something serious could have happened instead of beginning to check the equipment and electrodes. It is highly unlikely that a technical failure will occur and cause a change in the recorded potentials that might be confused with a biological cause for the change. The neurophysiologist should explain to the surgeon that a potentially serious event has occurred and then check the equipment and the electrodes for malfunction. The surgeon, not waiting for the completion of this equipment check, should immediately begin his/her own investigation to ascertain whether a surgically induced injury has occurred. If it is discovered that the change in the recorded potentials was caused by equipment malfunction, the surgeon can then be apprised of this; thus, the only loss that the incident would cause is a few minutes of the surgeon's time. If such an occurrence is regarded as a "false alarm," then the price for tolerating such "false alarms," namely that the operation might be delayed unnecessarily for a brief time, seems small compared to what could occur if one chose to check the equipment before alerting the surgeon.

If the cause of the change in the recorded neuroelectrical potentials was indeed a result of an injury that was caused by surgical manipulation of neural structures and appropriate action was not taken immediately by the surgeon, precious time would have been lost. This would occur if the neurophysiologist had assumed that the cause of the change was technical in nature. Not only would the opportunity to identify the cause of the change be missed by taking the time to check the equipment first, but such a delay could also have allowed the change in function to progress, thus increasing the risk of a permanent neurological deficit. The opportunity to properly reverse the cause of the observed change in the recorded neuroelectrical potentials might be lost if action is delayed while searching for technical problems.

In accepting this way of performing intraoperative neurophysiological monitoring, it must also be assumed that everything is done that can be done to keep technical failures that could mimic surgically induced changes in the recorded potentials to an absolute minimum. Actually, high-quality equipment very seldom malfunctions, and if needle electrodes are used in the way described in the following chapters and care is taken when placing the electrodes, incidents of electrode failure will be rare.

There are factors other than surgical manipulations or equipment failure that can cause changes in the waveform of the recorded potentials (e.g., changes in the level of anesthesia, blood pressure, or body temperature of the patient). It is therefore important that the person who is responsible for the intraoperative neurophysiological monitoring be knowledgeable about how these factors could affect the neuroelectric potentials that are being recorded. The physiologist should maintain consistent and frequent communication with the anesthesiologist to keep informed about any changes in the level of anesthesia and changes in the anesthesia regimen that could affect the electrophysiological parameters that are to be monitored.

How to Evaluate Neurological Deficits

To assess the success of avoiding neurological deficits, it is important that patients be properly examined and tested both preoperatively and postoperatively so that changes can be verified quantitatively. In some cases, an injury is detectable only by specific neurological testing, whereas in other cases, injury causes impaired sensory function that is noticeable by the patient. Other patients might suffer alterations in neural function that are noticeable to the patient as well as others in everyday situations. It is therefore important that careful objective testing and examination of the patient be performed before and after operations to make accurate quantitative assessments of sensory or neurological deficits.

There is no doubt that the degree to which different types of neurological deficit affect individuals varies, but reducing the risk of any measurable or noticeable deficit as much as possible must be the goal of intraoperative neurophysiological monitoring.

AIDING THE SURGEON IN THE OPERATION

In addition to reducing the risk of neurological deficits, the use of neurophysiological techniques in the operating room can provide information that can help the surgeon carry out the operation and make better decisions about the next step in the operation. In its simplest form, this might consist of identifying the exact anatomical location of a nerve that cannot be identified visually or it might consist of identifying where in a peripheral nerve a block of transmission has occurred (11). In operations to repair peripheral nerves, intraoperative diagnosis of the nature of the injury and its exact location using neurophysiological methods have improved the outcome of such operations.

An example of a more complex role of intraoperative recording is the recording of the abnormal muscle response in patients undergoing microvascular decompression (MVD) operations to relieve hemifacial spasm (HFS) (12,13). This abnormal muscle response disappears when the facial nerve is adequately decompressed (14), and by observing this response, it is possible to identify the blood vessel or blood vessels that caused the symptoms of HFS as well as to ensure that the facial nerve has been adequately decompressed.

Electrophysiological guidance for placement of lesions in the basal ganglia and the thalamus for treatment of movement disorders and pain is absolutely essential for the success of such treatment. More recently, making lesions in these structures has been replaced by electrical stimulation deep brain stimulation

(DBS) and electrophysiological methods are equally important for guiding the placement of electrodes for DBS.

Implantation of electrodes for DBS and for stimulation of specific structures in the spinal cord no doubt will increase during the coming years. Such treatments are attractive in comparison with pharmacological (drug) treatment in that it has fewer side effects. Whereas a physician with a license to practice medicine can prescribe many complex medications, procedures such as electrode implantation for DBS require expertise in both surgery and neurophysiology and it must involve intraoperative neurophysiological recordings being performed adequately. This means that the need of people with neurophysiological knowledge and skills of working in the operating room will be in increasing demand for the foreseeable future.

There is no doubt that in the future we will see the development of many other presently unexplored areas in which intraoperative neurophysiological recording will become an aid to the surgeon in specific operations, and the use of neurophysiological methods in the operating room will expand as a means to study normal as well as pathological functions of the nervous system.

WORKING IN THE OPERATING ROOM

Intraoperative neurophysiological monitoring should interfere minimally with other activities in the operating room. If it causes more than minimal interference, there is a risk that it would not be requested as often as it should. There is so much activity in modern neurosurgical, otologic, and orthopedic operating rooms that adding activity that consumes time will naturally be met with a negative attitude from all involved and might result in the omission of intraoperative neurophysiological monitoring in certain cases. Careful planning is necessary to ensure that intraoperative neurophysiological monitoring does not interfere with other forms of monitoring and the use of life-support equipment.

How to Reduce the Risk of Mistakes in Intraoperative Neurophysiological Monitoring

The importance of selecting the appropriate modality of neuroelectric potentials for monitoring purposes cannot be overemphasized and making sure that the structures of the nervous system that are at risk are included in the monitoring is essential. Thus, monitoring SSEP elicited by stimulating the median nerve while operating on the thoracic or lumbar spine naturally could lead to a disaster, because it is the thoracic lumbar spinal portion of the somatosensory pathway that is at risk of being injured when only the cervical portion of the somatosensory pathway is being monitored.

Monitoring the wrong side of the patient's nervous system is also a serious mistake. An example of this is presenting the sound stimulus to the ear opposite the side on which the operation is being done while monitoring ABR. This kind of mistake could occur when earphones are fitted in both ears and selection of which earphone to be used is controlled by the neurophysiologist. A user mistake can cause the wrong earphone to be used. Because the ABR is not fundamentally different when elicited from the opposite side, such a mistake will not be immediately obvious, but it will naturally prevent the detection of any change in the ear or auditory nerve as a result of surgical manipulation. The possible catastrophic consequence of failing to detect any change in the recorded potentials when the auditory nerve is injured by surgical manipulation is obvious.

Generally speaking, if a mistake can be made by the action of the user (neurophysiologist), it will be made; it might be rare. Mistakes might be tolerated, depending on the consequences and the frequency of its expected occurrence. Mistakes can only be avoided if it is physically impossible to make the mistake. Thus, only by placing an earphone solely in the ear on the operated side can the risk of stimulating the wrong ear be eliminated. If earphones are placed in each ear, the risk of making mistakes can be reduced by clearly marking the right and left earphone and only having properly trained personnel operate the stimulus equipment. This will reduce the risk of mistakes but not eliminate mistakes.

In a similar way, monitoring the wrong side of the spinal cord could cause serious neurological deficits without any change in the recorded neuroelectrical potentials being noticed during the operation. When an operation involves the spinal cord distal to the cervical spine and stimulating electrodes are placed in the median nerve as well as in a nerve on the lower limb, the median nerve might mistakenly be stimulated when the intention was to elicit evoked potentials from the lower limb. This could happen if the stimulation is controlled by the user. The considerable difference between the waveform of the upper limb SSEP and that of the lower limb SSEP might make this mistake more easily detectable than when eliciting ABR when the wrong ear is being stimulated or when eliciting SSEP from the wrong side.

Reliability of Intraoperative Neurophysiological Monitoring

Like any other new addition to the operating room armamentarium, intraoperative neurophysiological monitoring must be reliable in order to be a tool that is used routinely. It is not unreasonable to assume that if intraoperative neurophysiological monitoring cannot always be carried out and, consequently, operations are done without the aid of monitoring, it might be assumed by the surgeon that it is not necessary at all to have such monitoring.

Reliability can best be achieved if only routines that are well thought through and that have been thoroughly tested are used in the operating room. The same methods that have been found to work well over a long time should be used consistently. New routines or modifications of old routines should only be introduced in the operating room after thorough consideration and testing. Procedures of intraoperative neurophysiologic monitoring should be kept as simple as possible. The KISS Principle (Keep it Simple [and] Stupid) (or Keep it Simple and Straightforward) is applicable to intraoperative neurophysiological monitoring.

Electrical Safety and Intraoperative Neurophysiological Monitoring

A final, but not inconsiderable, concern is that intraoperative neurophysiological monitoring should not add risks to the safety, particularly electrical safety, of any operation. Intraoperative neurophysiological monitoring requires the addition of complex electrical equipment to an operating room already crowded with a variety of complex electrical equipment. Electrical safety is naturally of great concern whenever electronic equipment is in direct galvanic contact with patients, but this is particularly true in the operating room, where many pieces of electrical equipment are operated together, often in crowded conditions, and frequently under wet conditions. The equipment and procedures used for intraoperative neurophysiological monitoring must, therefore, be chosen with consideration for the protection of the patient as well as of the personnel in the operating room from electrical hazard. Accidents can best be avoided when those who work in the operating room and who use the electronic equipment are knowledgeable about the function of the equipment and how risks of electrical hazards that are associated with specific equipment could arise. For the neurophysiologist, it is important to have a basic understanding about how electrical hazards could occur and to specifically have an understanding of the basic functions of the various pieces of equipment used in electrophysiological monitoring. The area of greatest concern in maintaining electrical safety for the patient is, naturally, the placement of stimulating and recording electrodes on the patient. It is particularly important to consider the safety of the equipment that is connected to electrodes placed intracranially for either recording or stimulation.

HOW TO EVALUATE THE BENEFITS OF INTRAOPERATIVE NEUROPHYSIOLOGICAL MONITORING

Naturally, it is the patient who can gain the most from intraoperative neurophysiological monitoring. Many of the severe postoperative neurological deficits that were common before the introduction of intraoperative neurophysiological monitoring are now rare occurrences. It is not only the use of intraoperative neurophysiological monitoring that has caused these improvements of medical care, but also better surgical techniques and various technological advancements have provided significant progress. There is no doubt that the introduction of microneurosurgery and, more recently, minimally invasive surgery has made operations that affect the nervous system less brutal than it was 25 yr ago, and even the last decade has seen steady improvements regarding reducing complications.

Assessment of Reduction of Neurological Deficits

It has been difficult to accurately assess the value of intraoperative neurophysiological monitoring with regard to reducing the risk of postoperative neurological deficits. One of the reasons for these difficulties is that it has not been possible to apply the commonly used scheme, such as double-blind methods, to determine the value of intraoperative neurophysiological monitoring. Surgeons who have experienced the advantages of intraoperative neurophysiological monitoring are reluctant to deprive their patients of the benefits provided by an aid in the operation that they believe can improve the outcome. The use of historical data for comparison of outcomes before and after the introduction of monitoring has been described in a few reports, but such methods are criticized because advancements in surgical technique other than intraoperative neurophysiological monitoring might have contributed to the observed improvement of outcome. Even more difficult to evaluate is the increased feeling of security that surgeons note while operating with the aid of intraoperative neurophysiological monitoring.

For the sake of evaluating future benefits from monitoring, it is important that all patients who are monitored intraoperatively be evaluated objectively before and after the operation and that the results obtained during monitoring be well documented.

Which Surgeons Benefit Most From Intraoperative Monitoring?

Surgeons at all levels of experience could benefit in one way or another from the use of intraoperative neurophysiological monitoring, but the degree of benefit depends on the experience of the surgeon in the particular kind of operation being performed. Whereas an extremely experienced surgeon might benefit from monitoring only in unusual situations or for confirming the anatomy, a surgeon with moderate-to-extensive experience might feel more secure and might have additional help in identifying specific neural structures when using monitoring. A surgeon with moderate-to-extensive experience will also benefit from knowing when surgical manipulations have injured neural tissue. A less experienced surgeon who has done only a few of a specific type of operation is likely to benefit more extensively from using intraoperative neurophysiological monitoring, and surgeons at this level of experience will learn from intraoperative monitoring and through that improve his/her surgical skills.

Even some extremely experienced surgeons declare the benefit from neurophysiological monitoring and appreciate the increased feeling of security when operating with the assistance of monitoring. Many very experienced surgeons are in fact not willing to operate without the use of monitoring.

In fact, most surgeons can benefit from intraoperative neurophysiological monitoring mainly by its help in reducing the risk of postoperative neurological deficits as well as by its ability to provide the surgeon with a feeling of security from knowing that he/she will know when neural tissue is being adversely manipulated. Most surgeons will appreciate the aid that monitoring can provide in confirming the anatomy when it deviates from normal as a result of tumors, other pathologies, or extreme variations.

RESEARCH OPPORTUNITIES

The operating room offers a wealth of research opportunities. In fact, many important discoveries about the function of the normal nervous system as well as about the function of the pathological nervous system have been derived from research activities within the operating room. Neurophysiological recording is almost the only way to study the pathophysiology of many disorders. Many important discoveries were made by applying neurophysiological methods to work in the operating room, but many discoveries were made before the introduction of intraoperative neurophysiological monitoring (15,16) and many studies were made in connection with intraoperative neurophysiological monitoring (14,17,18). Some studies have concerned basic research (19), whereas other studies have been directly related to the development of better treatment and better surgical methods (14,17,18); some studies have served both purposes (15,17,19–24).

3

Generation of Electrical Activity in the Nervous System and Muscles

Introduction
Unit Responses
Near-Field Responses
Far-Field Potentials
Effect of Insults to Nerves, Fiber Tracts, and Nuclei

INTRODUCTION

To understand why and how neuroelectrical potentials, such as evoked potentials, might change as a result of surgical manipulations, it is necessary to understand the basic principles underlying the generation of the neuroelectrical potentials that can be recorded from various parts of the nervous system. In this volume, we discuss electrical potentials that are generated in response to intentional stimulation and we describe how the waveform of such recorded potentials might change as a result of injury to nerves or nuclei. It is also important to understand the nature of the responses that might be elicited by surgical manipulations of neural tissue and from surgically induced injuries. Further, it is important to know where in the nervous system specific components of the recorded evoked potentials are generated, so that the exact anatomical location of an injury can be identified on the basis of changes in specific components of the electrical potentials that are being monitored.

The potentials that can be recorded from nerves and structures of the central nervous system can be divided into three large categories: unit (or multiunit), near-field, and far-field potentials.

Unit potentials are potentials recoded from single nerve fibers, nerve cells, or from small groups of nerve fibers or nerve cells (multiunit recordings). Such potentials can be either spontaneous activity that occurs without any intentional stimulation or evoked by some form of stimulation. Unit or multiunit responses are recorded by placing small electrodes (microelectrodes) in indirect contact with nerve fibers or nerve cells. Recording of such potentials have played important roles in animal studies of the function of the nervous system. These techniques have only recently been introduced for use in the operating room.

Near-field evoked potentials are recorded by placing a much larger recording electrode directly on a nerve, a nucleus, or a muscle, and these potentials represent the sum of the activity in many nerve cells or fibers in one of only a few structures. It is not always possible to record near-field potentials because it is not possible to place a recording electrode directly on the structure in question; instead, one often has to rely on far-field potentials.

Far-field potentials are recorded from electrodes that are placed at a (long) distance from the structures that generate the potentials that are being recorded. Whereas near-field potentials, such as those recorded by placing an electrode directly on a nerve, nucleus, or muscle, reflect electrical activity in that specific structure, far-field potentials are usually mixtures of

From: *Intraoperative Neurophysiological Monitoring: Second Edition*
By A. R. Møller
© Humana Press Inc., Totowa, NJ.

potentials that are generated by several different structures.

Far-field potentials have smaller amplitudes than near-field potentials and their waveforms are more difficult to interpret because they represent more than one generator. The generation of far-field potentials is complex and it is not completely understood. The contribution from such different structures depends on the distance from the recording electrode(s) as well as the properties of the sources. For example, only under certain circumstances can propagated neural activity in a long nerve generate stationary peaks in potentials recorded at a distance from the nerve. The far-field potentials generated by nuclei depends on the orientation of the dendrites of the cells in the nuclei. The contributions from different structures to recorded far-field potentials are therefore weighted with regard to factors such as the distance from the source and the rate at which the amplitudes of the recorded potentials decrease with distance to the source, which depends on the properties of the source.

Components of the evoked potentials from different sources might overlap, depending on whether they appear with the same, or different, latencies from the stimulus that was used to evoke the response. Therefore, the waveform of far-field potentials is usually different from that of near-field potentials and are generally more difficult to interpret than near-field potentials.

Because of their small amplitude, far-field evoked potentials are usually not directly discernable from the background noise that always exists when recording neuroelectrical potentials; therefore, it is necessary to add many responses using the method of signal averaging (described in Chap. 18) so that an interpretable waveform can be obtained. The use of signal averaging to enhance a signal (evoked response) that is corrupted by noise assumes that the waveforms of all the responses that are added are the same and occur in an exact time relation (latency) to the stimulus. This might not be the case when the neural system that is being monitored is affected by surgical manipulation, excess heat, or anoxia. The necessity to average many responses might distort the waveform if the responses being added change (slowly) over the time during which the data are being collected and averaged and, therefore, make the added response difficult to interpret. This is another reason why changes in far-field evoked potentials are more difficult to interpret than are changes in near-field potentials.

In this chapter, we discuss in greater detail the three categories of neuroelectrical potentials that are often recorded in the operating room: unit (multiunit), near-field, and far-field potentials.

UNIT RESPONSES

Unit potentials reflect the activity of a single neural element or from a small group of elements (multiunit recordings). Action potentials from individual nerve fibers and from nerve cells are recorded by placing microelectrodes, the tips of which could be from a few micrometer to a fraction of a micrometer in diameter, in or near individual nerve fibers. The waveform of such action potentials is always the same in a specific nerve fiber or cell body, regardless of how it has been elicited. Information that is transmitted in a nerve fiber is coded in the rate and the time pattern of the occurrence of such action potentials. That means that it is the occurrence of nerve impulses and their frequency (rate) that is important rather than their waveform.

The action potentials of nerve fibers are the result of depolarization of a nerve fiber. Usually, the electrical potential inside a nerve fiber is about –70 mV. When this intracellular potential becomes less negative (brought closer to zero, or "depolarized"), a complex exchange of ions occurs between the interior of the nerve fiber and the surrounding fluid through the membrane. When the electrical potential inside an axon becomes sufficiently less negative than the resting potential, a nerve impulse (action potential) will be generated and the depolarization propagates along the nerve fiber. This depolarization and subsequent repolarization is associated with the generation of an action potential (also known as a nerve impulse, nerve discharge, or nerve spike). In myelinated nerve fibers (such as those in mammalian sensory and motor nerves), neural propagation occurs along a nerve fiber by saltatory conduction between the nodes of Ranvier, which can be recognized as small interruptions in the myelin sheath that covers the nerve fiber. Unit potentials have the character of nerve discharges (spikes) and are recorded by fine-tipped metal electrodes that are insulated except for the tip.

The main use intraoperatively of recording of unit potentials is for guiding the surgeon in the placement of lesions in brain structure, such as the basal ganglia or thalamus, for treatment of movement disorders and pain. More recently, lesions have been replaced by implantation of electrodes for electrical stimulation (deep brain stimulation [DBS]), which have a similar beneficial effect as lesions but with the advantage of being reversible. The responses that are observed in such operations are either spontaneous activity that occurs without any intentional stimulation, or by natural stimulation of the skin (touch), or from voluntary or passive movement of the patient's limbs. For such purposes, usually multiunit recordings are made, using electrodes with slightly larger tips than those used for recording of the responses from single fibers or cell bodies. These responses represent the activity of small groups of cells or fibers.

NEAR-FIELD RESPONSES

Near-field evoked potentials are defined as potentials recorded with the recording electrode(s) placed directly on the surface of a specific neurological structure. Responses recorded from fiber tracts and nuclei are the most important for intraoperative monitoring, but recordings from specific regions of the cerebral cortex are also regarded as near-field evoked potentials.

Near-field evoked potentials are recorded by placing recording electrodes that are much larger than microelectrodes (gross electrodes) on the surface of a nerve, fiber tracts, a nucleus or a

specific part of the cerebral cortex. Such potentials reflect neural activity in many nerve fibers or cells, but typically only in a single structure. The responses are usually elicited by transient stimuli that activate many fibers of cells at about the same time. Such responses are known as compound action potentials (CAPs) because they are the sum of many action potentials. The potentials are graded potentials and their waveforms are specific for nerves and nuclei; the waveform changes in a characteristic way when the structure, from which recordings are made, is injured.

Responses From Nerves

Near-field potentials from nerves reflect the activity in many nerve fibers; hence, it is obtained as a sum of the action potentials of many nerve fibers. The CAPs recorded from a nerve or fiber tract reflect the propagation of action potentials along individual nerve fibers (axons). When a depolarization is initiated at a certain point along a nerve fiber, the depolarization propagates along the nerve fiber with a (propagation) velocity that is approximately proportional to the diameter of the axons of the nerve. The relation between neural conduction velocity (in meters per second [m/s]) and fiber diameter (in micrometers [μm]) is approx 4.5 m/s/μm *(25)*. Older data *(26)* indicate a slightly higher velocity: 6 m/s/μm. The conduction velocity of peripheral sensory and motor nerves typically ranges from 40 to 60 m/s. The auditory nerve has an unusually low propagation velocity of about 20 m/s *(27)*. Normally, depolarization of nerve fibers is initiated at one end of a nerve fiber (peripheral end of sensory fibers and central end of motor fibers), but neural propagation can occur in both directions of a nerve fiber, and it does so with about the same conduction velocity.

Initiation of Nerve Impulses. Initiation of nerve impulses in sensory nerves normally occurs through activation of sensory receptors *(28)*, and motor nerves are activated through motoneurons either in the spinal cord for somatic nerves or in the brainstem for cranial motor nerves *(29)*. In the operating room, sensory nerves are almost always activated by sensory stimuli and motor nerves might be activated by (electrical or magnetic) stimulation of the motor cortex or the brainstem. Peripheral nerves and cranial motor nerves are also activated by electrical stimulation. Such stimulation depolarizes axons at the location of stimulation of a nerve.

Natural Stimulation. Nerve impulses in sensory nerves are normally initiated by an activation of specialized sensory receptor cells that respond to a specific physical stimulation *(28)*. The frequency of the elicited action potentials in individual nerve fibers (discharge rate) is a function of the strength of the sensory stimulation. The time pattern of the occurrence of action potentials in a fiber of a sensory nerve also carries information about the sensory stimulus in the somatosensory and the auditory nerves, because the discharge pattern is statistically related to the time pattern of the stimuli, which means that the probability of the occurrence of a discharge varies along the waveform of the stimulus *(28)*. This neural coding of the stimulus time pattern is of particular importance in the auditory system, in which much information about sound is coded in the time pattern of the discharges in auditory nerve fibers. The ability of the auditory nervous system to use the temporal coding of sounds for interpretation of complex sounds, such as in speech, is important for the success of cochlear and cochlear nucleus prostheses *(30)*. In the visual system, the temporal pattern of nerve impulses seems to have little importance, as is also the case in the olfactory and gustatory sensory systems.

When sensory nerves are stimulated with natural stimuli, the latency of the response from a sensory nerve decreases with increasing stimulus intensity, and this dependence exists over a large range of stimulus intensities. One reason for this stimulus-dependent latency is the neural transduction in sensory cells (such as the hair cells in the auditory system), where the excitatory post-synaptic potential (EPSP) increases from below threshold at a rate that increases with increasing stimulus intensity and the EPSP thereby reaches the threshold faster when the stimulus intensity is

high, as compared to when it is low *(31)*. Another reason for stimulus-dependent latency is the non-linear properties of the sensory organs such as the cochlea (*see* Chap. 5) *(32)*.

Electrical Stimulation. Although sound stimuli (click sounds) is the most common stimulation for monitoring the auditory system, electrical stimulation of peripheral nerves is the most common way of stimulating the somatosensory system and for monitoring and intraoperative diagnosis of peripheral nerves. Electrical stimulation is also in increasing use for stimulation of the motor cortex for monitoring motor systems (transcranial electrical stimulation [TES]).

The electrical stimulation that is used to depolarize the fibers of a peripheral nerve use brief (0.1–0.2 ms long) electrical current impulses that are passed through the nerve that is to be stimulated. A negative current is excitatory because it causes the interior of the axons to become less negative, thus causing depolarization. This might sound paradoxical, but, in fact, a negative electrical current flowing through the cross-section of a nerve fiber will cause the outside area of that nerve fiber to become more negative than the inside area and, thereby, the interior of the axon will become more positive (less negative) than its outer surface—thus, depolarization occurs.

When a nerve is stimulated by placing two electrodes on the same nerve a small distance apart, the negative electrode (cathode) is the active stimulating electrode and the positive (anode) electrode might block propagation of nerve impulses (known as an anodal block) so that depolarization will only propagate in one direction, namely away from the negative electrode.

The amount of electrical current that is necessary to depolarize the axons of a peripheral nerve and initiate nerve impulses depends on the properties of the individual nerve fibers. Large-diameter axons have lower thresholds than nerve fibers with small diameters. The threshold also depends on the duration of the electrical impulses that are used to stimulate a nerve. The necessary current to activate nerve fibers

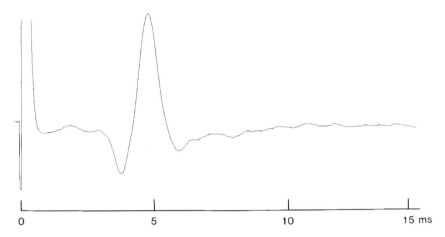

Figure 3.1: Monopolar recording from a long nerve of propagated neural activity elicited by electrical stimulation with a brief impulse of current passed through the nerve far from the location of recording. Note the stimulus artifact at the beginning of the trace. Negativity is shown as an upward deflection (as it is in all illustrations in this book).

decreases when the duration of the current impulses is increased, reaching (asymptotically) a duration where further increase in duration has little effect on the current needed to reach threshold. That occurs at shorter durations for large fibers than for axons of smaller diameter. The diameters of axons of a peripheral nerve can vary considerably and stimulation with impulses of certain duration and a certain intensity might therefore depolarize different populations of nerve fibers in a peripheral nerve.

Increasing the stimulus intensity does not change the way an electrical stimulus activates an individual axon, but it affects the number of axons that become depolarized. More axons will be depolarized when the stimulus strength is increased from below the threshold of the most sensitive nerve fibers. The anatomical location of a nerve fiber in relation to the stimulating electrodes is a factor, because the effectiveness of stimulation decreases with increasing distance.

When a normal peripheral nerve is electrically stimulated, supramaximal stimulation is usually desired, which means that the applied electrical stimulation should depolarize all axons of the nerve. It is a general rule to turn the stimulus current up approximately one-third above that which produces the maximal response amplitude. This might require a stimulus strength of 100 V (10–20 mA) when the stimulus duration is 0.1 ms and the stimulating electrodes are located close to a peripheral nerve. Nerves, the function of which is impaired, might require as much as 300 V (30–60 mA) in order to depolarize all fibers. In clinical settings, in which the patient is awake, it is not possible to reach supramaximal stimulus levels because of unacceptable pain that such stimulation incurs, but that is not a limitation in the anesthetized patient.

Activation of individual nerve fibers of a peripheral nerve by electrical stimulation with short impulses is an "all-or-none" process and, therefore, the latency of the response is less dependent, if at all, on the stimulus intensity. Only the number of nerve fibers that are activated depends on the stimulus intensity.

Monopolar Recording Compound Action Potentials From a Long Nerve. An electrode that is much larger than the size of individual nerve fibers record the sum of the nerve impulses of many nerve fibers (CAP). When a single electrode (monopolar) is placed on a nerve in which a depolarization has been initiated by a transient stimulation, the waveform of CAPs shows an initial (small) positive deflection that is followed by a large negative peak, and then followed by a small positive peak **(Fig. 3.1)**.

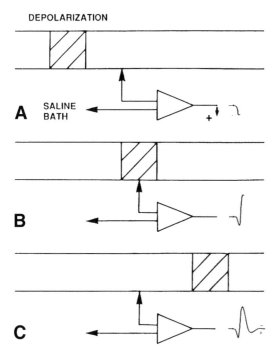

Figure 3.2: Illustration of how the CAP recorded from a long nerve by a monopolar electrode develops. The nerve is being stimulated electrically at a location to the far left (not shown), and the resulting area of membrane depolarization (marked by the crosshatched area) travels from left to right. The recorded electrical potentials that develop as the area of depolarization propagates along the nerve are shown to the right.

Monopolar recording from a long nerve in which a region of depolarization travels yields a CAP with a characteristic triphasic shape (**Fig. 3.1**). The initial positive deflection of the CAP occurs when the depolarization in the nerve approaches the location of the recording electrode (**Fig. 3.2A**). The large negative peak is generated when the depolarized portion of the nerve is directly under the recording electrode (**Fig. 3.2B**). The small positive deflection that follows is generated when the zone of depolarization moves away from the recording electrode (**Fig. 3.2C**). The width of the negative peak is related to the length of the depolarization and the propagation velocity of the nerve. A long area of depolarization or a slowly

moving region of depolarization yields a CAP with a wide negative peak.

In the example illustrated in **Fig. 3.1**, the potentials were recorded differentially between one electrode placed on a nerve and the other electrode—the reference electrode—placed at a distance from the recording electrode in the electrically conducting fluid that surrounded the nerve. This is an example of a monopolar recording of the CAP from a long nerve. The CAP occurs with a certain delay after the stimulus. The latency of the negative peak depicts the time it takes for the depolarization of the nerve fibers to travel from the site of stimulation to the site of recording.

Because recording of CAPs is done using differential recording techniques, it is the difference in the potentials recorded between two recording electrodes that is measured. To make a true monopolar recording, it must be assured that the reference electrode will not record any potential that is related to activity in the nerve. In real recording situations, this is often difficult to achieve because the reference electrode will also record evoked potentials, although of a lower amplitude than the active electrode will record.

The depolarization could have been initiated by electrical stimulation at a distance from the recording site. Similar depolarization could be initiated by natural transient stimulus such as that of a receptor that is innervated by the nerve. When a click stimulus is applied to the ear, a transient excitation of auditory nerve fibers occurs.

Effects of Temporal Dispersion of Action Potentials. When a nerve is stimulated by an electrical impulse and all the nerve fibers that discharge (depolarize) have identical properties so that the action potentials in all of the nerve fibers occur simultaneously, then the waveform of the CAP recorded by a monopolar recording electrode placed on a long nerve is mathematically described as the second derivative of the waveform of an action potential of an individual nerve fiber *(33)*. The action potentials of different nerve fibers elicited by electrical stimulation are assumed to arrive at the site of recording simultaneously, so that the action potentials of different nerve fibers coincide. In such a situation, the amplitude of the negative peak in the CAP is a measure of the number of nerve fibers that have been activated *(34)*.

The situation that exists when recording from mammalian peripheral nerves is different because such nerves are composed of nerve fibers with different conduction velocities. Therefore, the action potentials in individual nerve fibers do not occur exactly at the same time at a certain point along a nerve. The shape of the CAP, therefore, depends on the distribution of the arrival time of the discharges in the different nerve fibers at the site of recording. This, in turn, is a function of the conduction velocity and the length of travel of nerve impulses in the fibers that make up the nerve from which the recording is made. This means that the waveform of the CAP will reflect the distribution of the differing diameters of nerve fibers (conduction velocities) and the distance between the site of stimulation, and that of the recording.

Such time dispersion will broaden the recorded CAP compared to what it would have been if the action potentials in all the nerve fibers arrived at the recording site accurately aligned in time and the amplitude of the CAP will be lower than it would if all nerve impulses traveled at the same velocity. The mathematical description of the recorded CAP in such a situation is the convolution between the waveform of an individual action potential of a nerve fiber and the distribution of action potentials in the nerve fibers that make up the respective nerve *(34)*. This assumes that the waveforms of the action potentials of all nerve fibers are identical. In such a situation, it is the area under the negative peak of the CAP that is a measure of the number of nerve fibers that have been activated rather than the amplitude of the negative peak.

Depending on how great the dispersion is, the waveform of the CAP could differ from a triphasic waveform to a waveform with several peaks. If there are specific subgroups of nerve fibers in a nerve with similar conduction velocities, the

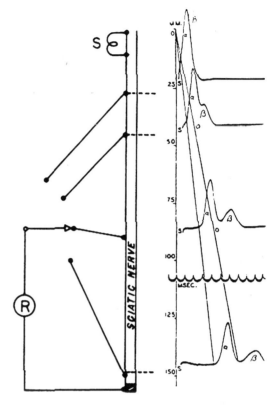

Figure 3.3: Recording of the CAP from a nerve in which there are groups of fibers with different conduction velocities. Recordings at different distances from the site of electrical stimulation (S) are shown. (Reprinted from: Erlanger J, Gasser HS. *Electrical Signs of Nervous Activity.* Philadelphia: University of Pennsylvania Press; 1937.)

activity in such subgroups might give rise to multiple peaks in the CAP. The late peaks moves further away from the initial peak when recorded at a longer distance from the location of stimulation **(Fig. 3.3)**. The effect on the waveform of the recorded CAP from a nerve with subgroups of nerve fibers with different conduction velocity is dependent on the size of the variations in neural conduction velocity in the individual nerve fibers and the distance between the site of stimulation and the site of recording **(Fig. 3.3)**.

Not all nerve fibers of a peripheral nerve contribute equally to the CAP; depending on the recording situation, some nerve fibers might contribute more than others. The mathematical solution of the generation of the CAP from a peripheral nerve might therefore require that different weighting factors be applied to the contribution to the CAP from different populations of the nerve fibers that makes up a peripheral nerve.

Determining the Number of Active Nerve Fibers. In the operating room, the task is not to determine the absolute number of active nerve fibers but, rather, to obtain an estimate of how many nerve fibers of a specific nerve have been rendered inactive as a result of surgical insults. The area of the negative peak in the CAP offers an accurate measure of the number of nerve fibers that have been activated. Because it is the change in the number of active nerve fibers that is of interest in connection with intraoperative monitoring, measuring changes in the amplitude of the negative peak provides a sufficiently accurate measurement for most tasks in the operating room although this measure also include the effect of increased dispersion because of the increased difference in the conduction velocity of individual nerve fibers.

An increase in the latency of the response and/or change in waveform of the recorded CAP are perhaps the two most important indicators of injury to a nerve, and these measures are therefore used extensively in intraoperative monitoring as indicators of injury to a nerve or fiber tracts. Monitoring the amplitude of the CAP is also important in intraoperative monitoring because of its relation to how many fibers are activated and how close together in time the action potentials of individual nerve fibers appear.

Bipolar Recording From a Nerve. Bipolar recording from a long nerve can be realized by placing a pair of recording electrodes that are connected to the two inputs of a differential amplifier close together on the nerve in question (**Fig. 3.4**). The output of the differential amplifier will be the difference between the potentials that are recorded by each individual electrode. A bipolar recording from a nerve in which neural activity is propagated produces a waveform that differs from that of monopolar recordings.

DEPOLARIZATION

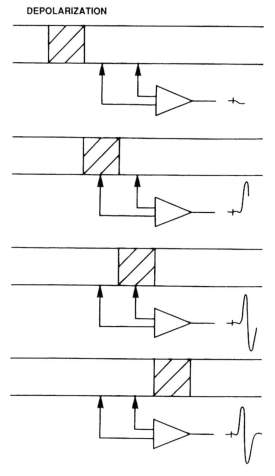

Figure 3.4: Bipolar recording from a long nerve, illustrated in the same way as the monopolar recording in **Fig. 3.2**. The two electrodes are connected to the two inputs of the differential amplifier in such a way that a negative potential at the electrode closest to the recording site (left-hand electrode) will result in an upward deflection (inverting input).

Two such electrodes act as two monopolar electrodes that are placed on a nerve and the output of the amplifier is the difference between these two "monopolar" recordings. When a wave of depolarization approaches the electrodes, the one closest to the depolarization will record a larger positive potential than the electrode that is further away (**Fig. 3.4**). A large negative potential will be recorded by the electrode that is close to the site of stimulation when the region of depolarization reaches the site of that electrode, and an upward (negative) deflection in the output of the differential amplifier will be produced. As the area of depolarization reaches the second electrode, the output of the amplifier will be a downward deflection because a large negative potential will be subtracted from a positive potential recorded by the electrode closest to the stimulation site. When the depolarization progresses further along the nerve, the output of the differential amplifier might show a small, upward deflection, because the second electrode records a positive potential while the first electrode records a smaller positive potential.

A bipolar electrode placed on a long nerve generally records only propagated neural activity. Passively conducted electrical potentials will appear at both electrodes with the same amplitude and exactly the same waveform and thus not generate any output of the differential amplifier that is connected to the bipolar electrodes. Propagated activity, on the other hand, will appear at the two electrodes with a certain time delay and therefore generate a noticeable output at the differential amplifier. This means that the output of the differential amplifier (that is connected to such a pair of electrodes that are placed close together on a long nerve) would be equal to the difference between the potentials recorded by one of the electrodes and their delayed replicas, the delay being the time it takes for the propagated neural activity to travel the distance between the two electrodes. If the distance is 2 mm and the propagation velocity is 20 m/s or 20 mm/ms (as it approximately is in the intracranial portion of the auditory nerve in man), the delay would be 1/10 ms (100 μs). The waveform and amplitude of the recorded potentials that appear at the output of the differential amplifier to which the input of such a pair of electrodes are connected will thus depend on the distance between the two recording electrodes in relation to the length of the area of the nerve that is depolarized.

*The waveform of the recorded potentials will change in a specific way when the distance between the two electrodes is varied. **Figure 3.5** shows the waveform of a simulated bipo-*

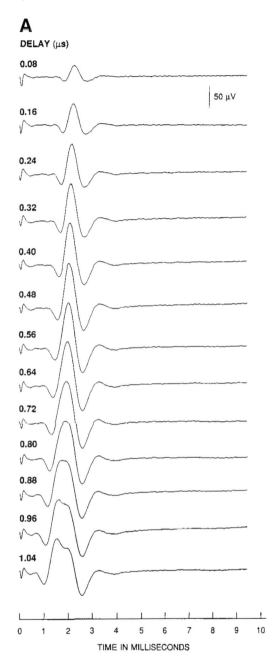

A

DELAY (μs)

| 50 μV |

TIME IN MILLISECONDS

Figure 3.5: *(Continued)*

lar recording during which the distance between the two electrodes was varied. This simulation was realized by subtracting the response recorded by a monopolar recording electrode from the same response after it

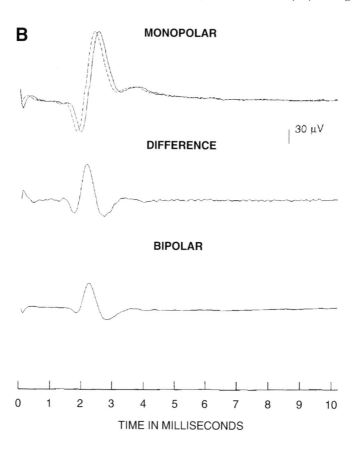

Figure 3.5: (A) Simulated bipolar recording from a long nerve on which the distance between the recording electrodes was varied. **(B)** Comparison between an actual bipolar recording (lower tracing) and a simulated bipolar recording using one of the bipolar electrode tips as a monopolar electrode (middle tracing). The upper tracing shows the monopolar recording together with a time-shifted version (dashed lines). The reference electrode was placed a long distance from the monopolar recording. (Reprinted from: Møller AR, Colletti V, Fiorino F. Click evoked responses from the exposed intracranial portion of the eighth nerve during vestibular nerve section: bipolar and monopolar recordings. *Electroenceph. Clin. Neurophysiol.* 1994;92:17–29, with permission from Elsevier.)

had been delayed. The delay was varied to simulate different distances between two electrodes. It was assumed that a bipolar recording electrode records the difference between the potentials that are recorded at two locations along a nerve and that the only difference between the potentials recorded by two such electrodes would be that they appear with a small difference in latency, the amount of which would be equal to the distance between the two electrodes divided by the propagation velocity.

If there is a difference between such calculated (simulated) bipolar recordings and actual bipolar recordings **(Fig. 3.5B)**, it would mean that either the bipolar electrodes recorded other potentials than the propagated neural activity or that the propagated neural activity had undergone a change while it traveled the distance between the two tips of the bipolar electrode so that it appeared with different waveforms or amplitudes at the two electrodes. The latter seems unlikely, and it might be justified to assume that any difference between actual and simulated bipolar recordings is a result of both of the bipolar recording electrodes picking up passively conducted neural activity. A difference in the actual recorded bipolar response vs that calculated on the basis of recording from only one electrode and shifting that recording in time could occur if the two electrode tips were placed on slightly different parts of the nerve (i.e., the two tips of the bipolar electrode not being properly aligned with regard to the course of the nerve fibers of the nerve) or because the two electrodes were different in size or geometry.

Unfortunately, it is often more difficult in practice to use bipolar recordings from a nerve when monitoring neural conduction intraoperative and, therefore, many operations limit the use of bipolar recording electrodes. (For more details about practical arrangements for recording from nerves, *see* Chap. 4.)

Responses From Muscles

Individual muscle fibers are organized into motor units, which are groups of muscle fibers that are activated by the same motor endplate. When a single fiber of a motor nerve is electrically stimulated, motor endplates are activated and the motor units that are innervated by that fiber will contract. Transmission of impulses from a motor nerve to a muscle is chemical in nature. The neural activity in the motor nerve causes the release of a transmitter substance (acetylcholine), which, in turn, releases calcium ions that causes muscle fibers to contract and the generation of electrical events that are similar to those generated in single nerve fibers. Because the process that occurs in the muscle endplates takes 0.5–0.7 ms, the earliest electrical activity that can be recorded from the muscle is delayed relative to the arrival of the neural activity at the muscle endplate. The electrical events that can be recorded in connection with contraction of muscles are EMG potentials or compound muscle action potentials (CMAPs). The CMAPs are equivalent to the CAPs recorded from a nerve. It is important to note that such muscle potentials are

abolished by the paralyzing agents that are used in many anesthesia regimens. Use of such agents makes recording of EMG potentials impossible. Muscle relaxants used in connection with anesthesia are of two types, namely substances that block transmission in muscle endplates (the curare type of substances) and succinylcholine, which causes a constant depolarization of the muscle endplates and thereby prevents muscle contractions. Such drugs therefore cannot be used when recordings of muscle activity are to be done as a part of intraoperative monitoring (*see* Chaps. 10 and 11).

The EMG potentials and CMAPs can be recorded by placing electrodes on the surface of the skin close to a muscle or from needle electrodes placed in a muscle. The use of needle electrodes for recording EMG potentials is usually preferred for intraoperative monitoring, because it is more specific and yields larger and more stable potentials than recordings from surface electrodes, which also are likely to include responses from several muscles. Recording from surface electrodes makes it difficult to differentiate the responses from individual muscles compared with recording differentially from a pair of needle electrodes placed in the same muscle. EMG recordings can be done by placing a single electrode on or in a muscle (monopolar recording) or by placing two electrode in a specific muscle (bipolar recording). These two forms of recordings produce EMG potentials with different waveforms when a muscle is activated by a single electrical impulse applied to its motor nerve **(Fig. 3.6)**.

Responses From Fiber Tracts

The neural activity that propagates in individual nerve fibers in a fiber tract in the central nervous system is similar to that in a peripheral nerve, namely as a series of neural discharges. Recording directly from fiber tracts in the spinal cord is done in intraoperative neurophysiological monitoring of the motors system where direct recordings from the corticospinal tract is done routinely (*see* Chap. 10).

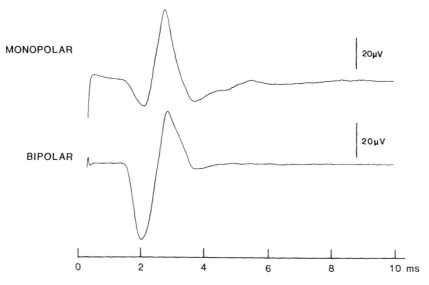

MONOPOLAR

20µV

BIPOLAR

20µV

| | | | | |
| 0 | 2 | 4 | 6 | 8 | 10 ms

Figure 3.6: Comparison between the waveform of EMG potentials that are recorded by a single electrode (monopolar recording) and a pair of electrodes (bipolar recording).

Response From Nuclei

The near-field response from clusters of nerve cells (nuclei) is more complex than that from a nerve or a nerve tract, because the nerve cells of a nucleus generate different kinds of electrical potentials. Generally, a nucleus generates two distinctly different kinds of electrical potentials when activated by a transient volley of neural activity in the nerve or fiber tract that serves as its input. One kind of potentials is fast and one is slow. When recorded by a monopolar electrode, the initial component of the response to transient activation is a sharp, positive–negative complex, which is usually followed by a slow potential **(Fig. 3.7A)**. Several peaks might be riding on the slow potential **(Fig. 3.7B)**. The slow potential is generated by dendrites and the sharp peaks that are riding on that slow wave are generated by firings of cells (somaspikes). The duration of the initial sharp peaks of the response is about the same as that of the CAP recorded from a nerve (0.5–2 ms). These initial fast components are generated when neural activity in the fiber tract that serves as the input to the nucleus reaches the nucleus.

Recordings from the cuneate nucleus of the cat *(37)* have helped understand how nuclei can generate near-field potentials **(Fig. 3.7B)**. The initial fast potentials are generated by the termination of the dorsal column fibers in the nucleus and this component can be recorded with similar waveform from the entire surface of a nucleus **(Fig. 3.7A)**. The size and the polarity of the slow potential, however, depends on the location on a nucleus from which it is recorded **(Fig. 3.7A)**. The slow potential is assumed to be generated by dendrites and it has the property of a dipole. An electrode placed on one side of a nucleus will record a negative slow potential (top recording in **Fig. 3.7A**), whereas an electrode placed on the opposite side the electrode will record a positive potential (bottom recording in **Fig. 3.7A**). Placed in between these two locations, the electrode will record very little of the slow potential **(Fig. 3.7A)**; only the initial positive–negative deflection is seen.

When the recording electrode is placed close to cell bodies, it records a positive potential because the electrode has been placed close to a source of current. A negative potential is recorded when the electrode is placed away from the cell bodies but close to their dendritic trees, because the electrode is then close to a "current sink." When a recording

A

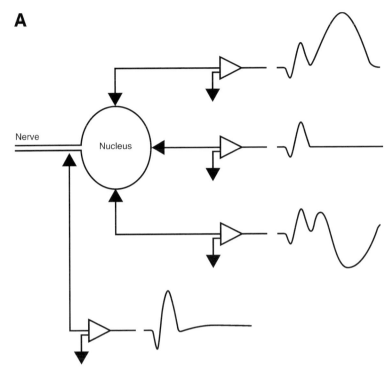

Figure 3.7: *(Continued)*

electrode is passed through a nucleus the polarity of the recorded slow potential will reverse at a certain point along the track of the recording electrode **(Fig. 3.7B)** *(37)*. This is why the generator of evoked potentials from a nucleus is often likened with that of a dipole source, being positive in one end and negative in the other end. If the recording electrode is placed at the same distance from these two ends of this imaginary dipole, it will not record any response because the positive and negative contributions are equal **(Fig. 3.7A)**.

The amplitude and the distribution of the potentials on the surface of a nucleus depend on the internal organization of the nucleus. Nuclei in which there is an orderly arrangements of the cells with dendrites pointing in the same direction produce responses of higher amplitude than nuclei in which the dendrites point in different directions.

Typical examples of the responses from nuclei of the ascending auditory pathway (the cochlear nucleus and the inferior colliculus in man) in response to click stimulation are seen in **Fig. 3.8A,B**, respectively. Recordings from sensory nuclei in the monkey *(38)*, man *(39)*, and from the ventro-posterior thalamus of the cat *(40)* all have a similar wave shape.

The sharp peaks that often are seen riding on the slow potentials in recordings from the surface of a nucleus are assumed to be generated by somaspikes. These sharp peaks occur with longer latencies than the initial positive–negative defection because of the delay in synaptic transmission in the nucleus.

FAR-FIELD POTENTIALS

The response that can be recorded from an electrode placed at a long distance from a nerve or a nucleus that is surrounded by an electrically conductive medium is known as a far-field response. For the purpose of intraoperative

B

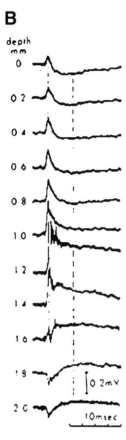

monitoring, recording far-field potentials is done when it is not possible to place electrodes directly on the active structures. Generally, the amplitudes of far-field potentials are much smaller than those of near-field potentials, and the waveforms of far-field potentials differ from those of near-field potentials. Far-field potentials often have contributions from several different sources. If these sources are activated sequentially, the contributions will appear in the recorded potentials with different latencies because of the delays in neural transmission. Contributions from sources that are activated simultaneously might not be easily discernable in the recordings because they are likely to overlap in time.

Most theories about how far-field potentials are related to the electrical activity of nerves, fiber tracts, and nuclei have been based on the concept that different neural structures can be regarded as independent generators of electrical activity in a way similar to that of a dipole. This means that nerves, fiber tracts, and nuclei can be viewed as sources of electrical current that at any given time are positive at one anatomical location and negative at another. When this theory is applied to the electrical activity that is generated by a nerve, the dipole in question is not stationary but moves along the nerve with the propagation of the neural activity in the nerve. The dipoles of nuclei are mainly stationary but might change after the initial activation because different parts of a nucleus might be activated sequentially in response to a transient stimulus.

The amplitude of the potentials that can be recorded from an electrode placed on the scalp in response to transient stimulation of a sensory system such as the auditory system depends not only on the strength of the dipoles that represent the neural activity in the different structures of the auditory pathways but also on the

Figure 3.7: Responses that can be recorded from the surface of a nucleus. (**A**) Schematic of the potentials that may be recorded from the surface of a sensory nucleus in response to transient stimulation such as a click sound for the auditory system. The three waveforms shown refer to recordings at opposite locations on the nucleus and in between to illustrate the dipole concept for describing the potentials that are generated by a nucleus. The waveform of the response that can be recorded from the nerve that terminates in the nucleus is also shown. (Reprinted from: Møller, AR. *Neural Plasticity and Disorders of the Nervous System.* Cambridge: University of Cambridge Press; 2005, in press, with permission from University of Cambridge Press.) (**B**) Schematic illustration of the responses that might be obtained from the cunate nucleus to stimulation of the median nerve at the wrist. The recording electrode was passed through the nucleus and the traces to the right show the recorded potentials at different

Figure 3.7: *(Continued)* locations. (Reprinted from: Andersen P, Eccles JC, Schmidt RF, Yokota T. Slow potential wave produced by the cunate nucleus by cutaneous volleys and by cortical stimulation. *J. Neurophys.* 1964;27:71–91, with permission from Elsevier.)

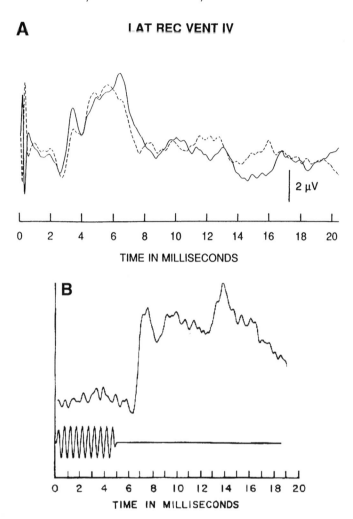

Figure 3.8: Typical response from nuclei recorded by a monopolar electrode. (**A**) The recordings obtained from the surface of the cochlear nucleus in a patient undergoing an operation to relieve HFS. The stimuli used to elicit the response were click sounds. (Reprinted from: Møller AR, Jannetta PJ, Jho HD. Click-evoked responses from the cochlear nucleus: a study in human. *Electroenceph. Clin. Neurophysiol.* 1994;92:215–224, with permission from Elsevier.) (**B**) Responses recorded from the exposed inferior colliculus in a patient operated on to remove a pineal body tumor. The responses were elicited by 2-kHz tone bursts. (Reprinted from: Møller AR, Jannetta PJ. Evoked potentials from the inferior colliculus in man. *Electroenceph. Clin. Neurophysiol.* 1982;53:612–620, with permission from Elsevier.)

(three-dimensional) orientation of these dipoles in relation to the placement of the recording electrodes. The distance from the recording electrodes to the structures in question naturally also plays a role, as does the electrical properties of the medium between the recording site and the active neural structures. The electrical resistance of the skull bone affects far-field potentials recorded from the brain from electrodes placed on the scalp.

Although various recording techniques are discussed later in this book (Chap. 4), some basic principles of recording far-field evoked potentials must be mentioned here. Ideally, when recording far-field potentials, one of the two recording electrodes connected to a differential amplifier should be placed as close to the source as possible (even though this location might be at a considerable distance), and the other recording electrode (often called the "reference electrode" or the "indifferent electrode") should be placed as far away from the source from which the recordings are being made so that it records as little as possible of the potentials that are generated by the part of the nervous system that is being studied (*see* Chap. 4). The best way to achieve that is to place the reference electrode outside the head (noncephalic reference) *(43–45)*. Using such a noncephalic reference makes interpretation of the potentials easier, and it provides better correspondence between the far-field potentials and the near-field potentials, thus facilitating identification of the neural generators of the different components of far-field potentials. However, it is not always possible to achieve this ideal situation, and in many instances, both of the two recording electrodes that are connected to a differential amplifier will record considerable evoked potentials from the system that is being tested and the recording will show the difference between the potentials that appear at the two locations where the recording electrodes are placed.

Nerves and Fiber Tracts

The neural activity that is propagated in a nerve or a fiber tract does not always generate stationary peaks in a far-field recording. This is because the neural depolarization that is elicited by a single transient stimulation propagates continuously along the nerve and that does not generate any stationary peaks in a far-field recording unless certain conditions are filled *(46)*: (1) The propagated activity stops such as it does when a nerve terminate in a nucleus, (2) a nerve is bent *(47)*, or (3) the electrical conductivity of the medium that surrounds the nerve in question changes *(48–50)*. Stationary peaks in far-field potentials can therefore be produced when a nerve or a fiber tract passes through a bony canal

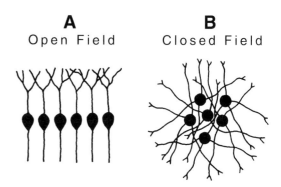

A Open Field   **B** Closed Field

Figure 3.9: Two different types of organization of cells in a nucleus: **(A)** open field; **(B)** closed field. (Modified from ref. *51*.)

from one fluid-filled space to another such as occurs when the spinal cord passes through the foramen magnum.

Nuclei

A nucleus can be regarded as one or several stationary electrical dipoles with a certain orientation in space. If the neuron's dendrites are all oriented in nearly the same direction, the (slow) far-field potentials that are generated by these dendrites will be large **(Fig. 3.9)**. The cerebral cortex is one example of a neural structure with a highly organized dendritic field, in which large dendritic trees point in nearly the same direction **(Fig. 3.9A)**, resulting in a large far-field potential being recorded. In a nucleus in which the cell bodies are in the center with the dendrites pointing in all directions **(Fig. 3.9B)**, the amplitudes of the far-field potentials will be small and might not be measurable at all. Such a nucleus is said to have a closed electrical field. A seemingly paradoxical situation might therefore arise in which a nucleus, despite the fact that it might have a large near-field potential, might not contribute measurably to the far-field potentials because of its internal organization, whereas another nucleus in which many dendrites point in the same direction might contribute significantly to the far-field potentials, although it might produce smaller near-field potentials *(51)*. In practice, it is difficult to find nuclei with an internal organization of just one such type; most nuclei have an organization that is somewhere between these two extremes. Discharges of the cell bodies in a nucleus might produce a sharp peak in the far-field potential (somaspikes).

EFFECT OF INSULTS TO NERVES, FIBER TRACTS, AND NUCLEI

The changes in the recorded neuroelectric potentials that are caused by changes in function of specific parts of the nervous system are the basis for interpreting the results of intraoperative neurophysiological monitoring. Various forms of surgical insults to nerves and nuclei results in characteristic changes in recorded neuroelectric potentials, which can make it possible to diagnose different forms of injury.

The Injured Nerve

The responses (CAP) from injured nerves have a different waveform than that recorded from a normal nerve. It is important to understand the meaning of these differences for proper diagnosis of injuries to peripheral nerves. (Trauma to peripheral nerves is discussed in detail in Chap. 13.)

Most forms of insults to a nerve reduce its conduction velocity, thus increasing the latency of the CAP recorded proximal to the injury when elicited by stimulation at a location that is distal to the recording site. If neural conduction in a fraction of the nerve fibers of a nerve is blocked, the amplitude of the negative peak in the CAP decreases. Similar changes in the CAP might occur when nerves are subjected to mechanical manipulation or injury from, for instance, heating such as might occur from electrocoagulation near the nerve. The magnitude of the decrease in amplitude of the negative peak is a measure of approximately how large is the fraction of the nerve fibers that have ceased to actively conduct nerve impulses. If the conduction velocity in different nerve fibers is affected differently, temporal dispersion of the nerve impulses will cause the negative peak of the CAP to become broader because the action potentials in different nerve

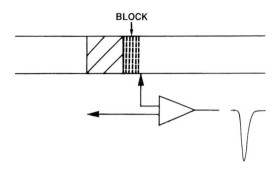

Figure 3.10: Monopolar recording from an injured nerve in which the propagation of a zone of depolarization stops before it reaches the recording electrode.

fibers will appear at different times at the site of recording.

Stretching of a nerve can increase the neural conduction time (decrease the conduction velocity) of all nerve fibers or a fraction of the fibers of a nerve. The decreased conduction velocity causes the latency of the CAP to increase. The waveform of the recorded CAP might become more complex and have multiple peaks as a result of insults to a nerve if the injury causes different groups of nerve fibers to have different degrees of prolonged conduction times.

If a total conduction block in all nerve fibers in a peripheral nerve occurs between the stimulation site and the recording site, it will abolish the negative peak of the CAP that is recorded by a monopolar recording electrode because the depolarization caused by the stimulation will not pass under the recording electrode as it does normally. A total conduction block causes the initial positivity in the CAP to dominate the recorded waveform **(Fig. 3.10)**. This is known as the "cut-end" potential. Likewise, a single positive deflection will be recorded if the recording electrode is placed beyond the end point of a nerve. Thus, for the CAP recorded from a nerve where the neural conduction is blocked by, for instance, crushing of the nerve so that the propagation of the zone of depolarization no longer passes under the recording electrode, the waveform of the recorded potentials changes from the typical triphasic shape to a single positive deflection.

If the site of injury occurs beyond the location of the (monopolar) recording electrode, little change in the recorded potentials might be seen. Such a situation could occur, for example, when recording evoked potentials from the peripheral portion of the auditory nerve (at the ear) in response to click stimulation during operations in which the intracranial portion of the auditory nerve is being surgically manipulated. No change in the response recorded from the distal portion of a nerve is likely to be detected even after the occurrence of a severe injury to the proximal (central) portion of the nerve or even severance of the proximal portion of the nerve (*see* Chap. 6).

The Injured Nuclei

Insult to nuclei can cause complex changes in the recorded evoked potentials. Synaptic transmission is more sensitive to insults such as anoxia and cooling than is the neural conduction in nerves and fiber tracts. That means that such injuries will affect the slow potentials that can be recorded from a nucleus, leaving the fast initial positive–negative deflection unaffected.

4

Practical Aspects of Recording Evoked Activity From Nerves, Fiber Tracts, and Nuclei

INTRODUCTION

Intraoperative neurophysiological monitoring employs methods and techniques similar to those currently used in the clinical neurophysiology laboratory, but there are several important differences between recording sensory evoked potentials and electromyographic (EMG) potentials for diagnostic purposes in the clinic and for doing so in order to detect changes in neural function during an operation. The operating room is usually regarded to be an electrically hostile environment, which differs from the clinical neurophysiological laboratory where recording of EMG responses and sensory evoked potentials such as auditory brainstem response (ABR), somatosensory evoked potentials (SSEP), and visual evoked potentials (VEP) are usually done in electrically and acoustically shielded rooms. In the operating room, many other kinds of electronic equipment are connected to the patient. Equipment that is used to monitor the patient's vital

From: *Intraoperative Neurophysiological Monitoring: Second Edition*
By A. R. Møller
© Humana Press Inc., Totowa, NJ.

parameters, for electrocoagulation, drilling of bone, and so forth might interfere with neurophysiological monitoring. In the clinic, however, usually only the equipment used for the recordings in question is connected to the patient. Therefore, knowing how to identify and reduce electrical interference is another important matter in connection with intraoperative monitoring (discussed in detail in Chap. 17).

Another difference between work in the operating room and in the clinical physiological laboratory is related to the fact that in the operating room, it is difficult to correct the placement of electrodes, earphones, and other equipment on the patient after the patient is draped. This, of course, puts great importance on the correct placement of electrodes for recording neuroelectric potentials and for electrical stimulation, as well as of other devices involved in stimulation (such as earphones) before the operation begins.

Reducing the potential for making mistakes is of critical importance when performing intraoperative neurophysiological monitoring. Because the results of monitoring must be available immediately, there are few possibilities for correcting mistakes.

Advanced planning and organization is essential for successful execution of any form of intraoperative neurophysiological monitoring. It is of significant importance that everything that is needed for monitoring is available and brought into the operating room before the operation begins, including spares of sterile items that might become contaminated during the operation. Using a checklist reduces the risks of making potential mistakes.

Everything that will be needed for the monitoring to be performed should be prepared and ready well in advance of the operation. The computer and the amplifiers should be set up for the particular recording to be done in each individual case, so that the collection of data can begin immediately after placement of the electrodes and the earphones.

The fact that neurophysiological monitoring equipment that is used in the operating room is constantly moved in and out of operating rooms exert strain on equipment especially cables and connectors. This makes it important to bring the equipment into the operating room well in advance of the beginning of an operation so that the equipment can be checked and possible malfunction be corrected before it is to be used.

PREPARING THE PATIENT FOR MONITORING

Patients who are to be monitored intraoperatively must have specific preoperative tests done. When sensory evoked potentials are to be monitored, preoperative assessment of the patient's sensory functions must be obtained before the operation. If auditory evoked potentials are to be monitored, the patient must have a hearing test, including pure tone audiograms and speech discrimination tests, before the operation. If SSEPs are to be monitored intraoperatively, the patient must have similar recordings of SSEP done preoperatively. In a similar way, if motor systems are to be monitored, it must be made sure that the patients preoperatively have the motor functions that

are to be monitored. Quantitative assessment of these motor functions must be done before the operation.

Before the patient is brought to the operating room, it must be planned what to monitor and how to do that, and placement of electrodes for recording and stimulation must be planned in detail. When the patient is brought to the operating room, the monitoring team should introduce themselves and briefly explain what they are going to do and why that is important for the patient. It is naturally better to do that the evening before if the patient is in the hospital at that time.

Careful planning of the details of the intraoperative monitoring makes it possible to apply electrodes for recording and stimulation promptly when the patient has been put to sleep. In this way, the necessary setup and patient preparations are performed without interference from, or delay to, the rest of the surgical team. In some cases, it is possible to place the stimulating and recording electrodes before the patient is put to sleep.

Recording and Stimulating Electrodes

Several different types of electrodes are used for electrical stimulation and for recording of near-field and far-field potentials, and all have advantages and disadvantages. Needle electrodes that are applied percutaneously are often used but also surface electrodes that are applied to the skin are commonly used. Which type of electrode is chosen depends on factors such as safety concerns and the possibility of obtaining reliable stable recordings over a long period of time. Surface electrodes take a longer time to apply than needle electrodes but can conveniently be applied before the patient is brought to a sleep. However, the electrode wires then have to be taped to the patient so they are not affected by moving the patient to the operating table.

Regardless of the type of electrodes that are chosen, it is important that all electrodes stay in place throughout the entire operation, because it is often not possible to gain access to the location where they were applied after the sterile drape has been placed. If recording or stimulating electrodes are to be applied after the patient has been anesthetized, it is also important that the electrodes can be applied quickly so that precious operating time is not wasted. At this time, before the operation begins, there are usually other preparations, such as shaving the head or preparing the skin, that must be done by the operating room staff, and there is usually enough time to place even a large number of needle electrodes in different locations while these other preparations are being done. Surface electrodes can be applied before the patient is anesthetized and even before the patient is brought into the operating room so that this task does not interfere with other activities involving the patient.

Platinum needle electrodes (such as Type E2, Grass Instruments Co., Braintree, MA) are suitable for recordings as well as to deliver electrical stimulation. It is important to observe the risks of acquiring potentially serious diseases in the operating room through contact with blood and accidentally acquired needle punctures. Therefore, it is recommended to use disposable needle electrodes. If platinum reusable needle electrodes are used, they must be cleaned and prepared according to the manufacturer's recommendations and handled carefully after use for the safety of the operating room personnel.

When placed percutaneously to record from the body surface and secured with a good quality plastic adhesive tape (such as Blenderm™; 3M, St. Paul, MN), needle electrodes provide stable recording and electrical stimulation for many hours and such electrodes are practically impossible to remove from the skin unintentionally. It is rare to have a needle electrode come off accidentally during an operation. The impedance of needle electrodes might be slightly higher than that of some types of surface electrode. Usually, this does not create any problems and the impedance of needle electrodes rarely increases noticeably during an operation.

The most common malfunction of electrodes is caused by the electrode becoming partly or completely disengaged from the patient. This increases the electrode impedance, electrodes that are used for recording will pick up more electrical interference; therefore, a sign that an electrode is coming loose is the display of an increased noise level on a recording channel. Determination of which one of the two electrodes that are connected to a differential amplifier is faulty can be made by using the option provided by most modern amplifiers to measure electrode impedance. A malfunctioning electrode has a higher than normal impedance.

Adverse effects of using needle electrodes in the form of infection or postoperative marks on the skin are very rare. Within a few days after the operation, it is usually impossible to identify the sites where the needle electrodes had been placed.

When using needle electrodes during operations, it is important that the electrocautery equipment used during the procedure be of high quality and an efficient return electrode pad be placed on the patient (usually the thigh). If the return connection is faulty, any electrodes placed on the patient that are in contact with grounded (electronic) equipment might carry some of the high-frequency current that is used for electrocautery back to the electrocautery generator. This might cause burns where the electrophysiological recording electrodes are placed on the skin (and possibly lead to destruction of the electronic recording equipment as well). The degree of skin injury is inversely related to the surface area of the electrodes, and because needle electrodes have a much smaller area than surface electrodes, the burns can be expected to be more severe when needle electrodes are used. Nevertheless, intraoperative monitoring in several thousand patients, sometimes with as many as 20 electrodes placed on the same patient, this author has never seen any burn marks from electrodes or any indication that excessive current had passed through the recording electrodes, despite the fact that the recording electrodes in nearly all of these patients were in place during the first phase of the operation, when high-powered monopolar electrocautery is used for cutting purposes.

Before the recording electrodes are applied to the patient and connected to the respective amplifiers, the power to the amplifiers should be switched on, because electrical surges might result from switching recording amplifiers on, and if the patient is connected to the amplifier at that time, these electrical surges might be harmful. In the same way, equipment should not be turned off before all electrodes have been removed from the patient.

When needle electrodes are used, they must be removed carefully from the patient when the operation is completed in order to avoid injury to the patient's skin. This is naturally of particular importance when electrodes are placed in the face. Needle electrodes should be removed one at a time, first removing the adhesive tape that holds them in place and then pulling the needle out while gently pulling the wire in the opposite direction in which the needle was inserted. With some experience, this can be done in a short time, even in cases in which many electrodes are placed in the face or in other places on the body. Disposable needle electrodes should be disposed of in a safe way in order to minimize the possibility of anyone being stuck by electrode needles that have been inserted into a patient. Reusable needles should be dropped in a solution of sodium hypochlorite (Clorox) for a few minutes. It is practical to place a bucket with Clorox solution under the operating table so that the needle electrodes can be dropped into the bucket immediately after they are removed from the patient without being touched. Afterward, the electrodes can be washed, rinsed, and then sterilized (either using an autoclave or gas sterilization) in accordance with the manufacturer's directions.

When handling needle electrodes, it must always be assumed that any patient can have a disease, such as hepatitis B or C, HIV, and so forth, that can be transmitted through bloodborne pathogens. The same precautions as taken when handling hypodermic needles used for injection purposes must be taken when handling needle electrodes. The person who places

and removes needles from patients before and after intraoperative monitoring must be adequately trained in handling infected needles and informed about the protocols that must be followed.

Earphones

Earphones used when recording auditory evoked potentials can be placed while other activity involving the patient is in progress. When miniature stereo earphones are used, they should be secured in the ear with adhesive tape in a watertight fashion to prevent fluids from reaching the ear canal. The earphone should be placed so that the sound-emitting surface of the earphone faces the opening of the ear canal. Before an earphone is placed in the ear, the ear canal should be inspected. In some elderly persons, the ear canal opening is nearly a narrow slit that might occlude when an earphone is placed in the ear. A short plastic tube of a suitable diameter placed in the ear canal can hold it open before the earphone is placed in the ear. When insert earphones are used, this is not a problem because the ear canal will be kept open by the tube that is inserted in the ear canal that conducts the sound to the ear. When insert earphones are used, it is important that the tube that is inserted in the ear canal fits well and that it is well secured so that it is not accidentally pulled out during the operation. The person who is to apply the earphones to the patient should inspect the patient's ear beforehand to assess any special needs.

Light Stimulators

Commercially available goggles with built-in light-emitting diodes are used in the clinic but are not suitable for use in the operating room. Contact lenses with light-emitting diodes are a better option to stimulate the visual system for recording VEPs. Only flash stimulation can be used in the operating room. The pattern-reversal visual stimulators that are used clinically cannot be used intraoperatively, because it is not possible to focus the conventionally used checkerboard pattern on the retina of a patient who is anesthetized and draped for surgery.

Electric Stimulation of Nervous Tissue

Electrical stimulation of peripheral nerves and cranial nerves is perhaps the most common way of activating nervous tissue for monitoring purposes. For stimulating peripheral nerves, needles are suitable, and for transderm stimulation, surface electrodes can be used. Intracranial stimulation can be done using handheld stimulators; either monopolar or bipolar electrodes are used, depending on how specific the stimulation is anticipated. Some investigators have developed surgical instruments that work as electrical stimulators for the purpose of detecting when specific nervous tissue is manipulated with the surgical instrument (52).

Electrical stimulation of the motor cortex is in increasing use for monitoring motor systems. Most commonly used is transcranial electrical stimulation using electrodes placed on the scalp (see Chap. 10). The voltage used are in the ranges from 500 to 1000 V; this is much higher than what is used for the stimulation of nerves and special precautions are necessary to ensure safety. Various kinds of stimulating electrode have been used, but "corkscrew" types of electrode are probably the most commonly used types of stimulating electrode (see Chap. 10). Such stimulation can only be used in anesthetized patients because of the excessive pain that it would cause in an awake individual. In operations where the motor cortex is exposed, direct stimulation can be applied, which requires much less voltage.

Recordings from the exposed cerebral cortex are done for identifying the location of the central sulcus. For that purpose, plastic strips with a string of four to eight electrodes or fields of 4 × 4 or 8 × 8 electrodes are used and placed directly on the exposed cerebral cortex (Chap. 14).

The stimulators that deliver constant-current or (semi) constant-voltage impulses should be chosen depending on the circumstances. For stimulating peripheral nerves, constant-current stimulators are most suitable, and for intracranial stimulation, constant-voltage stimulators are most suitable. The choice of stimulator type is discussed in detail in Chap. 18.

Magnetic Stimulation of Nervous Tissue

Magnetic stimulation (transcranial magnetic stimulation) is used to stimulate peripheral nerves or central nervous system (CNS) structures such as the cerebral cortex. Magnetic stimulation involves applying an impulse or a train of impulses of a strong magnetic field to the structure in question. This is done by placing a coil through which a strong electrical current is passed over the structure that is to be stimulated. It is not the magnetic field that causes the activation of neural tissue but, rather, the induced electrical current. Magnetic stimulation has advantages over electrical stimulation in that it can activate nerve and brain tissue noninvasively (extracranially) and without causing any pain.

RECORDING OF NEAR-FIELD POTENTIALS

Near-field potentials can almost always be recorded from muscles and peripheral nerves, whereas near-field potentials from the CNS can only be recorded intraoperatively in special situations. Therefore, evoked potentials from the CNS are normally recorded at a distance from the sources, thus "far-field" potentials.

Recording From Muscles

Recording of electromyographical potentials is now the most common way of recording responses from muscles, although other methods that make use of measurements of movement of muscles have also been in use (53–56). Recordings of EMG potentials provide accurate information about which muscle is being activated and such recordings make it possible to detect muscle contractions that are too small to be detected visually. Recording EMG potentials also offers a quantitative way to assess not only if a muscle is being activated but also to what degree it is being activated. EMG recording permits accurate measurement of latencies, thus making it possible to determine neural conduction velocities (and particular changes in neural conduction velocity) during an operation. EMG recording thereby makes it possible to assess neural conduction in motor nerves and detect conduction block in portions of nerves.

Continuous monitoring of neural activity in motor nerves by recording EMG activity from muscles innervated by both spinal and cranial motor nerves is useful for detecting the effects of surgical manipulations of motor nerves. Monitoring of EMG activity can also detect muscle activity elicited by mechanical stimulation of motor nerves and neural activity that might occur as a result of injury to the respective motor nerve. Detection of such mechanically evoked EMG activity or activity caused by injury makes it possible to alert the surgeon so that the particular manipulation can be stopped and reversed, if possible. Such information can also help to avoid similar injury in the remaining course of the operation and in future operations.

Making the recorded EMG activity audible is important because it can relate information about manipulations of motor nerves to the surgeon directly. The character of the sounds that EMG signals emit provides important information about the nature of the effects of surgical manipulations on the function of the motor nerve. Listening to the EMG sounds helps distinguish between severe injury and benign stimulation of a motor nerve. Making the muscle responses audible can alert the neurophysiologist without having to continuously monitor a computer screen, and it makes it possible for the surgeon to hear the spontaneous muscle activity that often results from surgical manipulation of a motor nerve (such as the facial nerve) and that indicates that the manipulation is causing injury to the nerve.

Rapid feedback to the surgeon is also important when mapping the surgical field with an electrical stimulating handheld electrode to determine where a motor nerve is located. Such mapping of the surgical field is important when removing tumors that adhere to a motor nerve. It might be even more important for finding regions of a tumor that do not contain a motor nerve so that the tumor can be removed safely one section after another without fear of injuring a nerve.

Some commercial equipment have the option of allowing the EMG signal to trigger a tone signal intended to warn that the amplitude of the EMG potentials has exceeded some preset value. However, the unprocessed EMG signal contains much information that such tone signals cannot communicate. Having EMG activity trigger tone signals might also be confusing because other equipment in the operating room often generate similar "beeps" and it might be difficult to distinguish EMG-elicited "beeps" from that of equipment such as that used by the anesthesia team.

Electrodes that are used for recording EMG potentials from superficial muscles might be needle electrodes or surface electrodes. Needle electrodes tend to provide more stable recordings over a long time than surface electrodes. Needle electrodes can be placed more precisely than surface electrodes, and needle electrodes can reach muscles that are located beneath the body surface such as the extraocular muscles.

Monitoring the Function of Peripheral Nerves

In the operating room, the most common way of monitoring the function of peripheral nerves involves electrical stimulation of the nerves and recording of the compound action potential (CAP) from the nerves in question. Needle electrodes are suitable for both purposes. When recording from nerves that are surgically exposed other kinds of stimulating and recoding electrodes can be used (see Chap. 13).

Recordings From Fiber Tracts, Nuclei, and the Cerebral Cortex

Whenever it is possible to place recording electrodes close to a structure of the CNS, near-field potentials can be recorded. For intraoperative monitoring, near-field potentials have been recorded from the intracranial portion of the auditory nerve, the cochlear nucleus, the cerebral cortex, and the surface of the spinal cord to record from the corticospinal tract. Such recordings can be made by placing a single electrode on the structure in question. This allows recording of evoked potentials from specific portions of the nervous system without including the recordings of potentials from other parts of that same system that might also respond to the stimulus. Using bipolar recording electrodes provides more spatial specificity than using monopolar recording electrodes. This is important to consider when recordings are to be made from specific peripheral nerves, muscles, or nuclei of the brain and when the electrical activity of other adjacent structures might produce electrical activity that can also be recorded by the recording electrodes. However, it is not always practical or possible to place a bipolar recording electrode on the structure from which recording is to be made.

Electrodes for intracranial stimulation and recording are placed by the surgeon and the task of the monitoring team is therefore reduced to making sure that electrodes are available to the surgeon and that the recording electrode is properly connected to the amplifier via the electrode box. The monitoring team must be responsible for the way the intracranial electrodes are transferred to the sterile field. Although the electrodes and their connecting cables are located within the sterile field, the electrode box that is used to connect the electrodes to the amplifier is outside the sterile field. The cables connecting the intracranial electrodes to the electrode box must be carried in and out of the sterile field in a safe way. It is important that the cables be secured well so that the intracranial electrodes cannot be disengaged from the wound by an accidental pull on the cables that connect them to their respective electronic equipment.

The parts of these electrodes that have been in contact with body must be discarded, but all other parts can be cleaned carefully at the end of the operation and sterilized (gas) before being used again.

Sensory evoked potentials such as ABR and SSEP are commonly recorded modalities for intraoperative monitoring, whereas VEPs are monitored in fewer operations. Such potentials typically contain responses from many different sources, which makes interpretation more difficult than near-field potentials. Of practical importance is the fact that far-field potentials have a much smaller amplitude than near-field potentials and the amplitude is often smaller than that of the background activity. That requires the use of signal processing methods such as signal averaging and filtering (*see* Chap. 18).

Optimal Placement of Recording Electrodes

The interpretation of far-field evoked potentials depends on the electrode placement. Far-field sensory evoked potentials are traditionally recorded differentially from two electrodes that both record the evoked potentials in question, although to a different degree; this contributes to the difficulties in interpreting sensory evoked far-field potentials. A few investigators have used electrode placement where the evoked potentials that are recorded with one of the two electrodes is negligible (noncephalic reference).

It is practical to always use the same electrode montage for a particular type of monitoring. Interpretation of far-field sensory evoked potentials is complicated by the fact that several neural generators contribute to the response, and some of these components might overlap in time. Electrodes placed at different locations on the scalp will record the various components differently, not only because of the different distances to the individual sources but more so because of the orientation of the dipoles of these sources. This will naturally make an interpretation of the origins of the various components complex. These matters will be discussed in more detail in Chaps. 6–8.

RECORDING OF FAR-FIELD POTENTIALS

Far-field evoked potentials are recorded from electrodes placed on the surface of the body.

HOW TO ACHIEVE OPTIMAL RECORDINGS?

There are many ways that the time needed to obtain an interpretable recording can be shortened, the most effective of which involves proper electrode placement, optimal stimulation, and the use of optimal filtering of the recorded signals.

Several factors affect the time it takes to obtain an interpretable record. The following list summarizes the factors that are important for obtaining a clean interpretable record in as short a time as possible:

1. Decrease the electrical interference that reaches the recording electrodes.
2. Use optimal stimulus repetition rate.
3. Use optimal stimulus strength.
4. Use optimal filtering of the recorded potentials.
5. Use optimal placement of recording electrodes.
6. Use quality control that does not require replicating records.

We will discuss the effect of electrical interference from other equipment than that used directly in an operation in detail in Chap. 18. In this chapter, we will discuss the effect of electrical interference on recordings of evoked potentials.

Selection of Stimulus and Recording Parameters

Optimizing stimulation and selection of optimal recording parameters and reduction of electrical interference are all factors that can shorten the time it takes to obtain an interpretable record. However, these factors have received less attention than deserved. It is important that the recording strategy be planned ahead of the time when the operation begins and that recording and stimulation parameters be set before the patient is brought into the operating room. We will discuss how to select the optimal stimulus and recording parameters in the chapters that cover monitoring of the different sensory systems (Chaps. 6–8).

It would be ideal to be able to record responses that are clearly discernable from that of the background activity that always exists in recordings taken in the operating room. Normally though, special processing of the recorded responses must be performed in order to obtain an interpretable record, including signal averaging and appropriate filtering. The background activity can be electrical interference and/or biological signals such as EMG potentials from nearby muscles. Also, ongoing (EEG) activity is a source of interference that can obscure evoked potentials when recording from electrodes placed on the head. The equipment should be set up according to such requirements and appropriate parameters for amplification and filtering should be selected and set before placement of electrodes on the patient.

DISPLAY OF RESULTS

Modern equipment offers a wealth of different ways of displaying evoked potentials, such as "waterfall" displays that show successive records stacked on top of each other, and various forms of trend analysis, such as the change in amplitude and latency of specified components. However, probably the most useful way of displaying evoked potentials is a single curve that is superimposed on a similar recording obtained at the beginning of the operation (baseline).

The baseline recording should be stored in the computer so that it can easily be displayed and compared with the subsequent recordings in order to facilitate detection of changes in the recorded potentials. It is practical to use autoscaling of the recorded potentials so that the averaged potentials can be viewed on a full screen in order to detect changes in the waveform of the evoked potentials. When autoscaling is used, the amplitude must be displayed on the screen in the form of a number so that the amplitude of the baseline recording can be compared with the amplitudes of the averaged potentials that are recorded during the operation. (Using autoscaling makes the waveform of the recorded potentials appear on the screen as if it always had the same amplitude.)

Baseline recording of ABR, SSEP, or VEP should be made after the patient is anesthetized but before the operation begins, and it is best done while the sterile drape is being placed but before the use of electrocautery starts.

ELECTRICAL INTERFERENCE

One of the greatest differences between recording neuroelectrical potentials in the operating room and the clinical physiology laboratory is the presence of many sources of electrical and magnetic interference in the operating room. Some forms of such electrical interferences can be reduced with appropriate measures, whereas other kinds of interference cannot be reduced, so their effect on recordings of electrical potentials from the nervous system and muscles must be reduced by other means such as signal averaging and filtering (*see* Chap. 18). There are two main kinds of electrical interference that appear in an operating room. One kind is always present in a specific operating room, whereas the other kind occurs only occasionally.

Continuous Electrical Interference

Continuous interference signals should be reduced as much as possible at the source and that should be done well in advance of doing actual intraoperative monitoring. Ideally, the operating room should be examined when it is not in use and without any time constraints, such as late afternoon the day before monitoring is scheduled in an operating room in which the monitoring team does not have experience of monitoring (as described in Chap. 18).

Interference That Appears Intermittently During an Operation

Interference that can appear suddenly during an operation must be dealt with promptly. Its source must be identified and the interference eliminated with as short a delay as possible because monitoring cannot be done while the interference exist. The operation is

not going to stop and that means that the patient does not have the protection of intraoperative monitoring until the interference is eliminated and recordings resume. Such intermittent interference might be caused by any one of the numerous pieces of equipment used by the anesthesia team. It can be generated by the switching on of a blood warmer that had not been used previously in the operation but which gives rise to severe interference when it is on.

One example of such biological interference in intraoperative monitoring of neuroelectric potentials involves the level of anesthesia of the patient, which might vary during an operation and can fall so low that spontaneous muscle contractions occur. Such muscle contractions will cause interference in the recorded neuroelectrical potentials because the electrical potentials that are associated with muscle activity are likely to be picked up by the electrodes used to record the evoked potentials. These are just some examples of the many ways in which intermittent interference can cause problems in monitoring patients intraoperatively.

If intraoperative monitoring is going to be successful, it is necessary to identify the sources and the natures of interferences within a very short time. It is, therefore, important that the neurophysiologist observe not only the averaged potentials but also directly observe the recorded potentials continuously and that he/she be able to distinguish between external electrical interference and interference that is of a biological origin, such as muscle activity. Promptly remedying problems related to suddenly appearing interference is one of the most challenging tasks of a monitoring team. It is important that the person who does the neurophysiological monitoring has enough experience to be able to quickly identify the source of the interference.

The use of electrocoagulation is an example of a strong intermittent kind of electrical interference that, in most cases, makes it impossible to do recordings of neuroelectrical potentials. It cannot be avoided and the only way to reduce its effect is to exclude recordings when electrocoagulation is done. The fact that the electrical interference almost invariably exceeds the dynamic range of the amplifiers used to record sensory evoked potentials might make it necessary to take special precautions in addition to the normally used artifact rejection options that are included in equipment to be used in the operating room.

RELIABILITY OF INTRAOPERATIVE MONITORING

Another important difference between performing neurophysiological recording in the clinical neurophysiological laboratory and in the operating room is that in the clinic, there is always time to replace an electrode that has slipped off or to repair or replace a piece of equipment if it fails to function, and if this is not possible within a reasonable time, the patient can usually be rescheduled for the test or there could be another test room available where the test can be done. No such possibility exists during intraoperative neurophysiological monitoring: if some equipment malfunctions, it either has to be fixed within a very short time or the operation will continue without the aid of intraoperative neurophysiological monitoring. The most common problem of this type is that one or more of the electrodes used for the monitoring might stop functioning (having a high resistance). Also, the breakdown of any part of the electronic equipment used for monitoring might make it impossible to complete the intraoperative monitoring. In addition, in the operating room, the sudden appearance of electrical interference, the cause of which cannot be ascertained, will result in the neurophysiologist having to stop the intraoperative monitoring, whereas in the clinical laboratory, such an occurrence almost never occurs because electrical interference from other equipment is not a factor.

Because any one of these problems might make continued monitoring in the operating room more difficult or impossible, it is very important that the person who is actually performing the monitoring (neurophysiologist)

be prepared for a variety of problems and know beforehand how to solve each problem. The person who is responsible for intraoperative neurophysiological monitoring must have sufficient experience and knowledge to be able to identify sources of electrical interference and to locate malfunctioning electrodes or equipment.

Naturally, the highest-quality electronic equipment will provide the most reliable service, but it is important that backup electronic equipment be available for use within a very short time. Having spare cables and electrodes available in the operating room is important, and it is wise to have redundant electrodes placed on the patient where manipulation during the operation might occur. A common factor for all such problems is that they appear when not expected.

COMMUNICATION IN THE OPERATING ROOM

Many of the problems that can occur during monitoring can be identified and solved without delay if the neurophysiologist is communicating effectively and often with the anesthesiologist. Such interaction between the neurophysiologist and the anesthesiologist is important in intraoperative monitoring and it is often also beneficial to the anesthesiologist. For instance, an increase in spontaneous muscle activity as a result of a decrease in the level of anesthesia is often noticeable in electrophysiological recordings long before the level of anesthesia has dropped to a point at which actual movements of the patient can be observed. By relaying information about such electrophysiologically recorded muscle activity to the anesthesiologist, the neurophysiologist might forewarn him/her that the anesthesia level is becoming less than desired. Such information is obviously valuable to the anesthesiologist as well as to the surgeon because it could prevent the anesthesia level dropping so low that the patient can move spontaneously.

References to Section I

1. Brown RH, Nash CL. Current status of spinal cord monitoring. *Spine* 1979;4:466–478.
2. Grundy B. Intraoperative monitoring of sensory evoked potentials. *Anesthesiology* 198;58:72–87.
3. Grundy B. Evoked potentials monitoring. In: Blitt C, ed. *Monitoring in Anesthesia and Critical Care Medicine.* New York: Churchill-Livingstone; 1985:345–411.
4. Raudzens RA. Intraoperative monitoring of evoked potentials. *Ann. NY Acad. Sci.* 1982;388:308–326.
5. Sekhar LN, Møller AR. Operative management of tumors involving the cavernous sinus. *J. Neurosurg* 1986;64:879–889.
6. Møller AR. Electrophysiological monitoring of cranial nerves in operations in the skull base. In: Sekhar LN, Schramm Jr VL, eds. *Tumors of the Cranial Base: Diagnosis and Treatment.* Mt. Kisco, NY: Futura;1987:123–132.
7. Yingling C. Intraoperative monitoring in skull base surgery. In: Jackler RK, Brackmann DE, eds. *Neurotology.* St. Louis, MO: Mosby-Year Book;1994:967–1002.
8. Deletis V. Intraoperative monitoring of the functional integrety of the motor pathways. In: Devinsky O, Beric A, Dogali M, eds. *Advances in Neurology: Electrical and Magnetic Stimulation of the Brain.* New York: Raven; 1993:201–214.
9. Møller AR, Jannetta PJ. Preservation of facial function during removal of acoustic neuromas: use of monopolar constant voltage stimulation and EMG. *J. Neurosurg.* 1984;61:757–760.
10. Prass RL, Lueders H. Acoustic (loudspeaker) facial electromyographic monitoring. Part I. *Neurosurgery* 1986;19:392–400.
11. Kline DG, Judice DJ. Operative management of selected brachial plexus lesions. *J. Neurosurg.* 1983;58:631–649.
12. Møller AR, Jannetta PJ. Monitoring facial EMG during microvascular decompression operations for hemifacial spasm. *J. Neurosurg.* 1987;66:681–685.
13. Haines SJ, Torres F. Intraoperative monitoring of the facial nerve during decompressive surgery for hemifacial spasm. *J. Neurosurg.* 1991;74:254–257.
14. Møller AR, Jannetta PJ. Microvascular decompression in hemifacial spasm: intraoperative electrophysiological observations. *Neurosurgery* 1985;16:612–618.
15. Penfield W, Boldrey E. Somatic motor and sensory representation in the cerebral cortex of man as studied by electrical stimulation. *Brain* 1937;60:389–443.
16. Ojemann GA, Creutzfeldt O, Lettich E, Haglund MM. Neuronal activity in human lateral temporal cortex related to short-term verbal memory, naming and reading. *Brain* 1988;111:1383–1403.
17. Lenz FA, Dostrovsky JO, Kwan HC, Tasker RR, Yamashiro K, Murphy JT. Methods for microstimulation and recording of single neurons and evoked potentials in the human central nervous system. *J. Neurosurg.* 1988;68:630–634.
18. Lenz FA, Kwan HC, Martin RL, Tasker RR, Dostrovsky JO, Lenz YE. Single unit analysis of the human ventral thalamic nuclear group. Tremor-related activity in functionally identified cells. *Brain* 1994;117:531–543.
19. Lenz FA, Dostrovsky JO, Tasker RR, Yamashiro K, Kwan HC, Murphy JT. Single-unit analysis of the human ventral thalamic nuclear group: somatosensory responses. *J. Neurophysiol.* 1988;59:299–316.
20. Lenz FA, Byl NN. Reorganization in the cutaneous core of the human thalamic principal somatic sensory nucleus (ventral caudal) in patients with dystonia. *J. Neurophysiol.* 1999;82:3204–3212.
21. Ojemann GA. Effect of cortical and subcortical stimulation on human language and verbal memory. *Res. Publ. Assoc. Res. Nerv. Ment. Dis.* 1988;66:101–115.
22. Ojemann JG. Language and the thalamus: object naming and recall during and after thalamic stimulation. *Brain Lang.* 1975;2:101–120.
23. Ojemann JG, Ojemann GA, Lettich E. Neuronal activity related to faces and matching in human right nondominant temporal cortex. *Brain* 1992;115:1–13.
24. Penfield W, Rasmussen T. *The Cerebral Cortex of Man: A Clinical Study of Localization of Function.* New York: Macmillan; 1950.
25. Desmedt JE, Cheron G. Central somatosensory conduction in man: neural generators and

interpeak latencies of the far-field components recorded from neck and right or left scalp and earlobes. *Electroenceph. Clin. Neurophysiol.* 1980;50:382–403.

26. Gasser H. The classification of nerve fibers. *Ohio J. Sci.* 1941;41:145–159.
27. Møller AR, Colletti V, Fiorino FG. Neural conduction velocity of the human auditory nerve: Bipolar recordings from the exposed intracranial portion of the eighth nerve during vestibular nerve section. *Electroenceph. Clin. Neurophysiol.* 1994;92:316–320.
28. Møller AR. *Sensory Systems: Anatomy and Physiology.* Amsterdam: Academic; 2003.
29. Møller AR. *Neural Plasticity and Disorders of the Nervous System.* Cambridge: Cambridge University Press; 2005, in press.
30. Møller AR. Neurophysiological basis for cochlear and auditory brainstem implants. *Am. J. Audiol.* 2001;10:68–77.
31. Møller AR. Latency of unit responses in the cochlear nucleus determined in two different ways. *J. Neurophysiol.* 1975;38:812–821.
32. Møller AR. *Hearing: Its Physiology and Pathophysiology.* San Diego: Academic; 2000.
33. Lorente de No R. Analysis of the distribution of action currents of nerve in volume conductors. *Studies Rockefeller Inst. Med. Res.* 1947;132:384–482.
34. Goldstein Jr. MH. A statistical model for interpreting neuroelectric responses. *Inform. Control* 1960;3:1–17.
35. Erlanger J, Gasser HS. *Electrical Signs of Nervous Activity.* Philadelphia: University of Pennsylvania Press; 1937.
36. Møller AR, Colletti V, Fiorino F. Click evoked responses from the exposed intracranial portion of the eighth nerve during vestibular nerve section: bipolar and monopolar recordings. *Electroenceph. Clin. Neurophysiol.* 1994;92:17–29.
37. Andersen P, Eccles JC, Schmidt RF, Yokota T. Slow potential wave produced by the cunate nucleus by cutaneous volleys and by cortical stimulation. *J. Neurophys.* 1964;27:71–91.
38. Møller AR, Jannetta PJ, Burgess JE. Neural generators of the somatosensory evoked potentials: recording from the cuneate nucleus in man and monkeys. *Electroenceph. Clin. Neurophysiol.* 1986;65:241–248.
39. Møller AR, Jannetta PJ, Jho HD. Recordings from human dorsal column nuclei using stimu-

lation of the lower limb. *Neurosurgery* 1990;26:291–299.
40. Andersen P, Brooks CM, Eccles JC, Sears TA. The ventro-basal nucleus of the thalamus: potential fields, synaptic transmission and excitability of both presynaptic and postsynap-tic components. *J. Physiol. (Lond.)* 1964;174:348–369.
41. Møller AR, Jannetta PJ, Jho HD. Click-evoked responses from the cochlear nucleus: a study in human. *Electroenceph. Clin. Neurophysiol.* 1994;92:215–224.
42. Møller AR, Jannetta PJ. Evoked potentials from the inferior colliculus in man. *Electroenceph. Clin. Neurophysiol.* 1982;53:612–620.
43. Cracco RQ, Cracco JB. Somatosensory evoked potentials in man: farfield potentials. *Electroenceph. Clin. Neurophysiol.* 1976;41:60–66.
44. Desmedt JE, Cheron G. Non-cephalic reference recording of early somatosensory potentials to finger stimulation in adult or aging normal man: Differentiation of widespread N18 and contra-lateral N20 from the prerolandic P22 and N30 components. *Electroenceph. Clin. Neurophysiol.* 1981;52:553–570.
45. Møller AR, Jannetta PJ. Neural generators of the brainstem auditory evoked potentials. In: Nodar RH, Barber C, eds. *Evoked Potentials II: The Second International Evoked Potentials Symposium.* Boston, MA: Butterworth; 1984: 137–144.
46. Kimura J, Mitsudome A, Yamada T, Dickens QS. Stationary peaks from moving source in far-field recordings. *Electroenceph. Clin. Neurophysiol.* 1984;58:351–361.
47. Jewett DL, Deupree DL, Bommannan D. Far field potentials generated by action potentials of isolated frog sciatic nerves in a spherical volume. *Electroenceph. Clin. Neurophysiol.* 1990;75:105–117.
48. Kimura A, Mitsudome A, Beck DO, Yamada T, Dickens QS. Field distribution of antidromically activated digital nerve potentials: Models for far-field recordings. *Neurology* 1983;33:1164–1169.
49. Lueders H, Lesser RP, Hahn JR, Little JT, Klein AW. Subcortical somatosensory evoked potentials to median nerve stimulation. *Brain* 1983;106:341–372.
50. Stegeman DF, van Oosterom A, Colon EJ. Far-field evoked potential components induced by a propagating generator: computational evidence. *Electroenceph. Clin. Neurophysiol.* 1987;67:176–187.

51. Lorente de No R. Action potentials of the motoneurons of the hypoglossus nucleus. *J. Cell Comp. Physiol.* 1947;29:207–287.
52. Kartush J, Bouchard K. Intraoperative facial monitoring. Otology, neurotology, and skull base surgery. In: Kartush J, Bouchard K, eds. *Neuromonitoring in Otology and Head and Neck Surgery.* New York: Raven; 1992:99–120.
53. Jako G. Facial nerve monitor. *Trans. Am. Acad. Ophthalmol. Otolaryngol.* 1965;69:340–342.
54. Silverstein H, Smouha E, Jones R. Routine identification of the facial nerve using elec-trical stimualtion during otological and neurotological surgery. *Laryngoscope* 1988;98:726–730.
55. Shibuya M, Matsuga N, Suzuki Y, Sugita K. A newly designed nerve monitor for microneurosurgey: bipolar constant current nerve stimualtor and movement detector with pressure sensor. *Acta Neurochir.* 1993;125:173–176.
56. Sugita K, Kobayashi S. Technical and instrumental improvements in the surgical treatment of acoustic neurinomas. *J. Neurosurg.* 1982(57):747–752.

SECTION II

SENSORY SYSTEMS

Chapter 5
Anatomy and Physiology of Sensory Systems
Chapter 6
Monitoring Auditory Evoked Potentials
Chapter 7
Monitoring of Somatosensory Evoked Potentials
Chapter 8
Monitoring of Visual Evoked Potentials

Understanding the anatomy and physiology of sensory systems is a prerequisite for understanding the changes in recorded responses from sensory systems that might occur when the function of these systems are monitored in patients undergoing operations where sensory systems might be injured. Without understanding the anatomy of the systems that are being tested during various kinds of operation and their normal physiology it is not possible to evaluate changes that might occur during operations and relate such recordings to the potential risk of permanent postoperative deficits. The auditory and the somatosensory systems are the sensory systems that are most often monitored intraoperatively, and the visual system is monitored in operations to a lesser degree. The other sensory systems (olfaction and taste) have not been the object of intraoperative monitoring.

This section also includes chapters that describe the technique of monitoring both far-field and near-field sensory evoked potentials. Specifically, the technique of monitoring auditory brainstem responses (Chap. 6), somatosensory evoked potentials (Chap. 7), and visual evoked potentials (Chap. 8) are described. Monitoring of near-field evoked potentials from these three sensory systems is likewise discussed in these three chapter.

5

Anatomy and Physiology of Sensory Systems

The Auditory System
The Somatosensory System
Visual System

THE AUDITORY SYSTEM

Introduction

Knowledge about the anatomy and physiology of the auditory system is a prerequisite for understanding not only the normal function of the auditory system but also the changes in function that might result from surgical manipulations of the auditory nerve and other, more central structures.

This chapter describes the anatomy and physiology of the auditory system as applicable to intraoperative monitoring of auditory evoked potentials. The generation of far-field auditory evoked potentials (auditory brainstem responses [ABRs]) and near-field auditory evoked potentials (compound action potentials [CAPs]), from the auditory nerve and cochlear nucleus will be discussed. The practical aspects of hearing preservation in various types of operation will be discussed in detail in Chap. 6 using recordings of both far-field and near-field auditory evoked potentials.

The Ear

The ear consists of the outer ear, the middle ear, and the inner ear (cochlea), where the first processing of sounds occurs and where the sensory receptors are located (**Fig. 5.1**).

Sound Conduction to the Cochlea. The middle ear functions as an impedance trans-

From: *Intraoperative Neurophysiological Monitoring: Second Edition*
By A. R. Møller
© Humana Press Inc., Totowa, NJ.

former that facilitates transmission of airborne sound into vibrations of the fluid in the cochlea. This transformer action is the result of a difference between the area of the tympanic membrane and the area of the stapes footplate. The stapes footplate, which is located in the oval window, performs a pistonlike in–out motion that sets the fluid in the cochlea into motion. The middle ear cavity is filled with air and acts as a cushion behind the tympanic membrane. The proper function of the middle ear depends on the air pressure in the middle ear cavity being equal to the ambient pressure *(3)*. This is normally maintained by the opening and closing of the eustachian tube (**Fig. 5.1A**), which occurs naturally by the swallowing action. Because anesthetized individuals do not swallow, a negative pressure could build up in the middle ear cavity during anesthesia and that can cause a reduction in sound transmission for low-frequency sounds. Although the effect of such a reduction on the results of intraoperative monitoring of auditory evoked potentials has been discussed, there is no substantial evidence of any noticeable effect on the results of monitoring click-evoked auditory potentials. (For more details about the anatomy and physiology of the middle ear and the acoustic middle ear reflex, refer to books on the physiology of the ear—for instance, refs. *3* and *4*.)

The Cochlea

The cochlea is shaped like a snail shell and has three fluid-filled compartments (scalae), which are separated by the cochlear partition (or basilar membrane) and the Reissner's membrane

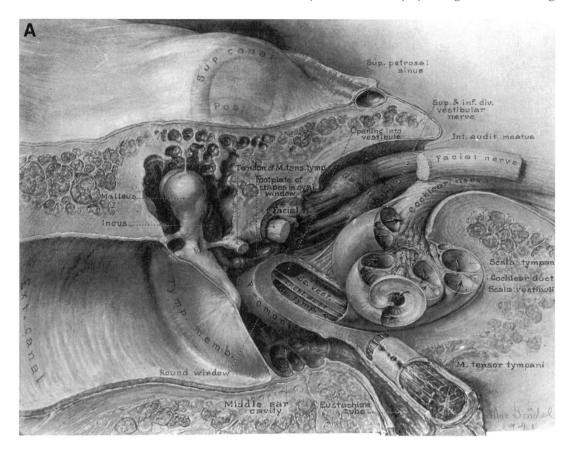

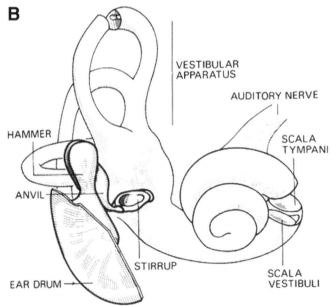

Figure 5.1: *(Continued)*

C

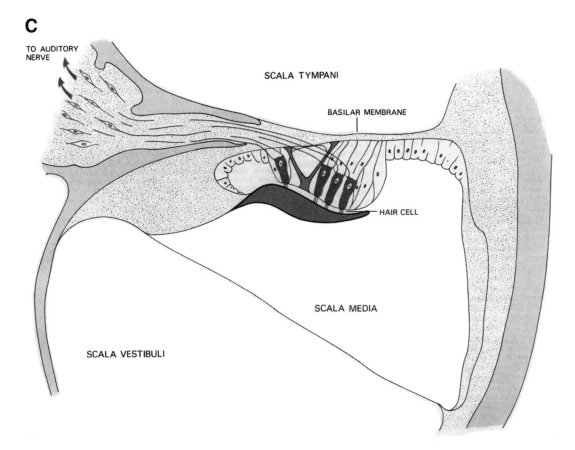

Figure 5.1: Anatomy of the ear: **(A)** cross-section of the human ear (reprinted from: Brodel M. *Three Unpublished Drawings of the Anatomy of the Human Ear.* Philadelphia, PA: W. B. Saunders; 1946); **(B)** Schematic drawing of the ear; **(C)** cross-sectional drawing of the cochlea illustrating the fluid-filled canals and the basilar membrane with hair cells (reprinted from: Møller AR. Noise as a health hazard. *Ambio* 1975;4:6–13, with permission from The Royal Swedish Academy of Sciences).

(Fig. 5.1C). The cochlea separates sounds according to their spectrum and transforms each sound into a neural code in the individual fibers of the auditory portion of the eighth cranial nerve (CN VIII).

Frequency Analysis in the Cochlea. The special micromechanical properties of the basilar membrane are the basis for the frequency analysis that takes place in the cochlea. The basilar membrane is set into vibration by the fluid in the cochlea, which, in turn, is set into motion by the in-and-out motion of the stapes footplate. The particular properties of the basilar membrane and its surrounding fluid make the motion of the basilar membrane like that of a traveling wave. This traveling wave starts at the base of the cochlea and progresses relatively slowly toward the apex of the cochlea, and at a certain point along the basilar membrane, its amplitude decreases abruptly. The distance that this wave travels before its amplitude decreases is a direct function of the frequency of the sound. A low-frequency sound travels a long distance before being extinguished, whereas a high-frequency sound gives rise to a wave that only travels a short distance before its amplitude decreases abruptly. Thus, a frequency scale can be laid along the basilar

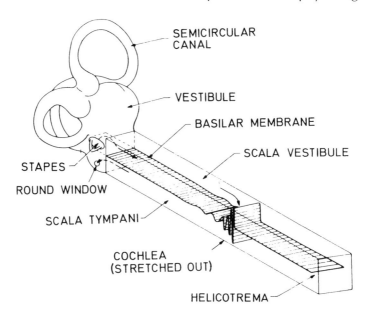

Figure 5.2: Schematic of an ear with the cochlea shown as a straight tube to illustrate the traveling wave. (Reprinted from: Zweig G, Lipes R, Pierce JR. The cochlear compromise. *J. Acoust. Soc. Am.* 1976;59:975–982, with permission from the Acoustical Society of America.)

membrane, with low frequencies at the apex and high frequencies at the base of the cochlea.

Each point on the basilar membrane can be regarded as being "tuned" to a specific frequency **(Fig. 5.2)**. The region of the basilar membrane, which is near the top (apex) of the cochlea, is tuned to low frequencies, and the frequency to which the membrane is tuned increases towards the base of the cochlea. The highest audible frequencies produce maximal vibration amplitude of the basilar membrane near the base of the cochlea.

The frequency tuning of the basilar membrane depends on the sound intensity *(6,7)*. The basilar membrane is more frequency selective for low-intensity sounds than high-intensity sounds as revealed by measuring the vibration amplitude of a single point of the basilar membrane when tones of different frequencies and different intensities are applied to the ear of an animal (guinea pig) **(Fig. 5.3)**.

Sensory Transduction in the Cochlea. Sensory cells, known as hair cells (because of their hair-like stereocilia), are located in rows along the cochlear partition. There are two types of hair cells—outer and inner—and they are arranged along the basilar membrane as one row of inner hair cells and three to five rows of outer hair cells **(Fig. 5.4)**. The human cochlea has approx 30,000 hair cells. The axons of the cochlear portion of CN VIII connect to the two types of hair cell in distinctly different ways: Each inner hair cell connects with several axons, whereas several outer hair cells connect with one nerve fiber *(9)* **(Fig. 5.5)** (for details, *see* ref. *3*). About 95% of the nerve fibers of the cochlear nerve connect to inner hair cells, whereas about 5% connect to outer hair cells.

The motion of the basilar membrane deflects the hairs on the hair cells. Deflection in one direction causes the intracellular potentials of the hair cells to become less negative (depolarization), whereas a deflection in the opposite direction causes hyperpolarization **(Fig. 5.5)**.

The intracellular potentials of inner hair cells control the discharge frequency of the individual auditory nerve fibers that terminate at their base; the deflection of the stereocilia thus controls the discharges of individual auditory nerve fibers. A depolarization of the hair

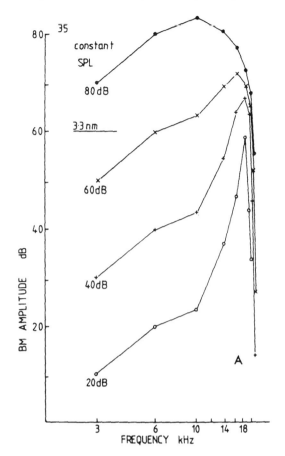

Figure 5.3: Frequency tuning of a point on the basilar membrane; the vibration amplitude of a point on the basilar membrane in a cat is shown as a function of frequency. (Modified from ref. *8*, which was based on ref. *7*.)

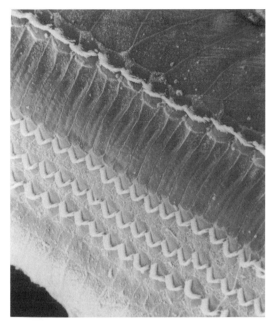

Figure 5.4: Scanning electron micrograph of hair cells along a small segment of the basilar membrane. (Courtesy of Dr. David Lim.)

cells causes the discharge rate to increase, whereas hyperpolarization has little effect or could cause a decrease in the discharge rate **(Fig. 5.6).**

Role of Hair Cells in the Motion of the Basilar Membrane. The functions of inner hair cells and outer hair cells are fundamentally different. Whereas the inner hair cells function as transducers, which makes the motion of the basilar membrane control the discharges of the individual auditory nerve fibers that connect to these hair cells, the outer hair cells function as "motors" that amplify the motion of the basilar membrane. The outer hair cells, as far

as we know, do not participate in communicating information about the motion of the basilar membrane to higher auditory nervous centers, as do the inner hair cells. The active motion of the outer hair cells inject energy into the motion of the basilar membrane and, thus, compensates for the frictional losses in the basilar membrane that would have dampened the motion of the basilar membrane. That improves the sensitivity of the ear by about 50 dB and it increases the frequency selectivity of the basilar membrane considerably, more so for weak sounds than for more intense sounds (*see* ref. *3*).

Because low-frequen sounds give rise to the largest vibration amplitude of the apical portion of the basilar membrane, a low-frequency sound will stimulate hair cells located in that region more than it will stimulate hair cells in other regions. In a similar way, high-frequency sounds will produce the largest vibration amplitude of more basal portions of the basilar membrane, thereby exciting the hair cells in that region to a greater extent than they do hair cells in other regions of the basilar membrane.

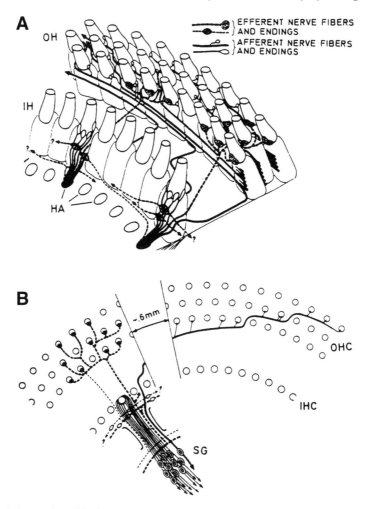

Figure 5.5: Schematic of hair cells located along the basilar membrane with their connections to the ascending fibers of the auditory nerve (solid lines). Also shown are the efferent fibers (dashed lines). OH: outer hair cells; IH: inner hair cells; HA: habenula perforate. (Reprinted from: Spoendlin H. Structural basis of peripheral frequency analysis. In: Plomp R, Smoorenburg GF, eds. *Frequency Analysis and Periodicity Detection in Hearing.* Leiden: A. W. Sijthoff; 1970:2–36.)

Otoacoustic emission is a sound generated by the cochlea as a result of the active function of the outer hair cells and it can be measured in the ear canal. The otoacoustic emission is increasingly becoming a valuable clinical test, but it has not yet been found to be of specific use in intraoperative monitoring.

Electrical Potentials Generated in the Cochlea. Several different types of electrical potentials can be recorded from the cochlea or its vicinity as a result of excitation of the hair cells. The cochlear microphonic (CM) potential follows the waveform of a sound closely (hence its name), and the summating potential (SP) follows the envelope of a sound. Excitation of the auditory nerve is the source of the action potentials (APs), which can best be elicited in response to click sounds or the sharp onset of a tone burst. Although all of these potentials can be evoked by the same sounds, each type responds best to specific types of sound. Thus,

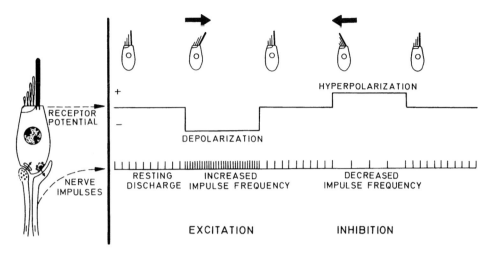

Figure 5.6: Schematic of the excitation of hair cells. The figure illustrates the function of hair cells in the lateral line organ of a fish. These hair cells are supposed to function in a way similar to that in the mammalian cochlea, but hair cells in the lateral line organ have kinocilia, whereas hair cells in the cochlea do not. (Reprinted from: Flock A. Transducing mechanisms in lateral line canal organ. *Cold Spring Harbor Symp. Quant. Biol.* 1965;30:133–146, with permission from Cold Spring Harbor Laboratory Press.)

the AP is most prominent in response to transient sounds, whereas the CM is most prominent in response to a pure tone of low-to-medium high frequency. The SP is most prominent when elicited in response to high-frequency tone bursts. **Figure 5.7** shows how the sharp onset of the tone burst elicits a prominent AP, and the CM from the sinusoidal wave of the tone is seen over the entire duration of the tone. The baseline shift seen during the tone burst is the SP (*see* ref. *3*). Clinically, these potentials are recorded from the cochlear capsule or the ear canal near the tympanic membrane, and in the clinic, they are known as electrocochleographical (ECoG) potentials (for details, *see* refs. *11* and *12*). These evoked potentials have gained some use in intraoperative monitoring.

Auditory Nervous System

The auditory nervous system consists of two main parts: the ascending system and the descending system. The anatomy of the ascending auditory pathway is more complex than that of other sensory systems such as the visual, olfactory, and somatosensory systems. Although the descending pathways are more abundant than the ascending pathways, much less are known about the descending pathways than the ascending pathways *(14)*.

Ascending Auditory Nervous System. There are two main, mostly parallel, ascending auditory pathways: the classical or lemniscal pathways and the nonclassical or extralemniscal pathways (also known as the nonspecific or polysensory pathways *[14]*). Much less is known about the nonclassical pathways than the classical pathways, both regarding their anatomy and their physiology.

CLASSICAL (LEMNISCAL) PATHWAYS. The most important nuclei of the ascending auditory pathway and its connections are shown in **Fig. 5.8**. The first relay nucleus of the ascending auditory pathway is the cochlear nucleus (CN). All fibers of the auditory nerve (AN) are interrupted in this nucleus, which has three main divisions: the dorsal cochlear nucleus (DCN), the posterior ventral cochlear nucleus (PVCN), and the anterior ventral cochlear nucleus (AVCN). Each fiber of the cochlear nerve bifurcates to terminate in the PVCN and the AVCN. The fibers that reach the

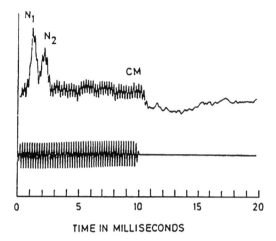

TIME IN MILLISECONDS

Figure 5.7: Different sound-elicited potentials that can be recorded from the round window of the cochlea. The recordings were obtained in a rat. The stimulus was a 5-kHz tone burst (10 ms). The cochlear microphonic appears as an oscillation with the frequency of the stimulus, the nerve action potentials appear as two upward peaks (N_1 and N_2), and the summating potential appears as the shift (upward) in the baseline recording that is seen during the time the stimulus was on. (Reprinted from: Møller AR. On the origin of the compound action potentials [N1N2] of the cochlea of the rat. *Exp. Neurol.* 1983;80: 633–644, with permission from Elsevier.)

PVCN send collateral fibers to the DCN. In that way, all auditory nerve fibers reach all three divisions of the CN.

The neurons of the CN connect to the central nucleus of the inferior colliculus (ICC) via several fiber tracts that cross the midline: the dorsal acoustic stria (DAS), the ventral acoustic stria (VAS), and the trapezoidal body. There are also connections from the CN to the IC that do not cross the midline. Some of the crossed fibers that originate in the CN reach the ICC without any synaptic interruption, whereas other connections from the CN are interrupted in the nuclei of the superior olivary complex (medial superior olivary nucleus [MSO], lateral olivary nucleus [LSO]) or the trapezoidal body (NTB). The fibers from these nuclei as well as those from the CN proceed to the ICC as the fiber tract of the lateral lemniscus (LL). Some

of the fibers of the LL reach the dorsal or ventral nuclei of the LL. All fibers that reach the ICC are interrupted in the ICC. The output fibers of the ICC form the brachia of the ICC and connect to the thalamic auditory relay nucleus, namely the medial geniculate body (MGB). The MGB furnishes auditory information to the primary auditory cortex (AI) (**Fig. 5.8**). (For details, *see* ref. *14*.)

The length of the different tracts of the ascending auditory pathways in humans are longer than those in the animals that are commonly used for studies of the auditory system. This means that the travel time throughout the ascending auditory pathways is longer than in animals, resulting in longer latencies of the different components of the auditory evoked potentials in humans compared with that in animals.

AUDITORY CORTEX. The auditory cortex in humans is located deep in Hechel's gyrus in the lateral fissure of the temporal lobe (Brodmann's area 41). The different areas are labeled AI (primary cortex) and all secondary cortices, anterior auditory field (AFF) and posterior auditory field (PAF). The AI area receives input from the MGB and sends a large fiber tract back to the MGB. These descending connections from the cerebral cortex to the MGB are important in connection with recent developments where the auditory cortex is stimulated electrically to treat hyperactive auditory disorders such as tinnitus and hyperacusis. The electrical stimulation that is applied to the cerebral cortex might have its effect by activating cells in the MGB via these descending pathways.

NONCLASSICAL (EXTRALEMNISCAL) PATHWAYS. Nonclassical pathways project to the secondary and association cortices, thus bypassing the primary auditory cortex. These pathways use the dorsal thalamus, whereas the classical pathways use the ventral thalamic nuclei. Intraoperative neurophysiological monitoring does not involve nonclassical pathways as far as is known. (For details, *see* ref. *14*.)

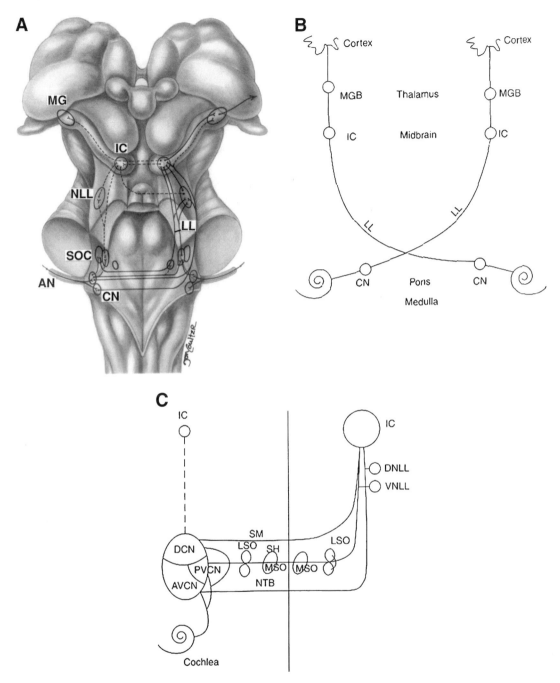

Figure 5.8: *(Continued)*

Physiology. The physiology of the auditory system is covered only briefly here; more detailed descriptions can be found in refs. *3* and *4.*

FREQUENCY TUNING. Frequency or spectral selectivity is a prominent feature of the response from single auditory nerve fibers. Each nerve

D

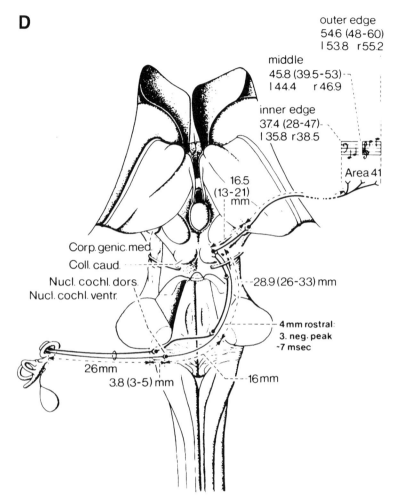

outer edge
54.6 (48-60)
l 53.8 r55.2

middle
45.8 (39.5-53)
l 44.4   r 46.9

inner edge
37.4 (28-47)
l 35.8 r38.5

Area 41

16.5
(13-21)
mm

Corp. genic. med.
Coll. caud.
Nucl. cochl. dors.
Nucl. cochl. ventr.

-28.9 (26-33) mm

4 mm rostral:
3. neg. peak
-7 msec

26 mm
3.8 (3-5) mm

16 mm

Figure 5.8: Anatomy of the ascending auditory pathway. **(A)** Illustration of how the main nuclei and fiber tracts are located in the brain. AN: auditory nerve; CN: cochlear nucleus; SO: superior olivary complex; LL: lateral lemniscus; IC: inferior colliculus; MG: medialgeniculate body. (Reprinted from: Møller AR. *Evoked Potentials in Intraoperative Monitoring*. Baltimore, MD: Williams and Wilkins; 1988, with permission.) **(B)** Schematic of the ascending auditory pathway. The pathways that ascend on the ipsilateral side are shown as dashed lines, whereas those that cross over to the other side are shown as solid lines. VCN: ventral cochlear nucleus; DCN: dorsal cochlear nucleus; IC: inferior colliculus; MGB: medial geniculate body; MGB: medial geniculate body. **(C)** Schematic of the pathways from the cochlear nucleus to the inferior colliculus. DCN: dorsal cochlear nucleus; PVCN: posterior ventral cochlear nucleus; AVCN: anterior ventral cochlear nucleus; LSO: lateral superior olive; NTB: nucleus of the trapezoidal body; MSO: medial superior olive; SH: stria of Held (intermediate stria); SM: stria of Monakow (dorsal stria); LL: lateral lemniscus; DNLL: dorsal nucleus of the lateral lemniscus; VNLL: ventral nucleus of the lateral lemniscus; IC: inferior colliculus. (From ref. *3.*) **(D)** Schematic of the ascending auditory pathway showing the length of the auditory nerve and the various fiber tracts. Results from 30 specimens. (Modified from: Lang J. Anatomy of the brainstem and the lower cranial nerves, vessels, and surrounding structures. *Am. J. Otol.* 1985;Suppl, Nov:1–19, with permission from Elsevier.)

fiber of the auditory nerve exhibits frequency selectivity based on the frequency selectivity of the cochlea (place code of frequency). Each nerve fiber is tuned to a specific frequency and so are nerve cells in the nuclei of the ascending auditory pathway. It is now believed that frequency tuning has its greatest importance for preparing sounds for temporal processing by separating the sound spectrum in bands of suitable sizes and that its importance for frequency discrimination is minimal.

Complex processing of information takes place in the various nuclei of the ascending auditory pathway, the nature of which is not completely understood, but for the most part it seems to enhance changes in amplitude and frequency of sounds.

The temporal pattern of a sound is coded in the timing of the discharges of single auditory nerve fibers. Temporal coding of sounds provides information about the spectrum of a sound, as does the place code that is represented by the tuning of various neural elements. Both place and temporal coding of auditory information are important for the discrimination of complex sounds such as speech and music. More specifically, the temporal coding is essential for speech discrimination; this is evidenced from the efficacy of cochlear implants that primarily code sounds by their temporal pattern, after separating the audible spectrum in only a few bands.

TONOTOPIC ORGANIZATION. Nerve fibers of the auditory nerve as well as those of nerve cells of these nuclei are arranged anatomically in accordance with the frequency at which their threshold is lowest (tonotopic organization). Thus, maps can be drawn on all neural structures of the classical ascending auditory pathway with regard to the frequency to which neurons respond best.

Descending Auditory Nervous System

Descending auditory pathways are abundant, and although the anatomy is relatively well understood, the function of these systems is not understood to any great detail.

Anatomy. Efferent pathways extend from the auditory cerebral cortex to the hair cells in the cochlea. These pathways have been regarded as several separate systems, but it might be more appropriate to regard the descending systems as reciprocal to the ascending pathways. The best known parts of these descending pathways are the peripheral parts. Thus, the auditory nerve contains efferent nerve fibers that originate in the superior olivary complex (SOC) and terminate mainly at the outer hair cells. These efferent fibers, also known as the olivocochlear bundle, consist of both crossed and uncrossed fibers. The efferent nerve fibers travel in the vestibular portion of the eighth nerve from the brainstem to Ort's anastomosis located deep in the internal auditory meatus where they shift over to the cochlear portion of the eighth nerve (for more details, *see* refs. *3* and *14*).

Physiology. The function of the descending pathways is poorly understood. The abundant descending system from the primary auditory cortex to the thalamus might function to change the way the thalamus processes sounds. Electrical stimulation of the primary auditory cortex might therefore affect the thalamus, and that is important when such stimulation is used to control tinnitus *(17)*. The olivocochlear bundles seem to influence outer hair cells, which are involved in "otoacoustic" emission. Therefore, measurements of otoacoustic emission can be used to investigate the function of this part of the efferent system.

Electrical Potentials From the Auditory Nervous System

For intraoperative monitoring, it is most important to know how the various nuclei of the ascending auditory pathways are connected and how these nuclei together with the fiber tracts that connect them produce electrical activity when the ear is stimulated with transient sounds.

The fact that the auditory nervous system has parallel pathways and that contributions from nuclei to the far-field potentials that are recorded from electrodes placed on the scalp depend on the architecture of the various nuclei are factors that are important for interpreting the responses used in intraoperative monitoring.

The function of the efferent system as well as matters regarding coding of complex sounds in the nuclei of the ascending auditory nervous system are probably of relatively little importance to the understanding of how neural activity in these structures contributes to the electrical activity that is recorded from electrodes placed on the scalp (ABRs). The sounds commonly used to elicit such responses are simple sounds, such as tone bursts and click sounds, and the complex processing that occurs in the auditory system of sounds such as speech and music probably does not affect the response to such simple sounds.

Auditory Brainstem Responses. Auditory brainstem responses (or brainstem auditory evoked potentials [AEPs]) are generated by the activity in structures of the ascending auditory pathways that occurs during the first 8–10 ms after a transient sound such as a click sound has been applied to the ear.

Typically, the ABRs are recorded between electrodes placed at the vertex (Cz) and the earlobe on the side that is stimulated. When the recordings are obtained in that way in a person with normal hearing is characterized by five or six (vertex-positive) peaks. These peaks are traditionally numbered consecutively using Roman numerals from I to VI *(18)* (**Fig. 5.9**). There is a certain distinct individual variation in the wave shape of the ABR—even in individuals with normal hearing. Pathologies that affect the auditory system *(19)* could result in abnormalities in the ABR that are specific for different pathologies. Hearing loss of various kinds could affect the ABR in a complex way. The waveform of the ABR also depends on three other key factors: the electrode placement used for recording the ABR, the stimuli used to elicit the responses and how the recorded potentials are processed (filtered).

When ABRs are recorded in the traditional way with one electrode placed on the vertex and another one placed on the earlobe or mastoid with each being connected to the input of a differential amplifier, both of these electrodes

are active (record sound evoked potentials). The potentials that are recorded by these two electrodes contribute to the recorded ABR. The mastoid (or earlobe) electrode contributes mainly to the first two (or three) peaks of the ABR, whereas the vertex electrode makes the greatest contribution to peak V. The standard way of displaying evoked potentials is to show negativity at the active electrode as an upward deflection. Because both electrodes are active, the ABR can be displayed in different ways, either with the vertex-negativity as an upward deflection (as shown in the middle curve of **Fig. 5.9**) or with vertex-positivity as an upward deflection (**Fig. 5.9**, top tracing). (Vertex-positive potentials shown as a downward deflection are associated with the vertex electrode being connected to the inverting input [G_2] of the differential amplifier.)

The fact that only the vertex-positive peaks in ABR are labeled (with Roman numerals) could imply that only vertex-positive peaks are important. This choice of labeling was, however, not based on any experimental evidence showing that the vertex-positive peaks of ABR are more important in diagnostics, nor was this choice in labeling related to the neural generators of these peaks. This arbitrary choice of labeling only the vertex-positive peaks of ABR is unfortunate because it focuses only on vertex-positive peaks while the vertex-negative peaks might be just as important for detecting functional abnormalities of the auditory system both in the clinic and in the operating room. (Studies of the neural generators of ABRs have supported the assumption that vertex-negative peaks are indeed important *[19]*).

Only a few studies have made use of the traditional way of labeling the different components of the ABR using "N" for negative peaks, followed by the normal value of the latency of the peak; conversely, positive peaks are labeled with a "P," followed by a number that is the peak's normal latency.

Because the convention of labeling the vertex-positive peaks of the ABR with Roman numerals has been used for a long time, we will also use this method for labeling ABR peaks in this volume.

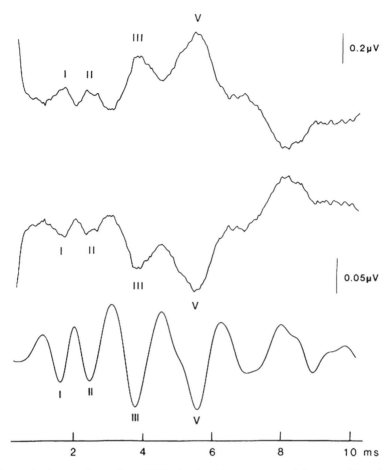

Figure 5.9: Typical recording of an ABR obtained in a person with normal hearing. The recording is the summation of 4096 responses to rarefaction clicks recorded differentially between the forehead and the ipsilateral mastoid with a band pass of 10–3000 Hz. The upper recording is shown with vertex-positivity as an upward deflection, and the middle curve is the same recording, but with vertex-positivity shown as a downward deflection. The bottom recording is the same recording, but after digital filtering (for details about digital filtering, *see* Chap. 8). (Reprinted from: Møller AR. *Evoked Potentials in Intraoperative Monitoring.* Baltimore, MD: Williams and Wilkins; 1988, with permission.)

Processing of ABR Can Change the Waveform. Recorded ABRs are always subjected to some forms of spectral filtering. Filtering can either be performed by electronic filters or by digital filters. Whereas some electronic filtering is necessary before the recorded responses are digitized for signal averaging to avoid aliasing (*see* Chap. 18), digital filters have advantages over electronic filters for enhancing the waveform of the ABR, as illustrated in **Fig. 5.9**. The top two ABR curves were not subjected to any filtering other than that rendered by the electronic filters that were built into the amplifiers. These electronic filters were set at rather "open" values; 10-Hz high pass and 3-kHz low pass, and the slope of the high-pass filter was 6 dB/octave and that of the low-pass filter was 24 dB/octave. The bottom response in **Fig. 5.9** shows the same response as that shown on the top after zero-phase digital filtering using computer programs *(3,20)*. The ABRs shown in the lower graph have a much clearer definition of the peaks than the ABRs that were only

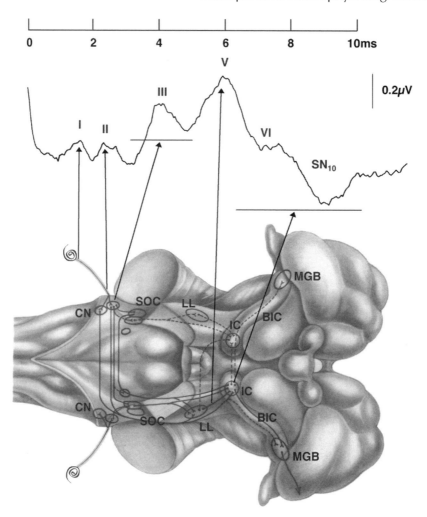

Figure 5.10: Schematic of the neural generators of the ABR. (Reprinted from: Møller AR. *Neural Plasticity and Disorders of the Nervous System.* Cambridge: Cambridge University Press; 2005, with permission from Cambridge University Press.)

subjected to electronic filtering. (The advantages and disadvantages of zero-phase finite impulse digital filtering are discussed later in this book [Chap. 6].)

Neural Generators of the ABR. Because of the (mainly) sequential activation of neural structures of the auditory pathways, the ABR consists of a series of components that are separated in time. The peaks and valleys that form the ABR therefore generally appear with different latencies in accordance with the anatomical location of their respective neural

generators. This depiction is a simplified description of the relationship between the different components of the ABR and the anatomy of the ascending auditory pathway; it can only serve as a first approximation because of the complexity of the ascending auditory pathway with its extensive parallel systems of neural pathways. Neural activation of some nuclei could therefore occur simultaneously, and the electrical activity of different nuclei and fiber tracts that is elicited by a transient sound could therefore overlap in time. **Figure 5.10** shows a schematic and simplified picture of our present concept of the neural generators of the human ABR.

Comparisons between ABR recordings made directly from the capsule of the cochlea in man (ECoG) have shown evidence that peak I in the ABR is generated by the auditory nerve (distal portion). The finding that the negative peak of the CAP recorded from the exposed intracranial portion of the auditory nerve in man has a latency close to that of peak II in the ABR *(22–24)* indicates that wave II is generated by the proximal portion of the auditory nerve. This has been supported by later studies *(25–27)*. This means that the auditory nerve in man is the generator of both peaks I and II of the ABR and that no other neural structure contributes to either of these two peaks.

Peak II might be generated because neural activity propagates in the auditory nerve where the electrical conductivity of the surrounding medium changes *(28,29)* or when the propagation of neural activity stops (as it does when it reaches a nucleus). The importance of the electrical conductivity of the medium that surrounds the auditory nerve intracranially has been shown in studies of patients undergoing operations in the cerebellopontine angle (CPA) *(30)*.

The auditory nerve in animals commonly used in experimental research only generates one peak in the ABR (peak I). Peak II in such animals is generated by the cochlear nucleus (see, for example, refs. 31–34). This difference between man and the animals commonly used in auditory research is the result of the auditory nerve being much longer in man (approx 26 mm [16,35]*) (Fig. 5.8D) than it is in such animals, including the monkey (8 mm in the cat* [36]*).*

Because the diameters of the fibers of the auditory nerve are relatively small, the conduction velocity in the auditory nerve is only about 20 m/s *(37)*. The time it takes for neural activity in the human auditory nerve to travel a distance of 2.6 cm from the ear to the brainstem is, therefore, a little more than 1 ms. [The average

diameter of axons in the auditory nerve in children is 2.5 µm with a narrow distribution in young individuals. With increasing age, the diameter increases and the variation becomes larger: 0.5–7 µm by the age of 40–50 yr *(38)*.]

The generators of the peaks of the ABR with latencies that are longer than that of peak II are more complex, and these peaks most likely have multiple sources. The high degree of parallel processing in the auditory nervous system could result in different structures being activated simultaneously. The consequences of this might be that an individual component of the ABR (e.g., peak IV) might receive contributions from fundamentally different structures of the ascending auditory pathway.

Intracranial recordings in patients undergoing neurosurgical operations have shown evidence that the earliest component in the ABR that originates in brainstem nuclei is peak III *(3)*. Although the cochlear nucleus is most likely the main generator of that peak *(39)*, there is evidence that the vertex-negative peak between peaks III and IV also receives contributions from the cochlear nucleus *(19,39)*. The contralateral cochlear nucleus might contribute to the ABR *(19,40)* through connections between the two cochlear nuclei.

Less is known about the source of peak IV than the sources of peaks I–III and V of the ABR. There is evidence that the source of peak IV is located deep in the brainstem (near the midline), maybe in the pons, the NTB, or the SOC *(19,41)* **(Fig. 5.10)**. Most likely, other structures contribute to peak IV, such as the cochlear nucleus and the distal parts of the lateral lemniscus. Peaks I–III receive input from only the ipsilateral side *(see* **Figs. 5.8** and **5.10**) *(19)*, whereas peak IV is likely to be the earliest positive peak of the ABR that receives contributions from contralateral structures of the ascending auditory pathway *(see also ref. 3)*. Peak IV might receive input from both sides of the brainstem.

Peak V of the ABR in man has a complex origin. There is evidence that the sharp tip of peak V is generated by the lateral lemniscus, where it terminates in the inferior colliculus *(42)*. There is also evidence from animal experiments *(34)* that the inferior colliculus itself generates only a very small far-field response, even though a large evoked potential can be recorded from its surface. The reason for this might be found in the anatomical organization of the inferior colliculus where its dendrites might point in a wide range of directions so that the nucleus generates a "closed field" *(43)*. The slow negative potential in the ABR in humans that occurs with a latency of about 10 ms (SN_{10}) *(44)* most likely represents postsynaptic potentials generated by the dendrites of the cells of the inferior colliculus. The amplitude of this component varies widely from individual to individual.

Studies in patients undergoing neurosurgical operations that included comparisons between the ABR intracranial potentials recorded from different locations along the lateral side of the brainstem have confirmed that peaks I–III receive contributions mainly from ipsilateral structures of the ascending auditory pathway, whereas peak V receives its major contributions from contralateral structures *(19)*.

Comparisons between the latencies of the different components of responses recorded intracranially and the vertex-positive and vertex-negative peaks of the ABR *(19,45)* also emphasize that it is not only the vertex-positive peaks of the ABR that have anatomically distinct neural generators but also the vertex-negative peaks. In fact, the vertex-negative peaks might be just as important as indicators of pathologies.

Some studies *(19)* have shown that the response recorded from the dorsal acoustic stria, on the floor of the fourth ventricle, generates a peak, the latency of which is slightly shorter than that of peak V. This indicates that if the lateral lemniscus is interrupted along its more rostral course (by surgically induced injury or by disease processes), the lateral lemniscus and maybe even the dorsal acoustic stria itself might generate a peak in the ABR that is indistinguishable from the normal peak V of the ABR (except for a slightly shorter latency than the normal peak V).

Little is known about the generators of peaks VI and VII, but they might be generated by neural firing in cells of the inferior colliculus (somaspikes) *(27,42,46)*.

THE SOMATOSENSORY SYSTEM

Introduction

Intraoperative monitoring of somatosensory evoked potentials (SSEPs) has mainly been used in operations on the spine, such as during fixation after trauma, corrective operations (e.g., scoliosis), and other operations on the spine where the spinal cord might be at risk of being manipulated. Monitoring in operations on the spinal cord such as resection of spinal tumors and during operations where there is a risk of ischemia as a result of compromised blood supply to the part of the brain that is involved in the generation of SSEP are also important. This section describes the anatomy and physiology of the somatosensory system that is important as a basis for intraoperative recordings of SSEP for monitoring the integrity of the somatosensory nervous system.

Sensory Receptors

The natural input to the somatosensory system is mechanical stimulation of receptors in the skin, muscles, and joints. These receptors respond to different forms of mechanical stimulation *(14)*, but that aspect is of minor importance for intraoperative monitoring where instead sensory nerve fibers are stimulated electrically.

Ascending Somatosensory Pathways

Information from sensory receptors of the body is conveyed by the fibers of the sensory parts of peripheral nerves to the spinal cord where they enter as the dorsal roots. The cell bodies of these fibers are located in the dorsal root ganglia. Sensory receptors of the head are innervated by cranial nerves (*see* Chap. 11). The nerve fibers that receive input from the body enter the dorsal horn of the spinal cord and ascend in the dorsal column of the spinal cord on the ipsilateral side to terminate in cells in the dorsal column nuclei **(Fig. 5.11)**.

Nerve fibers that innervate temperature and pain receptors also travel in peripheral nerves and enter the dorsal horn of the spinal cord, but these fibers terminate in cells in the spinal cord at segmental level. Pain and temperature systems are not monitored intraoperatively.

Dorsal Column System. The fibers of the dorsal column that originate in the upper portion of the body (thoracic and cervical segments) terminate in the neurons of the cuneate nucleus, whereas some of the nerve fibers that innervate receptors of the lower body terminate in the gracilis nucleus of the dorsal column nuclei. Information from muscle spindles and joint receptors in the lower body travels in the lateral fasciculi of the same side of the spinal cord. These fibers terminate in the nucleus Z, which is located more medially and rostral to the nucleus gracilis *(47)*.

This difference between the ascending pathways of the somatosensory system of the lower and upper body has important implications for the interpretation of the SSEP recorded in response to electrical stimulation of peripheral nerves of the lower limbs (peroneal or posterior tibial nerves) as well as when dermatomal stimulation is used, as we shall discuss later in this chapter.

When dermatomes of the lower body are stimulated electrically to elicit somatosensory evoked potentials, it is probably mainly skin receptors that are activated, and such neural activity will probably mainly travel in the dorsal column system.

Dorsal Column Nuclei. The nucleus cuneatus and the nucleus gracilis, together known as the dorsal column nuclei, are located in the caudal portion of the medulla. The nucleus Z is located slightly rostral and medial to the dorsal column nuclei. Fibers that leave the dorsal column nuclei and the nucleus Z cross over to the other side of the medulla to form the medial lemniscus. The medial lemniscus ascends in the brainstem, first near the midline and later more laterally, to terminate in the somatosensory nuclei (the ventral posterior lateral [VPL] nucleus) of the thalamus, which is the second main relay nucleus of the somatosensory system.

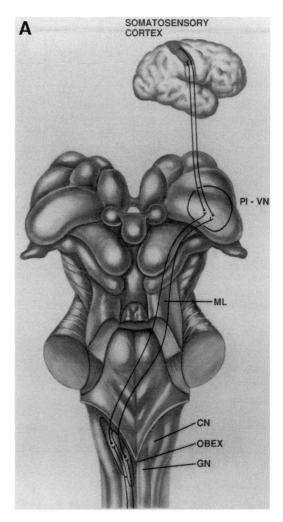

Figure 5.11: *(Continued)*

Organization of the Somatosensory Cortex. The primary somatosensory cortex receives its input from the ventrobasal nuclei of the thalamus **(Fig. 5.11B)** as third-order neurons. These neurons travel in the posterior limb of the internal capsule and disburse over the somatosensory cortex (postcentral gyrus of the parietal cortex) in a somatotopic fashion, with the legs represented closest to the midline, followed in the lateral direction by representation of the trunk, forearm, and hand **(Fig. 5.12)**. Secondary somatosensory cortices occupy large parts of the somatosensory cortical areas (for details, *see* ref. *14*).

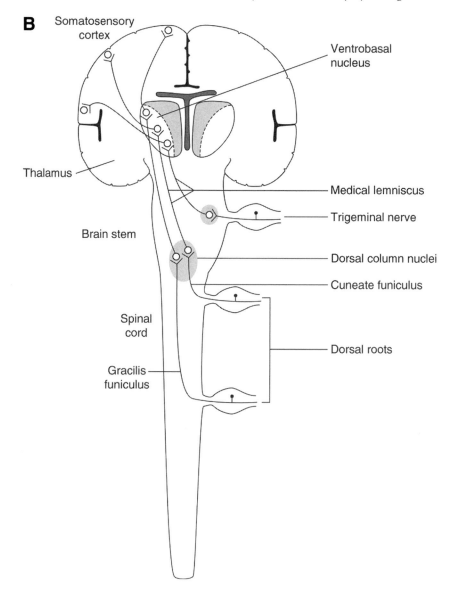

Figure 5.11: (A) Schematic diagram showing the neural pathway of the portion of the somatosensory system that travels in the dorsal column. GN: gracilis nucleus; CN: cuneate nucleus; Pl-VN: Posteriolateral ventral nucleus of the thalamus. (Reprinted from: Møller AR. *Evoked Potentials in Intraoperative Monitoring.* Baltimore, MD: Williams and Wilkins; 1988, with permission.) **(B)** Schematic showing the anatomical locations of the main components of the ascending somatosensory pathways. (Reprinted from: Møller AR. *Sensory Systems: Anatomy and Physiology.* Amsterdam: Academic; 2003, with permission from Elsevier.)

Anteriorlateral System. The axons of spinal neurons receive input from pain and temperature receptors ascend in the spinal cord on the opposite side from the anterior lateral system consisting of several different pathways, of which the spinothalamic tract is the best known. Other parts are the spinoreticular and spinoencephalic tracts. The anterior lateral

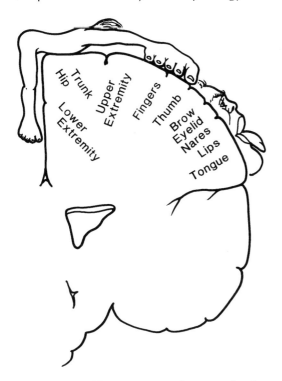

Figure 5.12: Somatotopic organization (homunculus) of the body surface on the somatosensory cortex by Penfield and co-workers. (From ref. *48.*)

system is an alternate pathway for somatosensory input from the body to the brain and it is similar to nonclassical pathways of other sensory systems *(14).* The ascending fibers of the anteriorlateral tracts originate from cells in the spinal cord at segmental levels. The system communicates deep touch, tickle, itch, temperature, and pain. (For more details, *see* ref. *14.*) The fibers of the anteriorlateral tracts travel on the contralateral side of the spinal cord to reach the thalamus. This system is concerned with less localized and more general tactile sensibility in contrast to the dorsal column system, which communicates fine touch and has an almost 1:1 synaptic ratio, thus providing for much more precise localization and discrimination.

The Trigeminal System. Tactile information from the face is mediated by the trigeminal system. The trigeminal nerve (fifth cranial nerve)

has its cell bodies in the trigeminal ganglion (ganglion of Gasser or semilunar ganglion), from where the central branches enter the sensory trigeminal nucleus that is located in the pons. The ascending fibers from that nucleus join the medial lemniscus on the contralateral side and extend to the thalamic nucleus (medial portion of the ventral posterior nucleus). The fibers from that nucleus project to the somatosensory cortex (postcentral gyrus), lateral to the projection of the hand (**Fig. 5.12**). The trigeminal nucleus has a large caudal–rostral extension in the brainstem, and the most caudal portion of the spinal nucleus of the trigeminal nerve is mainly concerned with pain and thermal sensations. This nucleus is probably involved in the generation of pain in patients with trigeminal neuralgia.

Electrical Potentials From the Somatosensory Nervous System

Recordings of evoked potentials from the somatosensory system play an important role in intraoperative monitoring both of the spinal cord and the brain. The somatosensory system generates several electrical potentials that are important for intraoperative monitoring and both near-field and far-field potentials are used in various kinds of monitoring of SSEPs.

Near-Field Evoked Potentials. Electrical stimulation of the median nerve gives a large response from the dorsal column nuclei that has a waveform that is typical for responses from a nucleus (**Fig. 5.13**). The response from the spinal cord to stimulation of the peroneal nerve gives a similar responses but contains a series of wavelets (**Fig. 5.14**) that indicate that the neural pathway that is activated has a large variation in fiber diameter and, therefore, that the neural activity that arrives at the level of the upper spinal cord is dispersed in time. Electrical stimulation of a peripheral nerve at the lower body that contains afferent fibers from both skin and proprioceptors activates the dorsal column system, nucleus gracilis, and the lateral funiculus and nucleus Z. The elicited volleys of nerve impulses arrives at the brainstem level more dispersed in time than

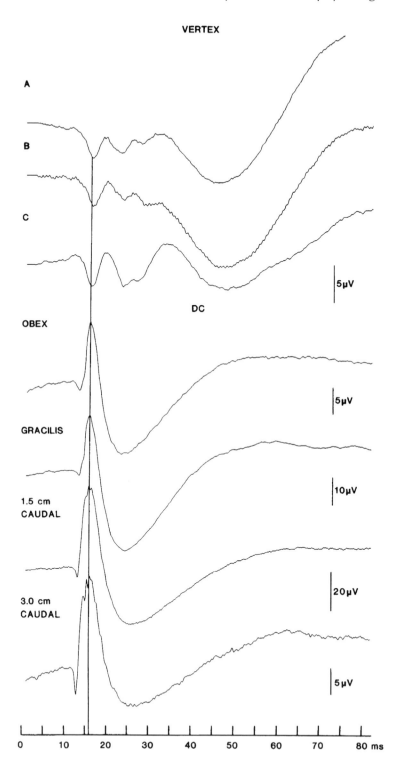

activity that is elicited from nerves on the upper limb.

*The stimuli used to evoke the responses shown in **Fig 5.13** and **5.14** were presented at a rate of 2 pps and the recording filters were set at 3–3000 Hz. Sampling intervals were 160 µs, and each recording had 512 data points. Negativity is shown as an upward deflection. The results were obtained in a patient undergoing microvascular decompression to relieve spasmodic torticollis.*

Far-Field Evoked Potentials. When peripheral nerves, such as the median or the posterior tibial nerves, are electrically stimulated for the purpose of recording SSEP, both the dorsal column system and the anteriorlateral system are most likely activated, but it is generally assumed that the anteriorlateral system is not represented to any noticeable degree in the responses that are recorded from electrodes on the scalp in response to electrical stimulation of the median nerve or the peroneal or posterior tibial nerves of the lower limb.

Upper Limb SSEP. SSEP recorded from electrodes placed on the scalp in response to electrical stimulation of the median nerve at the wrist have a series of peaks and troughs. The convention for labeling the peaks of the SSEP differs from that used for ABR and the positive peaks of the SSEP are usually labeled with a "P," followed by a number that is the normal latency of that peak. The negative peaks are labeled with an "N," followed by the normal latency in milliseconds.

The SSEPs in response to stimulation of the median nerve that are recorded from electrodes placed on the scalp over the contralateral somatosensory cortex in an awake or lightly anesthetized human are dominated by potentials that originate in the primary somatosensory cortex having a latency of approx 20 ms (N_{20}), but potentials with shorter latencies can also be identified (**Fig. 5.15**). The waveform as well as the amplitude of the recorded potentials depends on the placement of the recording electrodes. A negative peak with latency of 18 ms (N_{18}) can be recorded from large areas of the scalp on both sides. These peaks are preceded by a series of positive peaks (P_9,P_{11},P_{14}) that are best recorded from electrodes that are placed on the neck with a noncephalic reference (e.g., placed on the shoulder), but they can also be recorded from an electrode placed over the parietal region of the scalp and referenced to the upper neck (**Fig. 5.15**). Such electrode placement (contralateral–parietal to the upper dorsal neck) is practical for intraoperative monitoring and yields a clear representation of the $P_{13}–P_{16}$ peaks as well as the N_{20} peak (*see also* Chap. 10 for discussions of various recording techniques).

The two main negative peaks—N_{18} and N_{20}—are followed by a positive deflection (P_{22}), a large negative peak (N_{30}), and another positive deflection (P_{45}) that is broader than the P_{22} peak (not seen in **Fig. 5.15**). The N_{20}, P_{22}, and P_{45} are localized to the contralateral parietal region (3 cm behind C_3 or C_4), whereas the N_{18} and $P_{14}–P_{16}$ components can be recorded from large regions of the scalp, including that of the contralateral side (**Fig. 5.15**). Subtracting recordings

---

Figure 5.13: *(Opposite page)* Responses to electrical stimulation by an electrode placed over the median nerve at the wrist. **Upper curves:** far-field recordings (vertex–inion) obtained after the patient was anesthetized but before the operation began **(A)**, during direct recording **(B)**, and during closure **(C)**. **Middle curves:** recordings from the surface of the cuneate nucleus and the spinal cord using the opposite earlobe as a reference (DC). Stimuli were presented at a rate of 2 pps, and the recording filters were set at 3–3000 Hz. Sampling intervals were 160 µs, and each recording had 512 data points. Negativity is shown as an upward deflection. The results were obtained in a patient undergoing microvascular decompression to relieve spasmodic torticollis. (Reprinted from: Møller AR, Jannetta PJ, Jho HD. Recordings from human dorsal column nuclei using stimulation of the lower limb. *Neurosurgery* 1990;26:291–299, with permission from Lippincott, Williams and Wilkins.)

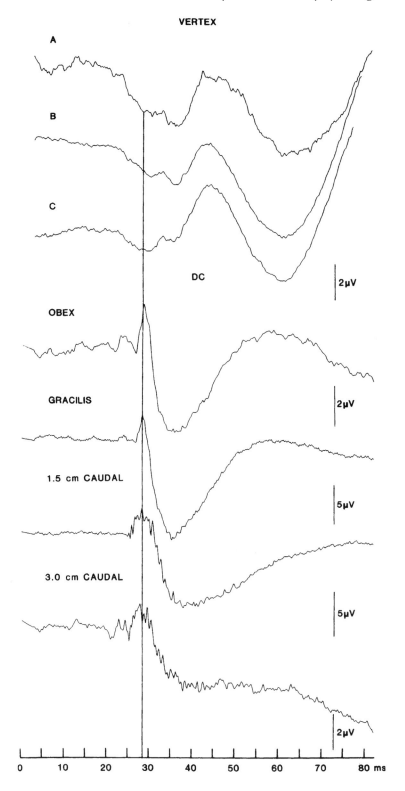

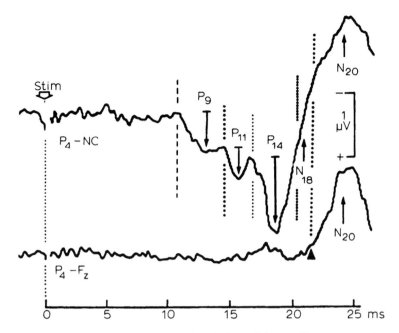

Figure 5.15: SSEP recorded in response to stimulation of the median nerve at the wrist: **(A)** non-cephalic reference; **(B)** frontal references. (Reprinted from: Desmedt JE, Cheron G. Central somatosensory conduction in man: neural generators and interpeak latencies of the far-field components recorded from neck and right or left scalp and earlobes. *Electroenceph. Clin. Neurophysiol.* 1980;50:382–403, with permission from Elsevier.)

from the ipsilateral and the contralateral sides makes the N_{20}, P_{22}, and P_{45} peaks appear more clearly (*see* Chap. 7).

Evoked potentials that are generated by the brachial plexus in response to electrical stimulation of the median nerve can be recorded by placing an electrode at Erb's point (Erb's point is found just above the mid-portion of clavicle). These potentials that are indicators of the degree of activation of the brachial plexus are valuable in intraoperative monitoring of SSEPs because their presence confirms that the electrical stimulation had properly excited the median nerve. Measuring the difference between the latencies of the different peaks in the SSEP and those of the potentials recorded from Erb's point eliminates the effect of changes in the conduction time of the median nerve in the arm (e.g., because of changes in temperature). If the absolute value of the latencies of the various peaks in the SSEP is used, a prolongation in the conduction time of the central portion of the somatosensory pathway cannot be distinguished from a prolongation in the conduction time of the median nerve. Another measure that eliminates the influence of neural conduction in the peripheral (median) nerve as well as that in the dorsal column is the frequently used

Figure 5.14: *(Opposite page)* Recording similar to those in **Fig. 5.13**, but obtained in response to electrical stimulation of the peroneal nerve at the knee from the gracilis nucleus. As in **Fig. 5.13**, the top tracings were obtained by recording from electrodes placed on the scalp (vertex–inion) before the operation began. (Reprinted from: Møller AR, Jannetta PJ, Jho HD. Recordings from human dorsal column nuclei using stim- ulation of the lower limb. *Neurosurgery* 1990;26:291–299, with permission from Lippincott, Williams and Wilkins.)

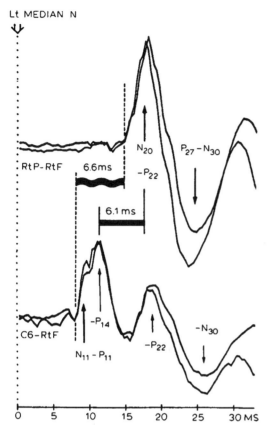

Lt MEDIAN N

Figure 5.16: Illustration of how the CCT is determined based on recordings of the SSEP with two different electrode placements: **(A)** recordings from a contralateral parietal location (behind C_3 or C_4) using a frontal reference; **(B)** recording from a noncephalic (spinal C_6) location using the same frontal reference as in **(A)**. The onset of the CCT is from the spinal entry of the neural activity. (Reprinted from: Desmedt JE. Somatosensory evoked potentials in neuromonitoring. In: Desmedt JE, ed. *Neuromonitoring in Surgery.* Amsterdam: Elsevier Science; 1989:1–21, with permission from Elsevier.)

central conduction time (CCT), which is the interval between the P_{14}–P_{16} and the N_{20} *(51)* **(Fig 5.16)**. (Further details on this subject are discussed in Chap. 7.)

LOWER LIMB SSEP. The SSEP elicited by stimulation of the posterior tibial or the peroneal

nerves at the knee do not exhibit as distinct early peaks as the SSEP elicited by median nerve stimulation. Because the nerve tracts involved in lower limb stimulation are much longer than those involved in median nerve stimulation, the latencies of the peaks in the lower limb SSEP are much longer than those of the peaks in the upper limb SSEP.

Recording of cortical responses elicited by lower limb stimulation might be done by electrodes placed on the midline scalp (at C_z 1) level (or, better, 3–4 cm posterior to C_z) using F_{pz} or the ipsilateral mastoid as reference **(Fig. 5.17)**. An electrode location 3–4 cm posterior to the C_z with a noncephalic reference placed on the upper neck is also often used. Recorded in this way, the response to stimulation of the posterior tibial nerve or the peroneal nerve is characterized by a series of peaks, which are assumed to be the result of successive excitation of neural structures that lead to the somatosensory cortex. The early positive peaks in the SSEP evoked by lower limb stimulation can only be recorded when the reference electrode is placed below the neck, and it is recorded best when it is placed on the knee or on the lower trunk (at the level of the T_{12} vertebrae).

The response from the popliteal fossa to stimulation of the posterior tibial nerve shows activation of the peripheral nerve that is being stimulated, similar to what is noted in recordings from Erb's point in upper limb SSEP and which indicates that proper stimulation has been applied to the respective (posterior tibial) nerve. Using a reference electrode placed on the upper neck, similar to that described for recording upper limb SSEP, might have advantages when recording potentials that are generated in the upper spinal cord and lower medulla **(Fig. 5.17)**. However, the amplitudes of such early components are small and individually variable. From experience, it is known that the earliest peaks in the lower limb SSEP (P_{17} and P_{24}) can only be recorded reliably from an electrode placed on the lower portion of the body, over the T_{12} vertebra or below the hip (e.g., on a lower limb). Such an arrangement might be

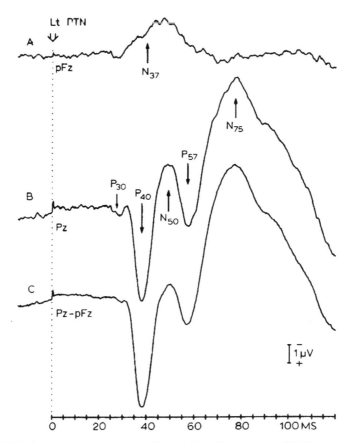

Figure 5.17: SSEP in response to stimulation of the left posterior tibial nerve using various locations for the recording electrodes. C_z, C_3, C_4, F_{pz}, F_z, and O_z refer to the international 10–20 system for placement of EEG electrodes *(53)*. **(A)** recordings from a frontal location, pF_z; **(B)** recording from a midline position, P_z. A noncephalic reference (on left shoulder) was used in both recordings. **(C)** The difference between the recordings in **(A)** and those in **(B)**, mimicking a differential recording between pF_z and P_z. (Reprinted from: Desmedt JE. Somatosensory evoked potentials in neuromonitoring. In: Desmedt JE, ed. *Neuromonitoring in Surgery.* Amsterdam: Elsevier Science; 1989:1–21, with permission from Elsevier.)

difficult to use for intraoperative monitoring because it often results in noisy recordings from electrical interference.

The temporal dispersion of the neural volley that is elicited by the electrical stimulation of peripheral nerves on the lower limbs is greater in older individuals and amplified by different kinds of neuropathy, such as those seen in diabetic patients or in postpoliomyelitis patients. Recording SSEP in response to upper limb (median nerve) stimulation usually can be done without difficulty in such patients, but recordings

of lower limb SSEP often fails because of such neuropathies.

The latencies of the individual components of the lower limb SSEP depend on the height of the individual in whom they are recorded to a much greater extent than what is the case for upper limb SSEP. Large differences in these latencies are seen in children *(54)*.

Neural Generators of the SSEP. The SSEP elicited by stimulation of the median nerve (upper limbs) and the peroneal or posterior tibial nerves (lower limbs) are fundamentally different and the neural generators of these two types of somatosensory evoked potential will be discussed separately.

UPPER LIMB SSEP. The introduction of the use of a noncephalic reference for recording upper limb SSEP *(55,56)* was a major breakthrough in studies of the neural generators of the SSEP studies, because it made it possible to identify the early components of the SSEP and enabled investigators to study the origin of these potentials in more detail *(50,56)*. Some of these studies compared recordings from the scalp with recordings from the ventral side of the spinal cord using a recording electrode that was placed in the esophagus.

The short latency evoked potentials in response to electrical stimulation of the median nerve are generated by the peripheral nerves, the spinal cord (the dorsal column fibers), and possibly by the medial lemniscus *(29,50,56,57)*, whereas the dorsal column nuclei seems to produce very small far-field potentials *(58)*.

Recordings from different locations along the spine have shown that the P_9 peak dominated at the spinal C_7 level, and it was concluded that P_9 peak of the scalp-recorded SSEP represented the neural volley that entered the spinal cord from the brachial plexus. Evidence was presented that the P_{11} peak is generated in the dorsal horn by neural structures that are not part of the ascending somatosensory pathway. These matters are important to consider when recordings of SSEP are used in intraoperative monitoring, because they mean that the P_{11} peak might be preserved, despite the fact that the ascending somatosensory tracts are compromised at the level of the foramen magnum.

The origin of the P_{14}–P_{16} peaks is not entirely clear. Some investigators (59) assumed that P_{14} was generated in the medial lemniscus. These results are supported by work by other investigators (60); yet, other investigators have arrived at different interpretations of the origins of the P_{13}–P_{16} peaks.

Some investigators (29) found evidence that P_{13} was generated more peripherally, namely where the dorsal column passes through the foramen magnum, and that P_{11} was generated by the dorsal root at the spinal C_2 level. It has been suggested that what these investigators (29) identified as P_{13} was, in fact, the same peak as what the other investigators (59) labeled P_{14}. The confusion between which peaks were P_{13} and P_{14} could have been a result of slightly different electrode placements and a small difference in the ways in which recordings were filtered by these two separate groups of investigators.

*Studies comparing the responses from the exposed surface of the dorsal column nuclei evoked by electrical stimulation of the median nerve in patients undergoing neurosurgical operations with those recorded from the scalp (SSEP) (49) **(Fig. 5.13)**, recorded simultaneously with the intracranial recordings, indicated that P_{14} is most likely generated by the fiber tract that terminates in the cuneate nucleus.*

Studies in the monkey (58) where the dorsal column nuclei were stimulated electrically and the elicited antidromic activity in the median nerve was recorded have provided accurate determinations of the neural conduction time in the median nerve. These experiments indicated that the initial components of the potentials that are recorded from the surface of the dorsal column nuclei reflect ascending activity in the dorsal column (58), thus supporting the assumption that the P_{14} peak in humans is generated by the termination of the dorsal column in the cuneate nucleus. Some investigators found evidence that P_{14} is generated by the medial lemniscus rather than the cuneate nucleus (57,60).

Most studies, however, agree that the dorsal column nuclei contribute little to the far-field potentials, possibly because the organization of these nuclei is such that they produce a closed, or nearly closed, electrical field *(43)* (see Chap. 2). This is similar to the conclusions regarding the neural generators of the ABRs, where the nucleus of the inferior colliculus was found to produce only a weak far-field.

The N_{18} peak that can be recorded over large regions of the scalp has a different source than the N_{20} peak. The N_{18} is generated by bilateral brainstem structures, whereas N_{20} is generated by the somatosensory cortex, thus specifically localized to the opposite side to that being stimulated. The N_{18} peak is assumed to be the result of excitatory postsynaptic potentials in several nuclei that receive input from the medial lemniscus, such as the superior colliculus (52,61). (It is important to keep in mind that fibers that constitute tracts such as the medial lemniscus have many collateral that connect to neurons in different parts of the central nervous system.) The N_{20} peak can only be recorded from a small area of the contralateral parietal scalp and it is assumed to be generated by the primary somatosensory cortex, where it represents the early response of the input from the thalamus (52). The generators of the components (positive and negative peaks) that follow N_{20} (P_{22}, N_{30}, and P_{45}) are not known in detail, but the generators of these components are assumed to be higher brain structures that receive input from the primary somatosensory cortex and secondary cortices and, perhaps, association cortices. These peaks are more individually variable and they are more sensitive to anesthesia than earlier peaks.

LOWER LIMB SSEP. The generators of the lower limb SSEP (elicited by stimulation of the tibial or the peroneal nerves) have been studied much less than the upper limb SSEP (elicited by stimulation of the median nerve). Likewise, the origins of the components of the lower limb SSEP are incompletely known. The N_{17} peak is assumed to be generated near the hip joint and the P_{24} peak is assumed to be generated at the level of the 12th thoracic vertebra. The P_{31} peak is probably generated where the spinal cord passes through the foramen magnum, and together with the P_{34} peak, these potentials might correspond to the P_{14}–P_{16} complex of the upper limb SSEP. The P_{34} peak is thus assumed to be generated by structures in the brainstem (medial lemniscus), but this peak could also be analo-gous to the N_{18} peak of the upper limb SSEP (62). The large negative deflection (N_{34}) following these positive peaks might be generated in the thalamus and brainstem structures. The lower limb response elicited by electrical stimulation of the posterior tibial nerve has a main positive peak with a latency of approx 40 ms (P_{40}) followed by a large negative peak at a latency of 45 ms. This negative peak is generally assumed to be generated by cortical structures and it is best recorded with an active electrode at the midline, 3–4 cm behind the C_z (52). A frontal reference is usually used for such recordings.

One reason that interpretation of the neural generators of the different components of the lower limb SSEP is less certain than for those of the upper limb SSEP is the more complex and diverse anatomical structures of the ascending somatosensory pathway from the lower portion of the body compared to that in the upper portion of the body. The early peaks in the SSEP evoked by lower limb stimulation are less distinct than those evoked by upper limb stimulation because of the greater temporal dispersion of the neural activity that arrives at the brain from the lower portion of the body (**Fig. 5.14**) because of the longer pathway than those of the upper limb SSEP. When nerve fibers have different conduction velocities, the temporal coherence of neural activity will decrease along such nerves. Therefore, long nerves tend to deliver less temporally coherent neural activity to central neural structures, than shorter pathways. Because the amplitudes of the various peaks in the far-field response depend on the degree of synchronization of neural activity (temporal coherence), such temporal dispersion results in the peaks becoming broader and smaller in amplitude compared to similar peaks in systems that have shorter pathways—such as the upper limb SSEP.

VISUAL SYSTEM

Introduction

Visual evoked potentials (VEPs) have been used in connection with intraoperative monitoring during operations in which the optic nerve or optic tract is involved, such as those to remove pituitary tumors, tumors of the cavernous sinus, and aneurysms in this area *(63)*. However, intraoperative monitoring of the visual system plays a much smaller role than monitoring of the auditory and somatosensory systems. The main reason for that is technical difficulties in presenting adequate stimuli to the eye of anesthetized individuals *(64,65)*. The adequate stimulus for the visual system is a change in contrast (for details, *see* ref. *14*) such as a reversing checkerboard pattern. The use of such a stimulus requires that the pattern be focused on the retina, which is not possible in an anesthetized patient. Therefore, flash stimulation is the only form of stimulation that can be used in an anesthetized patient and that is not an appropriate stimulus for evoking VEP (*see* Chap. 8).

The Eye

Light reaches the retina, where the sensory receptor cells are located, together with a neural network that processes the information from the receptor cells. Before it reaches the retina, light has passed through the conductive apparatus of the eye, consisting of the cornea, the lens, and the pupil. The optic apparatus of the eye projects a sharp image on the retina, where the light-sensitive receptors are located together with a complex neural network that enhances the contrast between areas with different degrees of illumination. The position of the eye is controlled by five extraocular eye muscles that are innervated by three cranial nerves (CN III, CN IV, and CN VI).

Much neural processing visual stimuli takes place in the neural network in the retina of the eye. This processing is also the basis for representation of differences in illumination over the visual field, and there are optic nerve fibers that have small excitatory fields that are surrounded by inhibitory areas, whereas others have inhibitory center areas that are surrounded by excitatory areas.

Receptors. There are two kinds of sensory cell (cones and rods) in the human retina. The outer segments of cones and rods contain light-sensitive substances (photopigment) *(14)*. The three different kinds of photo pigment in the cones, one for each of the three principle colors blue, green and red, provides the eye's color sensitivity (photopic vision). Rods are more sensitive than cones and provide vision in low light (scotopic vision).

Adaptation of the photoreceptors plays an important role for processing of information in the visual system, as it does in other sensory organs. Adaptation of the eye is a form of automatic gain control that adapts the sensitivity of the eye to the ambient illumination. The adaptation of photoreceptors provides most of the eye's automatic gain control. The pupil also provides some automatic gain control, the range of which varies among species.

Adaptation of the eye is often referred to as dark adaptation, which is the recovery of sensitivity that occurs after exposure to bright light. The first part of the dark-adaptation curve is steeper than the following segment and represents the dark adaptation of cones; the second segment is related to the function of rods. Light adaptation (the opposite of dark adaptation) is caused by exposure to bright light causing reduced sensitivity of the eye.

Ascending Visual Pathways

Two different afferent pathways have been identified: the classical and the nonclassical pathways, similar to that of the auditory and the somatic sensory systems *(14)*. In this volume, only the classical pathways known as the retinogeniculocortical pathway will be described. This pathway involves the lateral geniculate nucleus (LGN) of the thalamus and the primary visual cortex (striate cortex, V1) **(Fig. 5.18)**.

All visual information travels in the optic nerve (CN II) that enters the optic chiasm where the fibers reorganize to become the optic tract. From the optic chiasm the information travels in the optic tracts to the LGN in the thalamus, from which there are connections to the visual cortex (V1), which is located in the posterior portion of the brain.

The organization of the part of the optic nerve that belongs to the classical visual pathways is

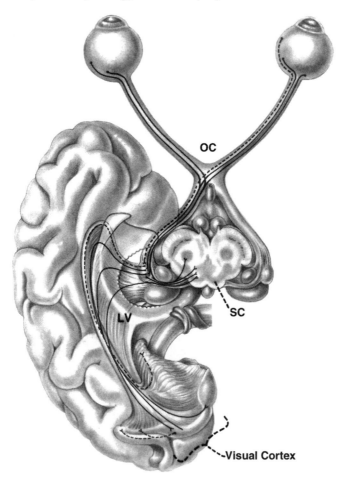

Figure 5.18: Schematic of the major visual pathways. OC, optic chiasm; SC, superior colliculus; LV, lateral ventricle. (Reprinted from: Møller AR. *Evoked Potentials in Intraoperative Monitoring.* Baltimore, MD: Williams and Wilkins; 1988, with permission.)

best illustrated by the effect on vision from visual defects that are caused by lesions of the optic nerve and the optic tract at different locations. If the optic nerve from one eye is severed, that eye will become totally blind. If the optic tract is severed on one side between the optic chiasm and the LGN in animals with forward-pointed eyes, the result is homonymous hemianopsia (the nasal field on the same side and the temporal field on the opposite eye will be blind), but the temporal field on the same side and the nasal field of the opposite eye will be unaffected. Midline sectioning of the optic chiasm causes loss of vision in the temporal field in both eyes (the crossed pathways), causing "tunnel vision."

Lesions at more central locations of the visual pathways such as the LGN or the visual cortex can cause complex visual defects such as scotoma that manifest by blind (black) spots in the visual fields. The spots that appear in the temporal visual field indicate a lesion that affects the contralateral side, whereas black spots in the nasal visual field are indication of lesions on the ipsilateral side (for details, *see* ref. *14*).

Visual Evoked Potentials

The VEP recorded from electrodes placed on the scalp are dominated by a positive peak with a latency of about 100 ms (P_{100}) *(66)*, and sometimes a small peak with a latency of 45–50 ms

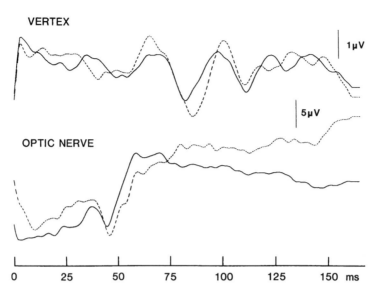

Figure 5.19: Recordings from an electrode placed directly on the optic nerve and from an electrode placed on the scalp at a location approximately overlying the visual cortex in response to stimulation with flashes of light delivered by a light-emitting diode attached to a contact lens. (Reprinted from: Møller AR. Electrophysiological monitoring of cranial nerves in operations in the skull base. In: Sekhar LN, Schramm Jr VL, eds. *Tumors of the Cranial Base: Diagnosis and Treatment.* Mt. Kisco, New York: Futura; 1987:123–132, with permission.)

and a negative peak with a latency of approx 70 ms (N_{70}) can be recognized.

Neural Generators of the VEP. Years of intensive research on coding in the visual system have resulted in an accumulation of a wealth of knowledge about the responses from single nerve cells in the visual cortex and the LGN as well as from the neural network in the retina. Information about the generators of the evoked response from the optic nerve and LGN is, however, sparse, and the relationship between the different components of the VEP and the potentials that can be recorded directly from the different parts of the visual system (near-field potentials) is poorly understood.

It is assumed that the N_{70} and P_{100} peaks are somehow generated in the visual cortex (striate cortex, area 17) *(14,67)*, but little is known about how these potentials relate to the normal

functioning of the visual system. The exact anatomical location of the generators of early components of the VEP is poorly understood. Intraoperative recordings from the optic nerve shows an early positive deflection with a latency of 75 ms, followed by a broad negative potential with a latency of approx 55 ms in response to short light flashes *(68)* **(Fig. 5.19)**. These potentials do not seem to have any corresponding components in the scalp recorded far-field potentials **(Fig. 5.19)**.

The reason that the optic nerve produces such a small far-field potential might be that the medium surrounding the optic nerve and the optic tract is relatively homogeneous with regard to electrical conductivity. The abrupt change in conductivity of the medium around the nerve, which is regarded to be a prerequisite for a nerve to generate stationary far-field peaks *(28,29,69)*, does not seem to exist for the optic nerve.

6

Monitoring Auditory Evoked Potentials

INTRODUCTION

The eighth cranial nerve (CN VIII) is at risk of being injured by surgical manipulations in microvascular decompression (MVD) operations to relieve trigeminal neuralgia (TGN), hemifacial spasm (HFS), glossopharyngeal neuralgia (GPN) *(70,71)*, and in connection with MVD operations of the eighth nerve in patients with tinnitus and disabling positional vertigo (DPV) *(72)*.

Preservation of auditory function during the removal of small vestibular schwannoma has recently improved because of advancements in operative techniques and through the introduction of intraoperative neurophysiological monitoring of the function of the ear and the auditory nerve *(73–78)*.

Intraoperative monitoring of the integrity of the intracranial portion of the auditory nerve during such operations is commonly done by recording the auditory brainstem response (ABR) from electrodes placed on the scalp. Direct recording

of the compound action potential (CAP) from the exposed eighth nerve has also been done during some MVD operations to monitor neural conduction in the auditory nerve *(71)*, and during operations to remove vestibular schwannoma, recordings of the ABR has been supplemented by recording the CAP from the exposed CN VIII *(73–76)*. Recording evoked potentials from the vicinity of the cochlear nucleus by placing the recording electrode in the lateral recess of the fourth ventricle *(39,45,77)* is an important addition to monitoring of the integrity of the auditory nerve. Recording from the vicinity of the cochlea (electrocochleography [EcoG]) has been done in operations for vestibular schwannoma *(79,80)*. In the following sections, the advantages and disadvantages of these different methods will be discussed and different ways to optimize such recordings will be described.

Recordings of the ABR have also been used to detect effects on the brainstem from surgical manipulations during operations on large vestibular schwannoma and on other types of mass that might occur in the cerebella pontine angle (CPA) *(68,75,81)*, as well as on tumors or other space-occupying lesions in the fourth ventricle.

From: *Intraoperative Neurophysiological Monitoring: Second Edition*
By A. R. Møller
© Humana Press Inc., Totowa, NJ.

The choice of acoustic stimuli and how they are presented, as well as the hearing status of the patient, might influence the way in which the recorded potentials change as a result of a specific surgically induced change in the function of the auditory system. Therefore, it is important to consider these factors in the interpretation of the results of intraoperative monitoring of auditory evoked potentials. Thus, all patients in whom intraoperative monitoring of auditory evoked potentials is to be done should have hearing tests performed preoperatively. Included in such tests should be, at the very least, pure tone audiometry, determination of speech discrimination (using recorded speech material), and the ABR. It is also preferable to include testing of the acoustic middle ear reflex. The results of such preoperative tests are a prerequisite to quantitatively assess a change in hearing status that might occur as a result of an intraoperative injury to the auditory nerve as well as to assess the value of intraoperative monitoring of auditory evoked potentials and the value of any modification in the usual surgical methods that might be made in an attempt to improve hearing preservation (*see* Chap. 19).

It is mainly changes in the latencies of specific components of the recorded evoked potentials (CAP from the auditory nerve, the cochlear nucleus, or the ABR) that are used as indications of injuries to the auditory nerve, but changes in amplitude of the recorded evoked potentials are valuable signs of surgically induced injuries *(82)*. Changes in CAPs recorded from the auditory nerve provide direct information about changes in the function of the auditory nerve, whereas interpretation of the intraoperatively recorded ABR is more complex because different neural generators contribute to the waveform of the ABR. As was discussed in the previous chapter, knowledge about the anatomy and function of the ear and the auditory nervous system and the neural generators of the ABR is important for correctly interpreting intraoperative changes in the ABR. ABRs were some of the earliest sensory evoked potentials to be used intraoperatively for the purpose of reducing intraoperative injuries to a part of the nervous

system. Recordings of the ABR was first used to for reducing the risk of intraoperative injury to the auditory nerve *(70,83)* and later other uses were introduced.

This chapter will discuss the practical aspects of hearing preservation in various types of operations using recordings of ABR or CAP directly from the auditory nerve or the vicinity of the cochlear nucleus.

AUDITORY BRAINSTEM RESPONSES

The technique used in recording ABRs for intraoperative monitoring is similar to that used clinically to obtain ABRs for diagnostic purposes. However, when recording ABRs intraoperatively, several modifications in this technique are necessary because of the special environment of the operating room and because, there, it is important to obtain an interpretable record in as short a time as possible. Because the purpose of intraoperative monitoring of ABRs is to detect changes that occur in the patient's auditory system during the operation, the recordings that are made during an operation must be compared with a baseline recording obtained in the same patient before the operation began, rather than with a standard ABR recording as is done when ABRs are used for clinical diagnostics. This influences the way the ABRs are recorded in the operating room and the way that the recorded potentials are processed.

How to Obtain an Interpretable Record in the Shortest Possible Time

The ABR obtained intraoperatively must be interpreted as soon as possible so that the cause of a change in the ABR can be identified with the shortest possible delay, so as to provide information to the surgeon if warranted.

Because the ABRs have much smaller amplitudes than the background of noise in the operating room (consisting of ongoing biological activity, EEG, and electrical interference), many responses must be added (averaged) to obtain an interpretable record. The time it takes to obtain an interpretable record therefore depends on the amplitude of the ABR in relation to the background noise (the signal-to-noise ratio) and how many responses can be added per unit of time, thus the repetition rate of the stimuli. The most important factors for obtaining an interpretable record in the shortest possible time are as follows:

1. The use of adequate stimulus strength.
2. The use of optimal stimulus repetition rate.
3. Optimal electrode placement.
4. Reduction of electrical noise that reaches the amplifiers.
5. Use of optimal filtering of recorded potentials.
6. Use of quality control that does not add to the time for data collection.

Stimulus Intensity. The stimulus intensity should be adequately high, without imposing a risk of causing noise-induced hearing loss (NIHL), so that the amplitude of the recorded ABR is as high as possible. Clicks at an intensity of 105 dB peak equivalent sound pressure level (PeSPL) have been used for intraoperative monitoring for many years without experiencing any problems. This intensity corresponds to the approx 65-dB hearing level (HL) (dB above the average threshold of hearing in individuals with normal hearing).

Stimulus Repetition Rate. When the stimulus repetition rate is increased, the number of responses that can be collected within a certain period of time increases. If the amplitude of the responses was independent of the repetition rate, then the time it would take to obtain an interpretable record would be inversely proportional to the repetition rate, thus a doubling of the repetition rate would shorten that time by a factor of two. However, this is only the case below a certain repetition rate, because the amplitude of the peaks decreases with increasing repetition rate above a certain repetition rate, diminishing the gain of increasing the repetition rate. Above a certain repetition, there would be no advantage to increasing the repetition rate.

The decrease in amplitude that occurs when the repetition rate is increased is minimal at low repetition rates, but it accelerates with increasing repetition rate (**Fig. 6.1A**). There are only small changes in the ABR when increasing the stimulus repetition rates from a few stimuli per second up to 20 pps (pulses per second). At a certain repetition rate, the reduction in amplitude of the recorded potentials outweighs the gain from producing more responses per unit time (**Fig. 6.1B**); if the repetition rate is increased beyond that critical rate, it will take a longer to obtain an interpretable record. Thus, there is a specific repetition rate that provides an interpretable record in the shortest possible time.

The optimal repetition rate is outside (above) the range of repetition rates for which data are available (up to approx 80 pps; **Fig. 6.1**). The relationship between repetition rate of the stimulation and the amplitude of the individual peaks of the ABR depends on the individual's age and hearing loss and it affects the different peaks differently. Peaks I–III are much more affected by an increased repetition rate than peak V, which is the most robust of the peaks of the ABR with regard to high repetition rate of the stimulus (84). Hearing loss of cochlear origin does not seem to affect the way that the amplitude of the ABR peaks decrease with increasing repetition rate of the click stimuli, but if the hearing loss is of retrocochlear origin, such as caused by an injury to the auditory nerve, then the amplitude of peak V deceases more rapidly with increasing repetition rate of the stimulus.

The amplitude of peak V times the repetition rate of the click stimuli in individuals with hearing loss of retrocochlear origin (presumably from injury to the auditory nerve) nearly reaches a plateau somewhere above 40 pps (85) (**Fig. 6.1B**). Similar results were obtained by others (86). On the basis of these results, it seems advantageous to use repetition rates of at least 50 pps, and perhaps as high as 70 pps. That is much higher than the commonly used repetition rate (10–20 pps) (85) (**Fig. 6.1**). (Because the time required to obtain an interpretable record when recording ABR in the clinic is not

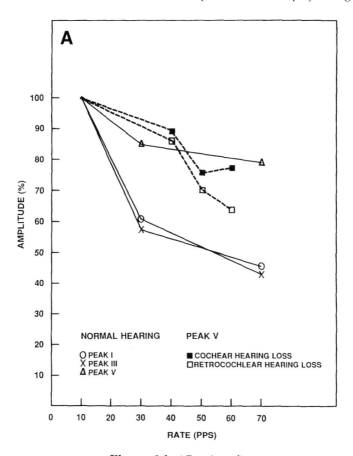

Figure 6.1: *(Continued)*

important, most clinical recordings of ABR employ a low repetition rate,10–20 pps.)

Because it is not completely known how disease processes that affect the ear and the auditory nerve can affect the relationship between stimulus repetition rate and the amplitudes of the various peaks, it might not be advisable to use repetition rates higher than 50 pps. When the repetition rate is increased, caution should be exercised because the risk of hearing loss increases accordingly, and it might not be advisable to use repetition rates higher than 40 pps if an intensity of 105 dB PeSPL is being used.

The fact that the latencies of the peaks of the ABR increase with increasing stimulus repetition rate is not important for the selection of the stimulus repetition rate for ABR in the operating room, because in the operating

room, the patient's own ABR is the reference (baseline), provided that the same repetition rate is used for monitoring as used for obtaining the baseline recording.

Sound Delivery. Several kinds of insert earphone are suitable for use in the operating room to deliver sound stimuli for recording ABRs. The miniature earphones used with, for instance, the Walkman™ type of tape recorder (Fig. 6.2) have a broad frequency response and can easily be fitted into the ear of a patient in the operating room. We have used such earphones (Realistic); Radio Shack, Ft. Worth, TX) routinely in the operating room for many years. The earphones are normally driven by rectangular waves of 100 μs duration. The sound system can be calibrated by

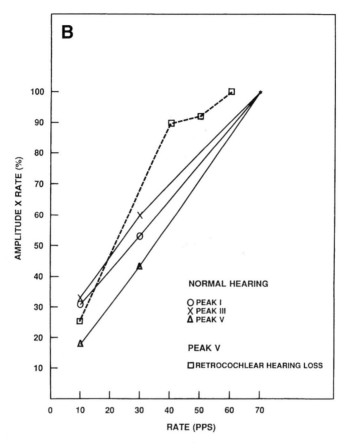

Figure 6.1: Decrease in the amplitude of peaks I, III, and V of the ABR as a function of the stimulus repetition rate (pps). **(A)** Solid lines are from patients with normal hearing (data from ref. *84*), and dashed lines (only peak V) are from patients with hearing loss of both cochlear origin (circles) and retrocochlear origin (crosses) (data from ref. *85*). The amplitude was normalized to 100% at 10 pps. **(B)** Same data as in **(A)**, but the amplitudes of the peaks were multiplied by the repetition rate and normalized to 100% at 60 and 70 pps.

measuring the sound pressure at the entrance of the ear canal by placing a 0.25-in. condenser microphone (Type 4135; Bruel and Kjaer, Naerum, Denmark) in the outer ear of an individual when the earphone is positioned in a way similar to that done during intraoperative monitoring. The condenser microphone can be placed under the earphone in such a way that it measured the sound pressure at the entrance to the ear canal.

*This type of earphone delivers a narrow sound impulse (**Fig. 6.3A**) and has a maximal sound output of approx 110 dB PeSPL, and they can deliver clicks of 105 dB PeSPL without any*

*noticeable differences in amplitudes or waveforms of rarefaction and condensation clicks (corresponding to approx 65 dB HL when presented at a rate of 20 pps). The frequency spectrum of the clicks that are generated by these earphones is relatively flat over a large range of frequencies (100–7000 Hz ± 8 dB, **Fig. 6.3B**), with a broad peak around 5 kHz when measured at the entrance of the ear canal. The dip at 10 kHz is caused by the fact that the spectrum of the electrical input to the earphone is a square wave of 100 µs duration. The spectrum of a square wave of 100 µs duration has a cutoff at 8000 Hz (6 dB) and its*

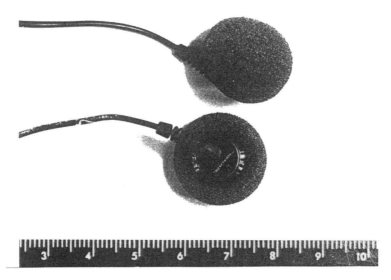

Figure 6.2: Miniature stereo earphone (Realistic; Radio Shack) (the scale is in centimeters).

energy is zero at 10 and 20 kHz causing the dips in the spectrum of the sound at these two frequencies *(Fig. 6.3B)*.

When such a miniature stereo earphone is placed in the ear of a patient, it should be placed so that its sound-radiating (flat) surface faces the ear canal and the earphone does not just rest in the pinna. This is particularly important to consider when such an earphone is placed in the ear of patients who have large outer ears (pinna), which is often the case in elderly men. The earphone must be carefully secured in place with several layers of a good quality plastic adhesive tape (e.g., Blenderm*R*; 3M, Minnesto Division/3M, St. Paul, MN) in such a way that fluid cannot reach the earphone just in case the area around the ear becomes wet. The cord to the earphone must be secured with adhesive tape to the side of the patient's face and to the head holder (or operating table) so that the earphone is not accidentally dislodged from the ear if the cable is accidentally pulled.

Some of the modern insert earphones usually have the transducer connected to the ear by means of a plastic tube of various lengths. When driven by the standard rec-

tangular wave of 100 µs duration, some earphones deliver a sound with a relatively flat spectrum up to approx 6 kHz, which is similar to the spectrum delivered by the earphones used in audiometry and those often also used in clinical ABR testing. The fact that insert earphones deliver sound through a long (plastic) tube results in a delay between the delivery of the electrical impulse that drives the earphone and the arrival of the sound at the ear. Sound travels at a speed of about 340 m/s, corresponding to a delay of 1 ms per 34 cm. Thus, the delay is slightly less than 1 ms for each foot of tubing. A delay of 1 ms makes the (electrical) stimulus artifact appear 1 ms ahead of the sound's arrival at the ear and thus reduces interference from the stimulus artifact with the ABR response.

Electrode Placement. The electrodes used for recording ABRs should be placed so that the amplitude of the recorded potentials will be as high as possible and so that the components of the ABR that are of interest will appear as clear as possible. The traditional way of recording ABRs is by connecting one of the two inputs of a differential amplifier to an

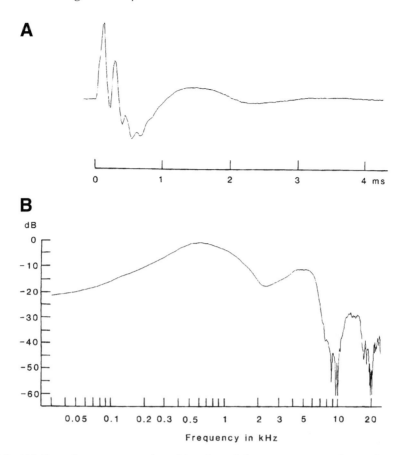

Figure 6.3: (A) Sound pressure produced by the miniature stereo earphone shown in **Fig. 6.2**, as measured at the entrance of the ear canal of an individual in whom the earphone was fitted in a way similar to that done in the operating room. The sound pressure was measured using a 0.25-in. condenser microphone (Type 4135; Bruel and Kjaer). The earphone was driven by rectangular pulses of 100 μs duration. **(B)** Spectrum of the sound at the entrance of the ear canal.

electrode placed on the vertex while the other input is connected to an electrode placed on the ipsilateral earlobe or on the mastoid.

We have noted advantages in recording ABRs on two separate recording channels recording differentially between electrodes placed at the vertex and on the dorsal upper neck (a noncephalic reference) and the other channel recording differentially from electrodes placed on the two earlobes. This way of recording ABRs provides a record in which peak V appears distinctly in the recording from the first channel and peaks I and III are better represented in the second channel than what can be seen in the traditional way of recording ABRs from electrodes placed at the vertex and on the ipsilateral earlobe. Recording in two independent channels offers two alternative ways to detect changes in auditory function during an operation and it makes it possible to continue monitoring using only one channel if one of the electrodes should malfunction during an operation.

RECORDING OF FAR-FIELD POTENTIALS AUDITORY POTENTIAL IN THREE ORTHOGONAL PLANES. *A different way to record sensory evoked potentials introduced involves recording from three pairs of electrodes placed orthogonally on the scalp (87–89). Each pair of electrodes is connected to the two inputs of three independent differential amplifiers. The recorded potentials are then plotted as a function of each other to form a three-dimensional display with time as a parameter. Such recordings provide additional information about the anatomical location of the neural generators of the various components of the ABR in the head, because they take into account the orientation of the different dipoles. There is, however, some uncertainty regarding the interpretation of the potentials when they are recorded in this way. This type of recording is not commonly used in intraoperative monitoring but has been used for research purposes in the operating room (30).*

TYPES OF ELECTRODE. When ABRs are recorded for clinical diagnostic purposes, it is convenient to use surface electrodes to record the responses, but in the operating room, needle electrodes are more suitable for several reasons:

1. Needle electrodes, when held in place with a good quality plastic adhesive tape (e.g., Blenderm[R]; 3M), provide a more stable recording over a longer period of time than do surface electrodes. Platinum subdermal electrodes (Type E2; Grass Instrument Co., Quincy, MA; or disposable electrodes that are available from numerous sources) are suitable.
2. Inserting needles takes much less time than placing surface electrodes on the skin. Because electrodes are usually applied in the operating room after the patient is anesthetized, any discomfort that a conscious patient might feel when placing such needles is not induced in the operating room.

All precautions should be taken to avoid failure of any recording electrodes during an operation. Thus, it is important that the electrodes be inserted properly and secured well so that they do not become dislodged should the electrode wires be accidentally pulled or the area where the electrodes are placed be disturbed during the operation. The electrode placed on the vertex for recording ABRs must be inserted deep in the tissue, and the wire must be drawn toward the forehead and placed under the hair as close to the skin as possible and then secured to the forehead with adhesive tape. When recording from a person with much hair, the drape can make the hair move, and if the electrode wire is resting on top of the hair, it too will move, thereby causing a noisy recording or even causing the needle electrode to be pulled out of the tissue. In operations in which skin incisions are made near the earlobe, the earlobe electrode might be pulled out if it is not sufficiently secured with adhesive tape or with sutures.

Reduction of Electrical Interference. Reducing electrical interference at its source is the most efficient way to improve recordings of evoked potentials of low amplitude, such as ABRs. This topic is treated in detail in Chap. 17 and will not be discussed here.

Processing of ABRs. The purpose of processing the recorded ABR is to obtain a record that is as clear as possible and to enhance features that are of interest. The techniques that are suitable for processing ABRs are similar to commonly utilized methods that are used to process other evoked potentials (for details, *see* Chap. 18).

Because it is mainly changes in the latency of peak V (and to some extent of peak III) that are used in connection with intraoperative monitoring, it is important that these peaks appear as clear as possible in the recordings. The purpose of processing recorded ABRs is, therefore, to enhance these peaks (III and V) so they can be clearly identified and their latency can be measured. This can be done by utilizing two methods: (1) averaging the responses to a sufficient number of stimuli and (2) suitable filtering of the responses. The latter can be done either at the same time that the responses are recorded using electronic filters or after the responses have been averaged using computer programs (digital filters) (*see* Chap. 17).

Display of ABRs in the Operating Room

When monitoring ABRs in the operating room, several tracings should be displayed, namely the digitally filtered averaged ABR recorded on two channels—one differentially between the vertex and the dorsal neck and the other differentially between the two earlobes. The filtered ABR should be superimposed on a baseline recording on both of these channels. It is also important to have a display of the output of the amplifiers of the ABR in order to be able to evaluate background noise. Suddenly occurring interference would only be detected by an increase in the number of rejected responses and that does not provide information about the kind of interference. Only by continuously observing the output from the amplifier can that be done (*see* Chap. 18 for details).

RECORDING OF NEAR-FIELD POTENTIALS

Recordings of near-field potentials from structures of the ascending auditory pathways in humans were first done for research purposes *(22–24, 39,42,90–92)*, but have later found practical importance in intraoperative monitoring, particularly for reducing the risk of injures to the auditory nerve *(73,74,76,93)*. Recordings from the exposed auditory nerve or from the surface of the cochlear nucleus is valuable in monitoring neural conduction in the auditory nerve *(78)*.

Direct Recording From the Eighth Cranial Nerve

Recording directly from the exposed CN VIII yields CAPs with amplitudes of a few microvolts in patients with normal hearing *(22–24,41)*. This method therefore provides a much more rapid way to detect injuries to the auditory nerve in MVD operations to relieve different cranial nerve compression disorders and in monitoring of operations to remove vestibular schwannoma *(22,73,74,76)*. This cannot be done

unless the intracranial portion of the eighth nerve becomes exposed during the operation, which occurs routinely in operations to remove vestibular schwannoma and in MVD operations on cranial nerves V, VII, VIII, and IX.

Recording of CAPs from the auditory nerve in such operations can be done by placing a recording electrode on the exposed eighth nerve. A fine, malleable, single-strand, Teflon-insulated silver wire (Type Ag 7/40T; Medwire Corp., Mt. Vernon, NY) *(22)* has been used by the author for many years. About 2 mm of the insulation is removed from the tip of this wire, and the bare wire is then bent over and a small piece of cotton is sutured to the tip using a 5-0 silk suture. The cotton is then trimmed using microscissors to produce the finished electrode shown in **Fig. 6.4**. It is important that the cotton be well sutured to the wire because the electrode is to be placed on the exposed eighth nerve and losing a piece of cotton in the CPA can have serious consequences. Shredded Teflon offers the same advantage as cotton but has a less adverse reaction if accidentally lost intracranially.

After the cotton wick is sutured to the silver wire, it is soldered to a PVC-insulated and electrostatically shielded wire that connects the electrode to the input of the amplifier (electrode box). In operations in the CPA, the recording electrode wire is tucked under one of the sutures that holds the dura open. In addition, the electrode wire is clamped to the drape near the wound to secure it in place.

The wire from the recording electrode should be connected to the inverting (G_2) inputs of a differential amplifier so that a negative potential will cause an upward deflection. The shield of the wire should be grounded to the iso-ground of the amplifier. The reference electrode for the intracranial recordings can be placed in the opposite earlobe. The recording electrodes should be interfaced with the differential amplifier through a suitable isolation unit that can ensure that the electrical current, which might flow from the amplifier to the recording electrode into the patient, will be well within the limits of safety.

The eighth cranial nerve is composed of the vestibular nerve and the auditory (or

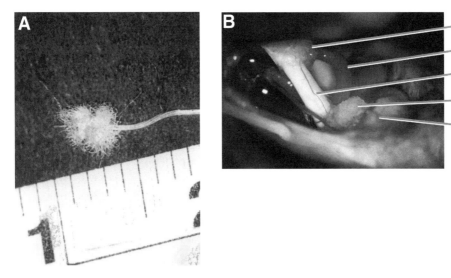

Figure 6.4: (A) The electrode used to record CAPs from the auditory nerve. The electrode is made from a Teflon-insulated silver wire with a the cotton wick sutured to its uninsulated tip. **(B)** The electrode in **(A)** placed on the exposed eighth cranial nerve to record CAPs from the auditory nerve.

cochlear) nerve. The arrangement of the different components of the eighth nerve is seen in cross-sectional view in **Fig. 6.5**, and the rotation of CN VIII is illustrated in **Fig. 6.6**. As seen from **Fig. 6.6**, the auditory nerve is located on the caudal side of the eighth nerve near the brainstem and anteriorventral to the eighth nerve near the porus acousticus.

The amplitude of the recorded potentials is largest when the recording electrode is placed on the auditory portion of the eighth nerve, but even when placed on the vestibular portion of the eighth nerve, the amplitude of the recorded potentials (CAPs) is normally several microvolts thus large enough to be visible directly on a computer screen (or after averaging only a few responses). The reason that potentials of such large amplitude can be recorded even when the electrode is placed on the vestibular portion of the eighth nerve is that the vestibular nerve is a good conductor of electrical current.

The CAP that can be recorded from the auditory nerve in a patient with normal or near-normal hearing—with the recording electrode placed on the nerve near the porus acousticus—has a triphasic waveform, with an initial (small) positive peak followed by a large

negative peak, which, in turn, is followed by another small positive peak (**Fig. 6.7A**). This is what might be expected when recording from a long nerve using a monopolar electrode (*see* p. 26). The waveform of the CAP depends on the placement of the electrode along the auditory nerve (**Fig. 6.7**).

The waveform of the normal CAP is essentially the same when using 2-kHz tone bursts as stimuli as when using clicks, but the changes in the responses as a result of pathologies affecting the ear or the auditory nerve might be different for click sounds than for tone bursts. The waveform of the CAP when recorded in the same way in patients with hearing loss (**Fig. 6.8**) might deviate noticeably from the waveform shown in **Fig. 6.7**.

Recording From the Vicinity of the Cochlear Nucleus

The value of monitoring directly recorded evoked potentials from the exposed auditory nerve is well documented. However, the difficulties in placing the electrode in the correct position on the eighth nerve are obstacles to the routine use of such directly recorded evoked potentials. The recording electrode

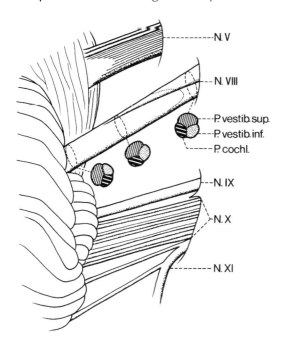

Figure 6.5: Schematic showing the CPA viewed from the dorsal side with a cross-section of the eighth nerve to illustrate the anatomical organization of the different portions of the eighth nerve. (Reprinted from: Lang J. Anatomy of the brainstem and the lower cranial nerves, vessels, and surrounding structures. *Am. J. Otol.* 1985; Suppl, Nov:1–19 with permission from Elsevier.)

must be placed proximal to the location on the nerve, where it is at risk of being injured and it might be difficult at times to keep the recording electrode in the correct position during an operation. These problems hamper the general use of recording directly from the auditory nerve.

Recording from the vicinity of the cochlear nucleus *(39,45)* can overcome many of the practical difficulties associated with recording directly from the exposed eighth nerve and it has similar advantages as recording the CAP directly from the eighth nerve *(77,78)*. The cochlear nucleus forms the floor of the lateral recess of the fourth ventricle *(77,96)*, and recording from the vicinity of the cochlear nucleus can be done by placing a recording electrode in the lateral recess of the fourth ventricle *(77,78)* **(Fig. 6.9A)**. The same type of

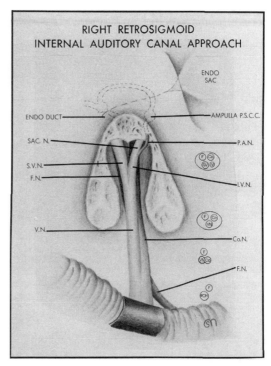

Figure 6.6: Drawing of the anatomy of the internal auditory canal as seen from a retrosigmoid approach. The posterior wall of the internal auditory meatus has been removed so that it appears as a single canal. IVN: inferior vestibular nerve; SVN: superior vestibular nerve; FN: facial nerve; VN: vestibular nerve; CoN: cochlear nerve. (Reprinted from: Silverstein H, Norrell H, Haberkamp T, McDaniel AB. The unrecognized rotation of the vestibular and cochlear nerves from the labyrinth to the brain stem: its implications to surgery of the eighth cranial nerve. *Otolaryngol. Head Neck Surg.* 1986;95:543–549, with permission from Elsevier.)

wick electrode as used to record from the exposed eighth nerve can be used for that purpose. The opening of the lateral recess of the fourth ventricle, known as the foramen of Luschka, is found just anterior to the entrance of the CN IX/CN X complex into the brainstem. The foramen of Luschka can be identified by locating the choroid plexus that normally protrudes from the foramen of Luschka. Elevating the cerebellum over the CN

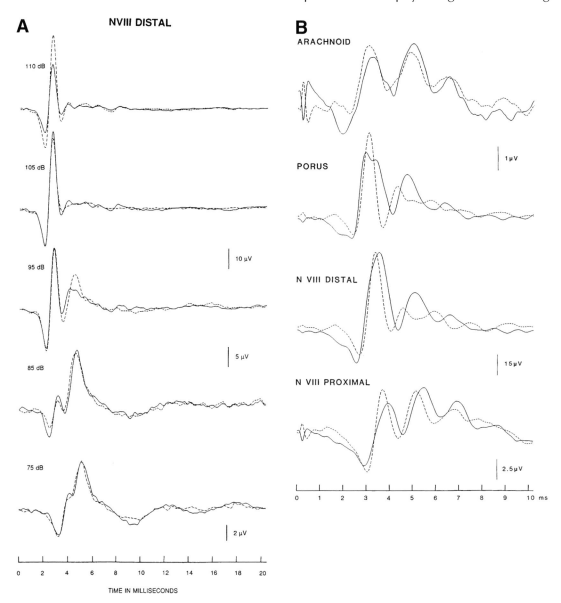

Figure 6.7: (**A**) Normal CAP recorded from the eighth nerve near the porus acusticus at different stimulus intensities (given in dB PeSPL). The responses were obtained in a patient undergoing MVD to relieve DPV, and the recording was made before manipulating the nerve. The sound stimuli were clicks delivered through a miniature stereo earphone (**Fig. 6.2**). (**B**) CAP recorded from different locations: near CN VIII (top tracing), from the porus acousticus, distally and proximally (near the brainstem). (Reprinted from: Møller AR. Direct eighth nerve compound action potential measurements during cerebellopontine angle surgery. In: Höhmann D, ed. *Proceedings of the First International Conference on ECoG, OAE, and Intraoperative Monitoring.* Amsterdam: Kugler, 1993:275–280, with permission from Kugler Publications.)

IX/CN X complex provides access to the foramen of Luschka. By following the choroid plexus into the lateral recess of the fourth ventricle, the recording electrode can be placed deep into the lateral recess *(77)*. The wire of the recording electrode should be tucked under the

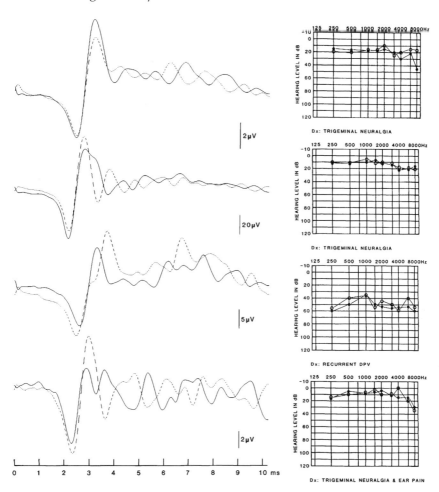

Figure 6.8: Examples of CAP recorded from patients with different degrees of preoperative hearing loss. The patients' preoperative hearing loss is shown by pure tone audiograms. (Reprinted from: Møller AR, Jho HD. Effect of high frequency hearing loss on compound action potentials recorded from the intracranial portion of the human eighth nerve. *Hear Res.* 1991;55:9–23, with permission from Elsevier.)

sutures that holds the dura open so that it cannot be easily moved during the operation (**Fig. 6.9A**). The opposite earlobe is a suitable location for the reference electrode for such recordings. It is practical to record ABRs and the potentials from the lateral recess simultaneously on different channels of the signal averager. The same stimuli as used to elicit ABRs are also suitable for eliciting these directly recorded potentials from the auditory nerve and the surface of the cochlear nucleus.

Recorded potentials from the surface of the cochlear nucleus consist of an initial sharp positive–negative deflection that is generated by the termination of the auditory nerve in the cochlear nucleus. This peak is followed by a slow wave that could last tenths of milliseconds (**Fig. 6.9B**).

Digital filters can be used to enhance the fast peaks of the responses and suppress the slow components (**Fig. 6.10**). Change in the stimulus intensity affects the fast (initial) and the (later) slow potentials differently. The amplitude of the main peak of the fast response, which occurs with a latency of approx 4 ms, decreases rapidly when the stimulus intensity is decreased,

A

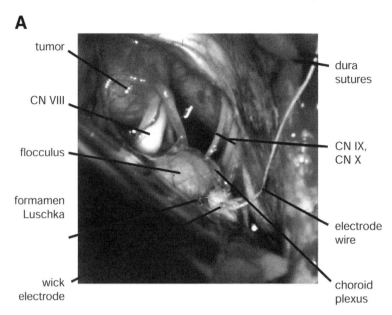

tumor

CN VIII

flocculus

formamen
Luschka

wick
electrode

dura
sutures

CN IX,
CN X

electrode
wire

choroid
plexus

Figure 6.9: *(Continued)*

whereas the slow components that dominate the unfiltered response only change slightly with decreasing stimulus intensity. It is not known which of these components—slow or fast—are the best indicator of injury to the auditory nerve, but it seems likely that the fast components (such as the peak at 4 ms) would be more sensitive to changes in neural conduction in the auditory nerve than the slow components.

It might sometimes be difficult to place the recording electrode deep in the lateral recess of the fourth ventricle, but it is not necessary to penetrate the foramen of Luschka with the recording electrode to obtain satisfactory recordings; merely placing the recording wick electrode on CN IX and CN X where they enter the brainstem will usually provide a satisfactory recording. The amplitudes of these potentials might be slightly lower than those recorded from an electrode placed deep in the lateral recess, but the potentials that are recorded from the entrance of CN IX and CN X in the brainstem are usually several microvolts and can thus be interpreted

after only a few hundred responses are added. It is easier to place the recording electrode in this location than it is to place it on the eighth nerve, and the recording electrode is away from the CN VIII, which is an advantage when monitoring operations for vestibular schwannoma.

Recordings from the lateral recess represent evoked potentials that are generated by structures located proximal to the location where the eighth nerve is often being manipulated, such as in MVD operations. Recordings from the lateral recess of the fourth ventricle are, however, perhaps of the greatest importance in connection with the removal of vestibular schwannoma in patients who have useful hearing preoperatively and in whom hearing preservation is being attempted during removal of the tumor.

Other Advantages of Recording Directly From CN VIII and the Cochlear Nucleus

Recordings of CAPs directly from the exposed eighth nerve or the vicinity of the cochlear nucleus during operations in the CPA has not only been valuable in reducing injuries

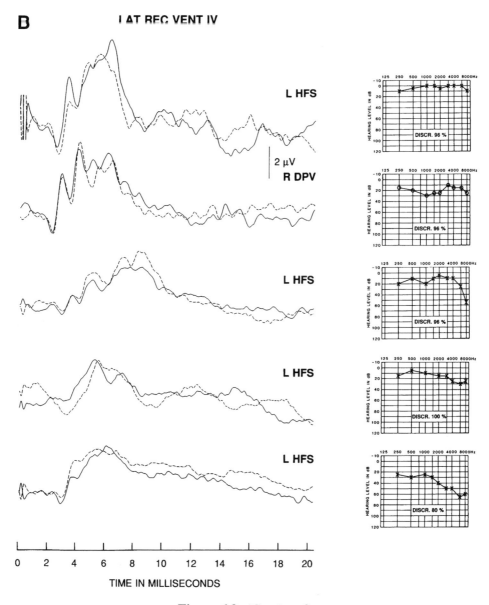

Figure 6.9: *(Continued)*

resulting from surgical manipulations in individual patients but has also contributed to our understanding of how injuries to nerves from surgical manipulations might occur. The ability to detect changes in neural conduction almost instantaneously has made it possible to detect such changes early enough to be able to identify exactly which step in an operation caused an adverse effect on neural conduction. Recordings of CAPs have provided information on how the auditory nerve might be injured by stretching and that it is highly sensitive to heat (from electrocoagulation). Experience has demonstrated that the auditory nerve can be seriously injured by the normal use of bipolar electrocoagulation when performed close to the auditory portion of CN VIII. The adverse effect on the auditory nerve is not caused by a spread of high-frequency current,

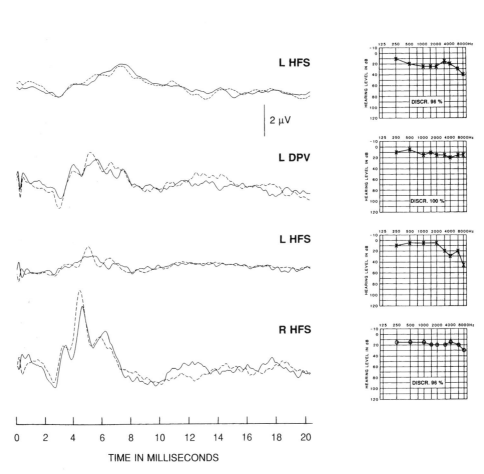

Figure 6.9: (A) Placement of the recording electrode in the lateral recess of the fourth ventricle. (Reprinted from: Møller AR. Monitoring techniques in cavernous sinus surgery. In: Loftus CM, Traynelis VC, eds. *Monitoring Techniques in Neurosurgery.* New York, NY: McGraw-Hill: 1994:141–155, with permission from McGraw-Hill, Inc.) **(B,C)** Examples of recordings from the vicinity of the cochlear nucleus in patients with varying degree of hearing loss.

which was a serious problem when monopolar coagulation was used, but rather by the spread of heat. Because all electrocoagulation is based on heating the tissue in question (e.g., a vein), such heat might spread to neural tissue located close to the site that is undergoing coagulation. Electro-coagulation using the bipolar technique might injure neural tissue from the spread of heat used to coagulate nearby tissue, even though the spread of high-frequency current might be negligible. These findings have prompted a change in the way electrocoagulation is done near the eighth nerve to use the lowest possible current and to do electrocoagulation in spurts of only a few seconds duration and allowing time for cooling of the tissue between periods of electrocoagulation. These changes in the way blood vessels are coagulated have reduced the risks of injury to neural tissue from electro-coagulation.

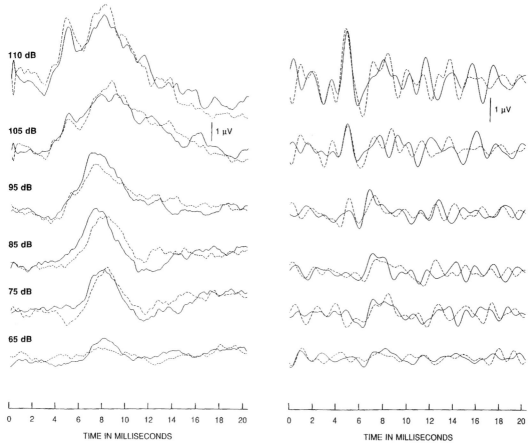

Figure 6.10: Typical recordings from the vicinity of the cochlear nucleus using the same electrode placement shown in **Fig. 6.9B**. **Left column:** Unfiltered responses; **right column:** same recordings after digital filtering to enhance the narrow peaks. These recordings were made consecutively and each record is the average of 250 responses. The dashed curves represent the baseline. (Reprinted from: Kuroki A, Møller AR. Microsurgical anatomy around the foramen of Luschka with reference to intraoperative recording of auditory evoked potentials from the cochlear nuclei. *J. Neurosurg.* 1995;82:933–939, with permission from Journal of Neurosurgery.)

PRACTICAL ASPECTS ON MONITORING AUDITORY EVOKED POTENTIALS IN VESTIBULAR SCHWANNOMA OPERATIONS

Most of the examples of results of intraoperative monitoring of auditory evoked potentials that were given earlier in this chapter were from monitoring of patients who underwent MVD of cranial nerves to relieve TGN, HFS, DPV, or tinnitus. It was shown that intraoperative monitoring of auditory evoked potentials could decrease the risk of hearing loss in such patients. MVD operations are rare, but similar methods to preserve hearing can be used in other operations in the CPA, such as those to remove vestibular schwannoma. Such operations are much more common than MVD operations. Diagnostic methods for identifying vestibular schwannoma continue to improve and such tumors can now be identified while still small. Many surgeons will recommend operation of small vestibular schwannoma in patients that have usable hearing to help retain

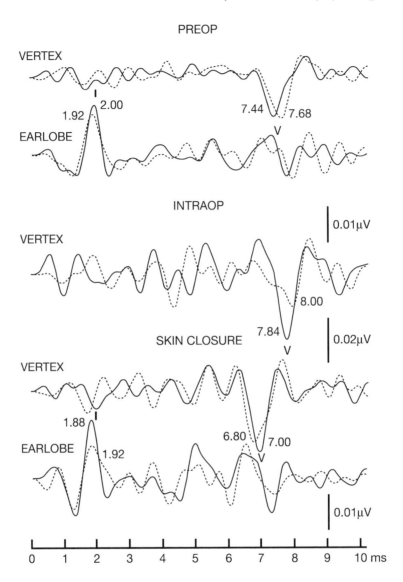

Figure 6.11: Samples of ABR recordings made on two channels from a patient undergoing removal of a vestibular schwannoma. The upper tracing shows potentials recorded from electrodes placed on the vertex and the upper neck, and the lower tracings were obtained by differential recordings between electrodes placed on the ear lobes. The stimuli were clicks presented to the ear on the side of the tumor at a rate of 20 pps. The recorded potentials were digitally filtered with a W50 filter (see p. 322).

the greatest degree of this sensory function. For that, intraoperative monitoring of the function of the auditory nerve is essential.

Auditory Brainstem Responses

An example of ABRs recorded during an operation to remove a vestibular schwannoma

in a patient who had good hearing before the operation (96% speech discrimination) is shown in **Fig. 6.11**. Despite variations in the ABR during the operation—there was an almost 1-ms prolongation of the latency of peak III in the early phase of the tumor resection procedure—the ABR obtained at the time of closure was remarkably similar to those obtained preoperatively (**Fig. 6.11**). Postoperatively, the patient had a speech discrimination score of 96%, and his pure tone audiogram showed no significant hearing loss (except at 4 and 8 kHz) as a result of the operation.

If peak I changes or disappears during an operation and there also is a change in all other peaks (or total obliteration of the ABR), it is a sign that the blood supply to the ear (cochlea) has been compromised. If peak I is largely unchanged while there are changes in both peaks III and V, it is likely that there has been injury to the intracranial portion of the auditory nerve, with the blood supply to the cochlea remaining intact. If there is a change in peak V but peak III is unchanged, there is reason to assume that the brainstem has been affected by surgical manipulations or that there is ischemia because of impaired blood supply. If it is not possible to clearly identify peak I, a judgment about the cause of a change in, for instance, peak V of the ABR cannot be made with certainty and the anatomical location of the injury will be less obvious.

Patients who undergo operations to remove vestibular schwannoma often have abnormal ABRs before the operation because the tumor affects the neural conduction in the auditory nerve, and the ABRs often have much smaller amplitudes than normal. This results in the need to average more responses in order to obtain an interpretable recording, consequently making it more difficult to use ABR to detect injury to the auditory nerve.

Patients undergoing operations to remove vestibular schwannoma are usually not paralyzed during the operation because the administration of muscle relaxants will prevent monitoring of the facial nerve, which is critical to preserving facial nerve function. The electromyographic (EMG) activity of the head muscles that might occur spontaneously when anesthesia drops to low levels, or when the facial nerve is manipulated acts as noise that contaminates the ABR recordings. This impairs the signal-to-noise ratio of the recorded ABR and, thus, increases the time required to obtain an interpretable record. There is, therefore, a great need to optimize the way

ABR is recorded and processed, such as utilizing optimal stimulus and recording parameters, aggressive filtering, and an efficient quality control system that does not require any additional time for data collection (p. 314). By taking these matters into proper consideration, it is possible to obtain an interpretable ABR and detect changes in the ABR by recording for about 1–3 min, at least in patients with a reasonably good ABR. These difficulties in obtaining interpretable ABR recording makes it important to be able to record CAP from the auditory nerve and the response from the cochlear nucleus, which have large amplitudes and, therefore, are not easily contaminated by EMG activity.

Recording CAP Directly From the Exposed Eighth Cranial Nerve

It is relatively easy to place a recording electrode on the proximal portion of the eighth nerve in operations on small vestibular schwannoma when there is a segment of the eighth nerve near the brainstem that is free of tumor (73–76). A click-evoked CAP recorded from the eighth nerve can provide a prompt indication of injury to the auditory nerve, thereby promoting the preservation of hearing. The same type of wick electrode as used in MVD operations (71) (**Fig. 6.5**) is suitable for this purpose, but removal of tumor mass often causes dislocation of the recording electrode when placed on the exposed CN VIII. The situation is even more apparant in operations on larger tumors where the tumor has reached the brainstem. In such operations, it is not possible to place an electrode on the proximal portion of the eighth nerve, at least not until some tumor has first been removed (because the eighth nerve in such cases is embedded in the tumor or is underneath it). Recording from the vicinity of the cochlear nucleus can, to a great extent, solve these practical problems.

Recording From the Vicinity of the Cochlear Nucleus

Auditory evoked potentials of large amplitudes can be recorded from the cochlear nucleus. That can be done by placing an electrode in the lateral recess of the fourth ventricle (foramen of Luschka) (39,77,78) (see p. 98).

Placing an electrode in the lateral recess of the fourth ventricle can be done even when operating on large vestibular schwannoma. More importantly, an electrode placed in or near the foramen of Luschka is far away from the operative field, and the electrode is not as easily dislocated as when placed on the CNVIII.

Recording From the Vicinity of the Ear (ECoG)

Some investigators have monitored auditory evoked potentials from the ear in operations to remove vestibular schwannoma *(98,99)*. For direct recording from the cochlear capsule, a recording electrode must be passed through the tympanic membrane, an invasive procedure that takes considerable skill to perform safely.

An electrode placed on the cochlear capsule will not only record CAPs from the distal portion of the auditory nerve, but it will also record the cochlear microphonic (CM) potential and the summating potential. These three different kinds of auditory evoked potential are known as the electrocochleographic (ECoG) potentials (**Fig. 6.12**). Only one of the components of the ECoG potentials is of interest in intraoperative monitoring for vestibular schwannoma, namely the CAPs from the auditory nerve. The CAPs from the auditory nerve that is recorded from the cochlea capsule usually have amplitudes within the range of several microvolts *(100)* and can therefore be evaluated with very little signal averaging (**Fig. 6.12A**). This makes it possible to detect changes in CAPs with practically no delays. When recorded from a wick electrode placed on the tympanic membrane (**Fig. 6.12B**) *(100)* or from an electrode placed in the ear canal, however, the amplitude of the CAP component is much less and a considerable number of responses must be averaged before an interpretable record can be obtained.

Unfortunately, there are several problems associated with the use of ECoG potentials recorded from the ear, or its vicinity, for intraoperative monitoring of hearing in patients undergoing vestibular schwannoma surgery. These problems are related to the fact that the CAPs recorded from the ear originate from the very distal portion of the auditory nerve where it exits the

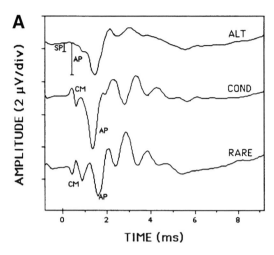

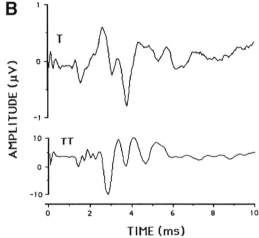

Figure 6.12: (**A**) Normal ECoG potentials recorded from the promontorium of the cochlea. The top tracing shows the response to clicks of alternating polarity, and the middle and lower tracings show the responses to condensation and rarefaction clicks, respectively. Note that negativity is shown as a downward deflection. (**B**) Comparison between ECoG potentials obtained from a wick electrode placed on the tympanic membrane (upper tracing) and on the promontorium (lower tracing). Note the much higher (about 10 times) amplitude of the response recorded from the promontorium than that recorded from the tympanic membrane. (Reprinted from: Winzenburg SM, Margolis RH, Levine SC, Haines SJ, Fournier EM. Tympanic and transtympanic electrocochleography in acoustic neuroma and vestibular nerve section surgery. *Am. J. Otol.* 1993;14:63–69, with permission from Elsevier.)

cochlea and, therefore, the ECoG potentials will not show change when the intracranial portion of the auditory nerve has actually been injured. In fact, the intracranial portion of the eighth nerve can be totally sectioned without any noticeable change in the CAP that is recorded from the ear. Because it is the intracranial portion of the auditory nerve that is most likely to be injured during removal of vestibular schwannoma, recordings of ECoG potentials are therefore not suitable for monitoring in operations for vestibular schwannoma because they do not detect injuries to the intracranial portion of the auditory nerve. Recording of ECoG potentials should not be used for hearing preservation in operations to remove vestibular schwannoma. Recording ECoG potentials makes it possible to detect if the blood supply to the cochlea has been compromised, but this can also be detected by methods that are useful in monitoring nerve conduction in the intracranial portion of the auditory nerve such as recording from the intracranial portion of CN VIII, the cochlear nucleus, or the ABR.

INTERPRETATION OF CHANGES IN AUDITORY RESPONSES

In the operating room, the task is to detect changes in auditory evoked potentials from a baseline recording done after the patient is brought to sleep but before the operations has begun. If possible, the observed changes should be related to specific manipulations such as stretching, compressing, or heating neural tissue and the anatomical location of the structures, the function of which has caused the changes, should be identified to the surgeon.

Interpretation of Changes in the ABR

Traditionally, it has been the latency of specific components (peaks) of the ABR that has been used to indicate surgically induced injuries to the auditory nerve. Because peak V of the ABR is the most prominent and most easily identified peak, it seems natural to use changes in the latency of this peak as an indication of injury to the auditory nerve. It has also often been assumed that any change in neural conduction of the auditory nerve is equally reflected in the latency of all ABR peaks that follow peak I. However, this is not necessarily true; therefore, there are reasons to monitor the latency of peak III instead. Peak III might be a more reliable (clean) indicator of changes in neural conduction of the auditory nerve than peak V. Often the vertex-negative peak between peak III and the peak IV–V complex is prominent, and in such cases, using this vertex-negative peak is just as suitable for monitoring purposes as peak III.

Changes in neural conduction of the auditory nerve might cause a smaller latency shift of peak V than of peak III. Peak V, therefore, might also be less sensitive to injury to the auditory nerve than peak III and, naturally, the CAP recorded intracranially from CN VIII or the cochlear nucleus.

If the latency of peak V increases but the latency of peak III remains unchanged, the interval between peaks III and V increases (increased interpeak latency [IPL] III–V). The reason for such a change is most likely changes in the function of structures of the ascending auditory pathways that are located rostral to the generators of peak III (the cochlear nucleus). Increased IPL III–V might also be caused by general changes in, for example, cerebral circulation or from changes in oxygenation from other causes. If this occurs in operations in the CPA, the anesthesiologist should be informed because such changes might be a result of cardiovascular changes or other changes that the anesthesiologist can correct.

Interpretations of CAP From CN VIII and the Cochlear Nucleus

Changes in the CAP that can be recorded directly from the proximal portion of the auditory nerve as a result of manipulation of the CN VIII are more easily interpreted than changes in the ABR. The CAP recorded from the CN VIII or the cochlear nucleus is probably more sensitive to small changes in the function of the auditory nerve than are the ABR. Recording of ABR is, however, the only way to detect injuries to the auditory nerve that might occur before surgical exposure of the eighth nerve.

Such changes might be caused by retraction of the cerebellum or surgical dissection to expose the auditory nerve.

The major advantage of recording directly from the exposed CN VIII is that changes in neural conduction in the auditory nerve can be detected almost at the moment they occur. The large amplitude of the CAP recorded directly from the auditory nerve allows the CAP to be viewed on a computer screen once a few responses have been added, making it possible to accurately identify which steps in an operation cause change in neural conduction in the auditory nerve. The rapid detection of change in neural conduction of the auditory nerve also provides a much better possibility to reverse a surgically induced changes in the function of the auditory nerve, thus increasing the effectiveness of intraoperative monitoring. Assessment of neural conduction in the auditory nerve on the basis of changes in the ABR takes a much longer time than from inspection of the CAP recorded directly from the auditory nerve.

The first CAP that is recorded should be used as a baseline to which successive recorded potentials can be compared. Any deviations in the components from the baseline recording should be regarded as a sign of an effect on neural transmission in the part of the auditory nerve that is located distal to the location of the recording electrode on the nerve.

The change in the CAP recorded from the auditory nerve, which could occur as a result of surgical manipulations or heating, is a more or less marked decrease in the amplitude of the main negative peak of the CAP, in addition to an increased latency. An increased amplitude of the initial positive peak (**Fig. 6.13**) indicates that a conduction block has occurred in many nerve fibers. The recordings shown in **Fig. 6.13** illustrate changes that occurred after heating of the auditory nerve by electrocoagulation. Shortly after the eighth nerve was exposed, the recorded CAP had the normal triphasic waveform, but after electrocoagulation of a nearby vein, it changed to a single positive peak, indicating that there was nearly total blockage of neural conduction in the auditory nerve.

Heating from electrocoagulation can cause changes in the waveform of the CAP recorded from the exposed auditory nerves (**Figs. 6.13** and **6.14**).

Examples of changes in the CAP caused by retraction of the cerebellum are seen in **Fig. 6.15**. The slight widening of the main negative peak in the CAP is an indication that the increase in latency (decreased conduction velocity) affected the different nerve fibers of the nerve differently. The small decrease of the amplitude of the negative peak indicates that almost all of the fibers of the auditory nerve were conducting nerve impulses. Changes in neural conduction that cause increases in the latency of the main negative peak with little change in amplitude indicate that the only effect of the surgical manipulation was an increase in neural conduction time (decrease in conduction velocity). We believe that this is what happens when the auditory nerve is stretched slightly to moderately. Provided that proper action is taken promptly to reverse the injury, such changes seem to be completely, or nearly completely, reversible so that the patient will not acquire postoperative hearing deficits when assessed by traditional measurements of hearing postoperatively.

In order to understand the nature of this kind of injury, the generation of the CAP from a long nerve, when recorded by a monopolar electrode, should be recalled. The initial positive deflection in the CAP is generated by a region of neural depolarization approaching the site of the recording electrode and the negative peak in the CAP is generated when the region of depolarization of auditory nerve fibers passes under the recording electrode (*see* Chap. 3, p. 26). The nearly disappearance of the negative peak (**Fig. 6.14**) can be explained by the region of depolarization never reaching the location on the nerve where the recording electrode is placed. The amplitude of the initial positive peak in the CAP, which is generated when the region of depolarization of nerve fibers approaches the recording electrode, is normally decreased because the negative peak that normally follows is pulling up the positive peak. When the amplitude of the negative peak decreases, this "pull" of the positive peak

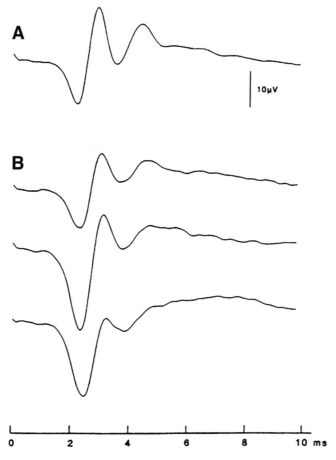

Figure 6.13: Typical alterations in the CAP recorded from the auditory nerve that resulted when heat from electrocoagulation was transmitted to the nerve. The sound stimuli were clicks at 110 dB PeSPL. (Reprinted from: Møller AR. *Evoked Potentials in Intraoperative Monitoring.* Baltimore, MD: Williams and Wilkins; 1988, with permission.)

upward decreases, and, therefore, the positive peak appears to have become larger in amplitude.

Changes that consist of broadening of the negative peak indicate that the latency of neural conduction has increased (decreased conduction velocity) unevenly for different nerve fibers (**Fig. 6.15**).

Less experience has been gained regarding the interpretations of recordings made from the vicinity of the cochlear nucleus than from recording from the auditory nerve. It is not known for certain which of the different components of the potentials that are recorded from the cochlear nucleus are most sensitive to changes in neural conduction in the auditory nerve. The slow components and the fast components decrease at different rates when stimulus intensity is decreased (*see* p. 101), which could mean that fast components are more sensitive to changes in neural conduction in the auditory nerve than the slow components. More experience is needed to resolve this question, but results from intraoperative recording during removal of a vestibular schwannoma such as those illustrated in **Fig. 6.16** seem to support this hypothesis. Whereas the amplitude of the slow components is largely unchanged, there is a considerable change in the amplitude of the fast components. The latencies of both the fast and slow components of these potentials, however,

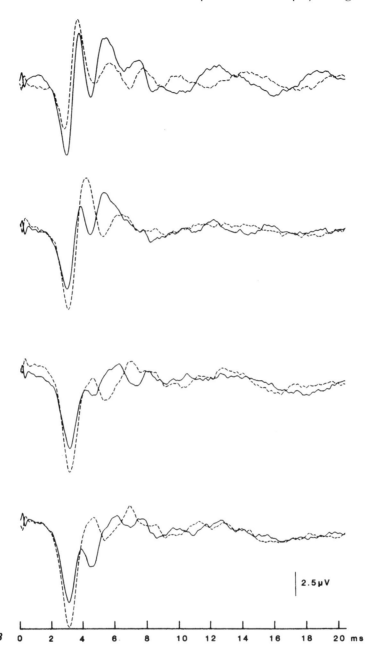

Figure 6.14: Examples of changes in the CAP recorded from the proximal portion of CN VIII as a result of surgical manipulations (probably heating). Solid lines are the responses to rarefaction clicks and dashed lines are the responses to condensation clicks.

were prolonged as a result of surgical manipulation. This indicates that the latencies of either slow or fast components might be valid indicators of changes in neural conduction in the auditory nerve (but perhaps not the amplitudes).

Relationship Between Changes in the ABR and in the CAP From the Auditory Nerve and the Cochlear Nucleus

The CAP recorded from the exposed CN VIII have specific relationships to the waveform

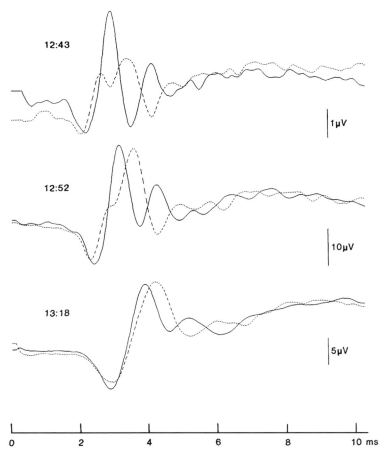

Figure 6.15: Examples of changes in the CAP recorded from the proximal portion of CN VIII as a result of surgical manipulations (stretching). Solid lines are the responses to rarefaction clicks and dashed lines are the responses to condensation clicks.

of the ABR. Surgical manipulations of the auditory nerve that causes changes in the waveform of the CAP recorded from the exposed CN VIII also causes changes in the ABR, but the changes in the ABR are less specific and, therefore, less interpretable (**Fig. 6.17**). Although there is an increase in latency and widening of the negative peak of the CAP after surgical manipulation of CN VIII indicating an uneven increase in neural conduction time of different auditory nerve fibers, similar information cannot be obtained from inspection of the ABR.

Surgically induced injuries to the auditory nerve do not necessarily result in the same change (prolongation) of the latency of the CAP recorded from CN VIII, or from the cochlear nucleus, or that of peaks III and V of

the ABR. The amplitudes of these two different kinds of auditory evoked potential do not necessarily change to the same degree as a result of injury to the auditory nerve.

One reason that the different components of the far-field response (ABR) might change in a different way than the near-field response (CAP from the auditory nerve or cochlear nucleus) is that the different components of the ABR are less dependent on the temporal coherence of neural activity than are the responses that are recorded directly from the auditory nerve.

The later peaks in the ABR are less dependent on temporal coherence of neural activity than the CAP recorded from CN VIII (**Fig. 6.15**). Thus, a large reduction in the coherence of neural activity in auditory nerve fibers, which manifests as a

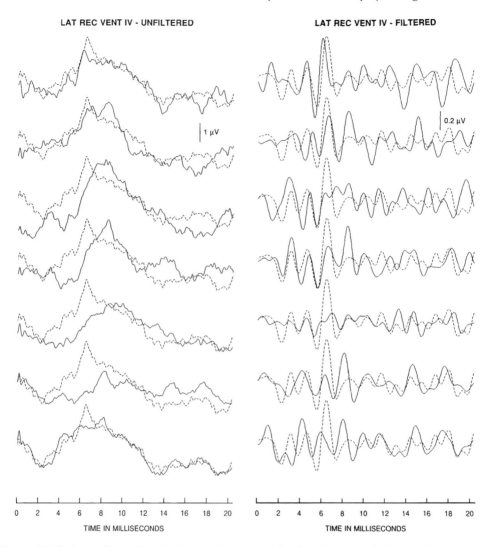

Figure 6.16: Recordings from the lateral recess of the fourth ventricle in a patient undergoing removal of a vestibular schwannoma (3 cm) before filtering (left column) and after digital filtering (right column, W50 filter, *see* p. 322). The dashed lines in all recordings are baseline recordings obtained before tumor removal. The patient had normal hearing before the operation and his hearing threshold and speech discrimination did not change noticeably after the operation.

large reduction in the response from the auditory nerve, might reduce the amplitude of the later peaks in the ABR to a smaller degree. This is why potentials recorded from the auditory nerve are probably more sensitive to surgically induced injuries, and these potentials might therefore be better suited for intraoperative monitoring during operations in which the eighth nerve is manipulated than recordings of the ABR.

Effect of Injury to the Auditory Nerve on the ABR

It has traditionally been the latency of the different components of the ABR that has been used as criteria for altered neural conduction in the auditory nerve. As discussed earlier, the amplitude of the CAP that can be recorded from a nerve is proportional to the number of nerve fibers that are conducting, and loss of

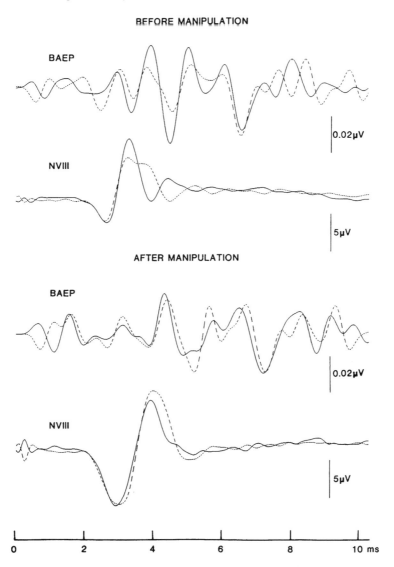

Figure 6.17: The ABR recorded simultaneously with the CAP from the eighth nerve. Each recording of the ABR represents about 2000 responses, and the averaged responses were filtered with a zero-phase digital filter (*see* Chap. 18). (The directly recorded responses from CN VIII were not digitally filtered.) (Reprinted from: Møller AR, Jannetta PJ. Monitoring auditory functions during cranial nerve microvascular decompression operations by direct recording from the eighth nerve. *J. Neurosurg.* 1983;59:493–499, with permission from Journal of Neurosurgery.)

conduction in some nerve fibers causes a decrease in the amplitude of the recorded CAP. This means that, presumably, also the amplitude of the different components of the ABR changes when neural conduction in the auditory nerve is altered. It would therefore be expected to be valuable to monitor amplitudes of the different components of the ABR in addition to monitoring latencies *(82)*.

One of the reasons why latency changes have been favored over amplitude changes as indicators of injury to the auditory nerve is that the latencies of ABR peaks are less variable than the amplitudes of the peaks. The reason for the greater variability of the amplitude of the different peaks is not known, but changes in recording conditions might contribute to this variability. The noise that is always super-imposed on ABR recordings also contributes to the variability of the amplitude of the compo-nents (peaks) of the ABR.

One reason for a decrease in the amplitude of the recorded ABR is, naturally, that the ampli-tude of the recorded potentials really decreases, but this is not the only reason. Another reason for a decrease in amplitude is associated with the use of signal averaging. When many responses are added, the amplitude of the resulting aver-aged recording will decrease if the latencies of the different components (peaks) of the ABR change during the time that the recorded poten-tials are being acquired, and the averaged response becomes less than the sum of the amplitudes of the same peak in the different recordings. A change in the latency of peaks in the ABR during the time the evoked potentials are being acquired also cause changes in the waveform of the averaged response, and the waveform of the averaged response will be dif-ferent than that of the waveform of the individ-ual responses that were added. These effects of the averaging process will increase when more responses are added and the more the ABR changes during the time of data acquisition.

It was mentioned earlier that excitation of the hair cells in the basal portion of the cochlea evokes more synchronized discharges than does excitation of hair cells that are located in the low-frequency (apical) portion of the basi-lar membrane and that excitation of low-frequency hair cells contributes little to the CAP and ABR elicited by wide-band click sounds. In a similar way, it might be assumed that loss of low-frequency nerve fibers might not affect the responses to wide-band click sounds noticeably, and it is possible that low-frequency hearing loss could escape detection by intraoperative monitoring when click sounds are used as stimuli.

The response generated by more centrally located structures of the ascending auditory path-way seems to be less affected by the temporal coherence of the neural discharges in the audi-tory nerve than are responses recorded directly from the auditory nerve. Thus, the later peaks of ABR, particularly peak V, is often seen to be less affected by injuries to the auditory nerve than earlier peaks. The amplitude of peak V is also less affected by changes in the intensity of the sound used to evoke the ABR than do ear-lier peaks. This means that CAPs recorded from the auditory nerve are likely to be more sensitive to injury of the auditory nerve than is peak V of the ABR. Whereas the CAP recorded from the auditory nerve usually have a much lower amplitude in patients with hearing loss caused by auditory nerve injuries, the ampli-tude of wave V in patients with such hearing loss might be close to that in patients with nor-mal auditory nerve function.

Relationship Between Auditory Evoked Potentials and Hearing Acuity

It is important to remember that changes in auditory evoked potentials do not measure changes in hearing. The effects on hearing threshold of injuries to the auditory nerve there-fore cannot be predicted directly on the basis of knowledge about the changes in the CAP recorded from the auditory nerve. Changes in neural conduction as revealed by changes in the CAP recorded from the exposed auditory nerve can be totally reversible, although studies in ani-mals indicate that the injury might be caused by a partial dislocation of the transition zone between the peripheral and central myelin of the auditory nerve (Obersteiner–Redlich zone [O–R zone]) *(21,101,102)*, which might be assumed to be irreversible and, thus, imply a permanent injury.

It is not known if deterioration of the earli-est peaks of the ABR with a preservation of peak V, after injury to the auditory nerve, means that the patient's hearing ability to understand speech will be impaired or if also peak V has to be noticeably affected before a functional change in hearing might occur. Patients in whom the intracranial portion of the auditory nerve had sustained surgically induced injury often have severely impaired

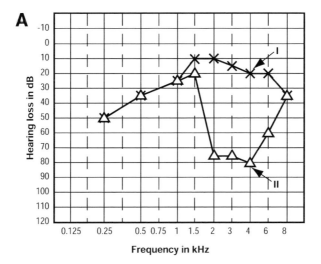

I: Pre-op   Discr.=96%   AS

II: 5 days post-op   Discr.=0%   AS

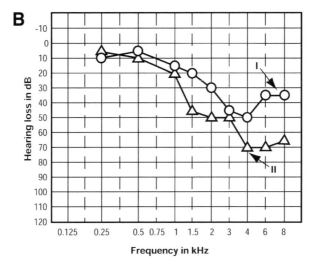

I: Pre-op   Discr.=80%   AS

II: 7 days post-op   Discr.=30%   AS

Figure 6.18: Pure tone audiograms obtained before and after operations where the auditory nerve had been manipulated, illustrating the effect on the tone threshold and speech discrimination from iatrogenic injury to the auditory nerve. **(A)** Data obtained in another patient before (I) and 5 d after (II) an operation in the CPA where the eighth cranial nerve was manipulated. The speech discrimination decreased from 96% before the operation to 0% after the operation. **(B)** Large changes in speech discrimination with relatively small changes in the pure tone audiogram: I: preoperative audiogram; II: audiogram obtained 7 d after an operation in the CPA where the eighth cranial nerve was manipulated. The speech discrimination decreased from 80 to 30% after the operation.

speech discrimination, with only a moderate reduction in hearing threshold, as revealed by pure tone audiograms (**Fig. 6.18**). This means that synchronization of neural activity in the auditory nerve can be impaired with only moderate effect on the pure tone threshold. Such patients also often have severe tinnitus.

Injuries to the auditory nerve from surgical manipulations often produce a greater loss in speech discrimination than would have been inferred from the threshold elevation to pure tones (pure tone audiograms) (**Fig. 6.18**) *(72)*. The likely reason is that slight injuries to the auditory nerve might cause reduced temporal coherence of neural firing in auditory nerve fibers without affecting the threshold of pure tones (according to the results of pure tone audiometry). Deterioration of the timing of neural discharges is known to affect the ability to discriminate speech.

The effects of injuries to the auditory nerve on everyday use of hearing (such as speech intelligibility) are not well described by the pure tone audiogram, because injury to the auditory nerve is likely to cause a considerable decrease in the speech discrimination score even when the pure tone threshold is only slightly affected, as indicated on a conventional audiogram *(103)*. Speech discrimination can deteriorate to a considerable degree with little or moderate changes of the pure tone audiogram *(21)*. Therefore, the pure tone audiogram alone is not a suitable measure of (functional) hearing loss in patients whose CN VIII has been injured and speech discrimination tests should be used to evaluate injuries to the auditory nerve *(103)*.

FACTORS OTHER THAN SURGICAL MANIPULATION THAT MIGHT INFLUENCE AUDITORY EVOKED POTENTIALS

Monitoring of the ABR and CAP from CN VIII or the cochlear nucleus is affected by the condition of the ear and the auditory nervous system of individual patients before the operation. Other factors such as operations done in the same region at earlier times, the patient's general health condition, and the presence of other disorders such as cardiovascular disorders are likely to affect auditory evoked potentials. Technical matters, such as the sound delivered to the ear, can also affect the auditory evoked potentials that are recorded during an operation.

Effects of Preoperative Hearing Loss on ABR and CAP From the Auditory Nerve

The presence of preoperative hearing loss might affect click-evoked ABR as well as the CAP that can be recorded from the exposed CN VIII or the vicinity of the cochlear nucleus. The effect depends on the degree and type of hearing loss. Hearing loss that is caused by an impairment of the conduction of sound to the cochlea (affecting the ear canal, tympanic membrane, middle ear) *(3)* affects the ABR and CAP from the auditory nerve and the cochlear nucleus in similar way, as does a decrease in the intensity of the stimulus sound. Different forms of conductive hearing loss might affect sound transmission for different frequencies differently and might thereby affect the recorded responses differently. Evoked responses from the auditory nervous system to broad-spectrum sounds, such as click sounds, might therefore differ from that of a person with normal hearing, even when the stimulus intensity has been elevated to compensate for the loss in sound transmission to the cochlea. The high-frequency spectral components of broad-band sounds (such as click sounds) are most important for eliciting auditory evoked responses. A low-frequency hearing loss of the conductive type therefore might not affect ABR noticeably and individuals with such hearing loss could have ABRs that are similar to those of individuals with normal hearing. The intensity of the click sound that is used to elicit ABR intraoperatively in a patient with conductive hearing loss should therefore only be increased if the hearing loss includes the high-frequency range of hearing (above 4 kHz). If a true conductive hearing loss involves the high-frequency range of hearing, the stimulus sound level can be increased by an amount equal to the conductive hearing loss for high frequencies

(4–8 kHz) in order to obtain an interpretable ABR recording. It is, however, unusual that conductive hearing loss extends to the high-frequency range of hearing.

A moderate sensorineural hearing loss caused by cochlear deficits has minimal effect on the ABR. Sensorineural hearing loss often occurs in elderly individuals (presbycusis) but could also be present in younger individuals, often caused by noise exposure (NIHL) or administration of ototoxic drugs such as aminoglycoside antibiotics. These factors all affect auditory sensitivity to sounds of higher frequencies more than it does to sounds of lower frequencies. Cochlear hearing loss is caused by loss of outer hair cells, primarily in the basal portion of the cochlea, thus mostly affecting high-frequency hearing affecting the cochlear amplifier, which is most important for sounds of low intensity, and usually not affecting cochlear function noticeably for sound levels, such as those used for recording auditory evoked potentials (3).

Whereas hearing loss of cochlear origin can affect the waveform of the ABR, there is no reason to increase the stimulus intensity used to elicit auditory evoked potentials in patients who have a cochlear type of hearing loss. Such hearing loss might also affect the CAP recorded from the exposed CN VIII to an extent depending on the severity of the hearing loss. The CAP that is recorded from patients with such hearing loss often has a more complex waveform than in individuals with normal hearing with several peaks (95,104).

Abnormalities in the waveform of the ABR and the CAP recorded from the exposed CN VIII in patients with hearing loss are less important when auditory evoked potentials are used for monitoring purposes than when they are used for clinical diagnostic purposes, because it is deviations from a baseline recording (done in the same patient) that are important in intraoperative monitoring. Nevertheless, it is important to know what type of hearing loss might be present before recording auditory evoked potentials and to have a preoperative ABR done so that it is known what might be expected in the operating room regarding the

waveform of the evoked potentials that are to be recorded intraoperatively.

In the extreme situation in which a patient's disorder of the ear or of the auditory nervous system is so severe that it is not possible to obtain an interpretable ABR recording from the patient before the operation, it will not be possible to perform intraoperative monitoring of auditory evoked potentials. If the person in charge of monitoring did not know before the operation that such a patient had a severe hearing loss, a tedious search for technical causes for the failure to obtain a reproducible ABR in the operating room would ensue. On the other hand, if the patient had a reproducible ABR preoperatively but it is not possible to obtain a response in the operating room, then it is obvious that the cause of the failure to obtain a reproducible ABR in the operating room is a technical problem that must be solved before the operation can begin.

Previous Injuries to the CN VIII

The ABRs recorded from patients with hearing loss caused by injury to the auditory nerve could have complex abnormalities, including increased interpeak latencies and waveforms of the recorded potentials that are different from that seen in patients with normal hearing. Injury to the auditory nerve is typically present in patients with vestibular schwannoma or in patients who have undergone surgical operations in which injury to the auditory nerve has occurred. Such conditions affects the ABR in a different way than do lesions to the cochlea. Injuries to the auditory nerve typically cause ABRs to have low amplitudes and complex waveforms. The CAP recorded from the exposed CN VIII in patients with an injured auditory nerve is likely to have complex waveforms (**Fig. 6.8**).

Slight injury to the auditory nerve might decrease the temporal coherence of discharges in different nerve fibers, because the conduction velocity in different fibers might be affected differently as a result of such injury. The complex waveform and low amplitude of the CAP in patients with an injured auditory nerve is a result of decreased coherence of discharges in the different nerve fibers that make up the auditory nerve.

Unknown Causes of Injury to the Auditory Nerve

Experience from intraoperative monitoring of auditory evoked potentials in MVD operations to of cranial nerves has shown that there might be causes for injury to the auditory nerve other than direct and known surgical manipulations or heating from electrocoagulation.

An example of such unknown cause of injury was a patient who lost hearing after an operation in the CPA during which there was no remarkable changes in the auditory evoked potentials. The ABR was not monitored in the operating room after the dura was closed because it was believed then that the risk of injury to the auditory nerve had passed when the dura was closed. However, the ABRs in this patient were recorded automatically to the end of the operation as a part of a research project. Examination of the records after it was discovered that the patient had suffered a total hearing loss revealed a steadily increasing latency of peak V of the ABR after the dura was closed (Fig. 6.19A). Obviously, something happened after closing the dura that caused the auditory nerve to be stretched or affected it in some other way. This experience taught us to always monitor the ABR until skin closure. On several occasions after this experience, once the dura was closed, large changes in the ABR were experienced in similar operations. In each of these patients, reopening the dura, releasing fluid, and irrigating the CPA caused the ABR to recover and, thus, seemingly resolve the problem; however, it was not possible to pinpoint the exact cause of these ABR changes. None of these patients suffered permanent hearing impairment.

In a similar operation in which there were large changes in the ABR during the operation because of operative difficulties, the latency of peak V of the ABR decreased toward normal values during the wound closure. This patient experienced a moderate postoperative hearing impairment, but the hearing improved within a 3-mo period.

Results of intraoperative monitoring of ABR have also shown evidence that irrigation of the CPA in the region of CN VIII can cause severe injury to the auditory nerve, possibly leading to permanent hearing impairment and even deafness. It was first believed that a strong beam of fluid from a syringe used for irrigation could injure the auditory nerve, but, later, it was found that even a low velocity pouring of saline into the CPA could injure the auditory nerve. These experiences changed the way irrigation in the CPA was done, and after these experiences, saline was gently poured on the cerebellum and never directly into the CPA.

These are examples of how intraoperative neurophysiological monitoring can improve operative techniques.

Masking of the Sound Stimuli by Noise From Drilling of Bone

Whenever auditory evoked potentials—either ABR or other types (e.g., those recorded from the proximal portion of the auditory nerve or the vicinity of the cochlear nucleus)—are monitored in connection with vestibular schwannoma operations, drilling of the porus acousticus to expose the eighth cranial nerve in the internal auditory meatus often results in changes in the ABR, and the response might even disappear totally. This can be because of injury to the auditory nerve either from the drilling itself or from heat caused by the drilling that might be conveyed to the auditory nerve. It is more likely, however, that the changes in the auditory evoked potentials that are seen during intensive drilling are caused by (acoustic) masking of the click stimuli, used to elicit the auditory response, by the noise produced by the drilling. This noise is transmitted to the cochlea through vibrations in the skull bone (bone conduction) rather than via the normal route for airborne sound, which is through the middle ear. Although sealing the ear canal will reduce the airborne noise that reaches the tympanic membrane, it will not reduce the noise from

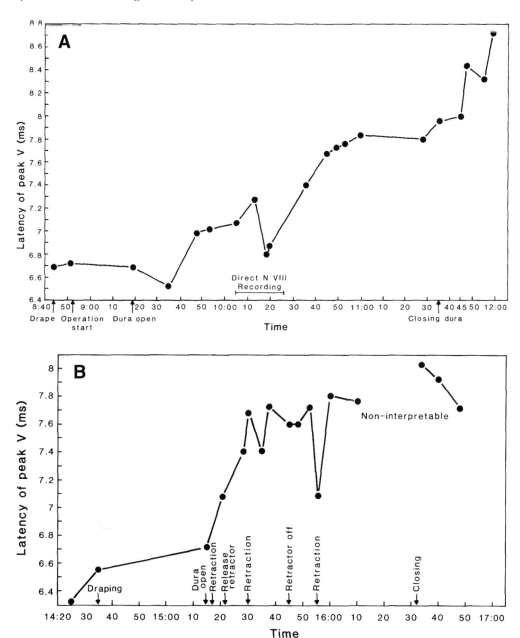

Figure 6.19: Changes in the latency of peak V during MVD operations to relieve cranial nerve disorders. **(A)** Results from a patient who was operated on to relieve HFS and who acquired a post-operative hearing loss that became partly resolved over a 3-mo period. **(B)** Graph similar to that in **(A)**, but showing an increase in the latency of peak V after the dura was closed. This patient lost hearing permanently. (Reprinted from: Møller AR, Møller MB. Does intraoperative monitoring of auditory evoked potentials reduce incidence of hearing loss as a complication of microvascular decompression of cranial nerves? *Neurosurgery* 1989;24:257–263.)

drilling that reaches the cochlea through bone conduction. In fact, a closed ear canal might enhance the transmission of bone-conducted sound to the cochlea, although this effect is slight.

Intensive drilling of the internal auditory meatus might cause impairment of the function of the cochlea similar to NIHL (temporary threshold shift). This might cause alterations in ABR to persist for some time after termination of the drilling. It has been debated whether permanent impairment in hearing could result from noise exposure resulting from such drilling of bone.

ABR AS AN INDICATOR OF BRAINSTEM MANIPULATIONS

Nuclei of the brain (gray matter) are more sensitive to ischemia and surgical manipulations than fiber tracts (white matters). Several components of the ABR have their generators in nuclei in the brainstem, and the recorded ABR therefore depends on the integrity of several nuclei, in addition to that of fiber tracts in the brainstem. Therefore, surgical manipulations and ischemia of the brainstem cause changes in the ABR; thus, recording of ABR is valuable in monitoring patients where the brainstem is surgically manipulated or when there are risks of ischemia of this part of the central nervous system.

The changes in the ABR that result from brainstem manipulation are more complex than those seen when the auditory nerve has been injured, and they are therefore more difficult to interpret. Which components of the ABR are affected depends on which parts of the brainstem that are manipulated. On the basis of knowledge about the neural generators of ABR, it is often possible to relate a certain change in the ABR waveform to specific anatomical structures. Thus, a change (increase) in the IPL of peaks III and V might be assumed to indicate an effect on the lateral lemniscus on the side opposite to the one that is being stimulated, and perhaps an effect on the nuclei of the superior olivary complex (SOC) on either side. Changes in the IPL of peaks I and III of the ABR indicate that lower brainstem structures at the level of the auditory nerve or cochlear nuclei, on the side that is being

stimulated, are being affected. A change in the IPL of peaks I–III is less likely to occur when the ear opposite to the operated side is being stimulated. There is, however, a possibility that manipulation of the brainstem might cause a stretching of CN VIII on the opposite side or affect the region of the pontomedullary junction of the brainstem causing changes in the IPL of peaks I–III in the ABR elicited by stimulating the ear opposite to the tumor. When it is not clear which side of the brainstem might be compressed or manipulated, it might be justified to record ABR elicited by stimulating both ears (one at a time, as it serves no purpose to stimulate both ears simultaneously).

Figure 6.20 shows the latencies of peak III and peak V of recordings from a patient undergoing an operation to remove a large clivus chordoma. The patient presented with hydrocephalus, hemisensory loss, and gait ataxia. There were large changes noted in the ABR during the operation that were interpreted to be the result of brainstem compression from this large tumor. During the course of the operation, wave V of the ABR, which was evoked by stimulating the ear opposite to the operative side, changed while the earlier peaks remained nearly unchanged, as did the ipsilateral response. Assuming that the main neural generator of wave V is the lateral lemniscus where it terminates in the inferior colliculus on the side opposite to the one being stimulated (27,42) (see p. 63), such change in the contralaterally evoked ABR might be assumed to be caused by manipulation or compression of the contralateral side of the brainstem overlying the lateral lemniscus.

The baseline recording of ABR that was obtained after the patient was anesthetized but before the operation began was normal. Shortly after the beginning of the operation, when a craniectomy was being performed, a large change in peak V of the contralateral-elicited ABR was noted (10:27). This change consisted of an increased latency of peaks III, IV, and V. In addition, the amplitudes of these peaks were reduced. The reduction in

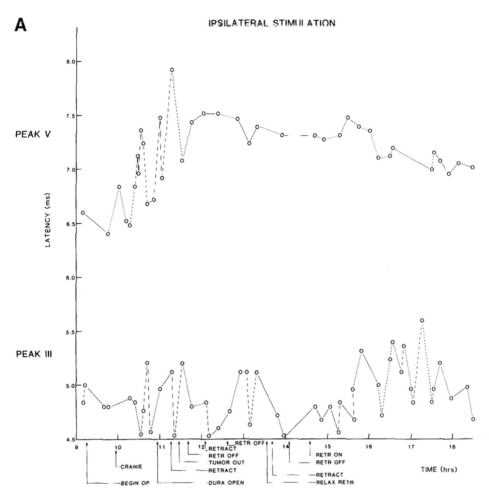

Figure 6.20: Latencies of peak III and V of the ABR recorded intraoperatively in a patient who was operated on to remove a large clivus cordoma. The stimuli were 2-kHz tonebursts of 1 ms duration, presented at a sound level of 95 dB and at a rate of 10/s. ABR was recorded between vertex and ipsilateral earlobe. (**A**) Response to ipsilateral stimulation. (**B**) Response to contralateral stimulation.

amplitudes remained after the dura was opened (at 11:00), when it was found that the cerebellum was tight; very little fluid was drained when the cerebellum was retracted, indicating that the tumor filled the entire space over the floor of the fourth ventricle. A part of the cerebellum was removed to release pressure (11:05). Retraction of the cerebellum resulted in a large change in the ABR (11:21). When the retraction was released (11:46), an improvement in ABR was seen, and at 12:20, when the patient's blood pressure increased, a further improvement in ABR occurred. The waveform of the

ABR improved, the latency decreased, and an increase in the amplitudes of the peaks was noted. Such improvements indicate that perfusion might have been insufficient before the blood pressure was elevated. This exemplifies another important application of ABR in such operations, namely to monitor adequate perfusion of the brainstem. Release of retraction at 12:23 resulted in further improvement.

*The ABR began to normalize when large portions of the tumor had been removed (15:30) in this patient (**Fig. 6.21**). At the end of the operation, the recorded ABRs were similar to*

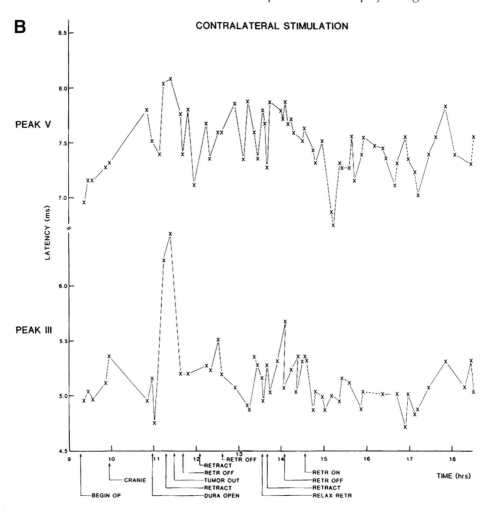

Figure 6.20: *(Continued)*

the baseline ABR obtained before the operation. SSEPs were also recorded in this patient, as were EMG responses from facial muscles, from the lateral rectus muscle (innervated by CN VI), and from the inferior rectus muscle (innervated by CN III). During the operation, spontaneous activity of these muscles was observed occasionally, probably brought about by manipulation of the respective nerves. The response to electrical stimulation of the respective cranial nerve was used to identify those nerves (see Chap. 5).

The example shown in **Fig. 6.22** illustrate the use of ABR not only to indicate that the

brainstem has been manipulated but also to determine the anatomical location where the manipulation had caused changes in function. Such topographical diagnosis of injury is naturally also of great importance when determining which surgical manipulation caused a change in ABR, so that that particular manipulation can be promptly reversed.

Large Vestibular Schwannoma and Skull Base Tumors

Operations on large vestibular schwannoma and tumors of the skull base might involve manipulations of the brainstem that can result in severe complications. The ABR elicited from the

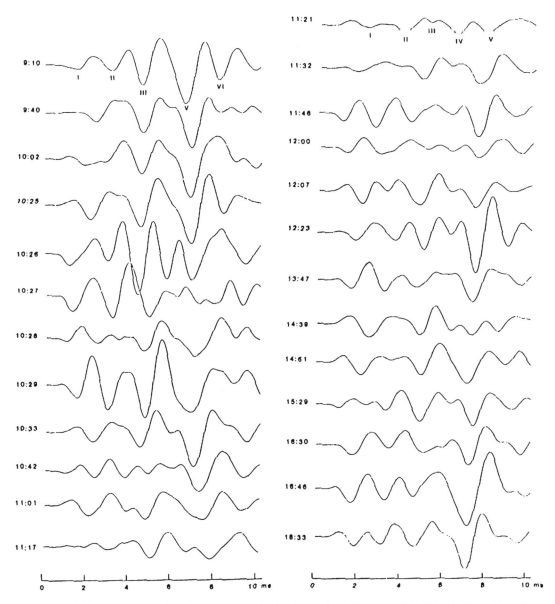

Figure 6.21: ABR recorded intraoperatively in the patient illustrated in **Fig. 6.20** and in whom a large clivus chordoma was removed. Stimuli were 2-kHz tone bursts of 1 ms duration, presented at a sound level of 95 dB SPL and at a rate of 19/s to the ear on the side of the tumor. The potentials were recorded differentially from the vertex and the ipsilateral earlobe. Each recording is the average of 2048 responses and each was digitally filtered using a W50 filter (*see* **Fig. 18.7**). (**A**) Response to ipsilateral stimulation; (**B**) response to contralateral stimulation.

opposite ear often change as a result of brainstem manipulations and brainstem compression, and these ABR changes occur earlier than, for example, cardiovascular changes *(105)*.

When used to monitor brainstem function, the ABR should be elicited by stimulating the ear opposite to the side of the tumor and recorded in the conventional way. Because patients with

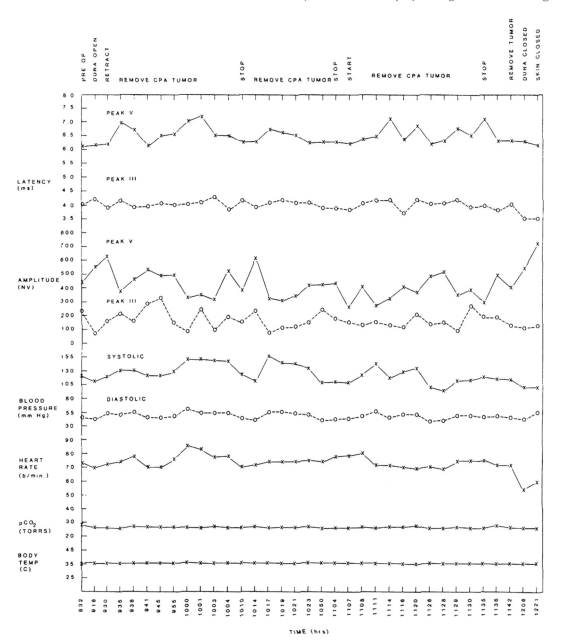

Figure 6.22: Change in the latency and amplitude of peaks III and V in the ABR in response to contralateral stimulation together with changes in cardiac parameter during an operation to remove a vestibular schwannoma. (Reprinted from: Angelo R, Møller AR. Contralateral evoked brainstem auditory potentials as an indicator of intraoperative brainstem manipulation in cerebellopontine angle tumors. *Neurol. Res.* 1996;18:528–540, with permission.)

large vestibular schwannoma usually do not have any usable hearing on the affected side, it is not helpful to record auditory evoked potentials elicited from the ear on the operative side.

Comparison Between ABR Changes and Cardiac Changes. In a study of patients undergoing removal of large vestibular schwannoma, ABR elicited from the contralateral ear was

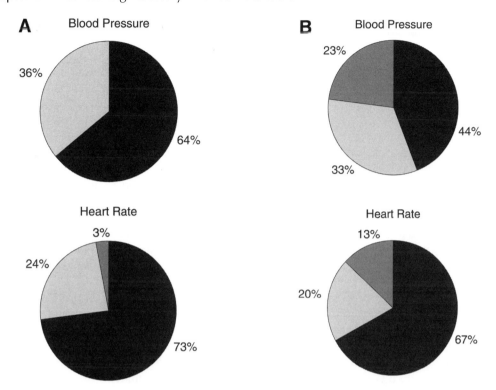

Figure 6.23: Comparison between ABR changes and changes in blood pressure and heart rate during the operation of a large vestibular schwannoma. **(A)** Percentage of manipulation conditions in which the latency of peak V of the ABR increased above the 95% confidence interval before, after, or at the same time as blood pressure and heart rate changed exceeds the 95% confidence interval. **(B)** Percentage of manipulation conditions in which the amplitude of peak V of the ABR decreased above the 95% confidence interval before, after, or at the same time as blood pressure and heart rate changed exceeds the 95% confidence interval. (Reprinted from: Angelo R, Møller AR. Contralateral evoked brainstem auditory potentials as an indicator of intraoperative brainstem manipulation in cerebellopontine angle tumors. *Neurol. Res.* 1996;18:528–540, with permission.)

*monitored (105). When the observed changes in ABR were compared to changes in blood pressure, it became evident that changes occurred generally in both ABR and blood pressure but that the changes occurred earlier in the ABR (**Fig. 6.22**). This supports the assumption that intraoperative monitoring of ABR is beneficial in operations in which the brainstem might be manipulated (75,105). Comparison of changes in blood pressure and heart rate with changes in the amplitude and latency of peak V of the ABR during the operation of a large vestibular schwannoma (105) have shown that the latency of peak V changed before changes in heart rate in 73% of the time and at the same time in 24% of the*

*time. In only 3% of the time did the heart rate change before the latency of peak V change (**Fig. 6.23A**). Changes in the latency of peak V occurred before changes in blood pressure in 64% and at the same time in 36% of the time. Changes in the amplitude of peak V was slightly less effective compared with changes in heart rate and blood pressure. The amplitude of peak V changed before blood pressure in 44% of the time and at the same time in 33%, and in 23% of the time, changes in the amplitude of peak V occurred after that the blood pressure had changed. Changes in the amplitude of peak V occurred before changes in heart rate in 67% of the time, at the same time in 20%, and after in 13%.*

These results showed clearly that intraoperative monitoring of the ABR elicited from the contralateral ear is an important indicator of brainstem manipulation and that it is a valuable supplement to the traditionally used indicators, namely change in heart rate and blood pressure.

OTHER ADVANTAGES OF RECORDING AUDITORY EVOKED POTENTIALS INTRAOPERATIVELY

Studies of the changes in auditory evoked potentials have provided information that has gained development of better surgical methods, thus being important not only for the individual patient in whom monitoring was performed. Thus, there are advantages of using direct recording of the CAP from the auditory nerve that exceed that of reducing the risk of hearing loss in the individual patient in whom monitoring is being done. If only recorded the ABR is available, it is not possible to relate the effects to specific surgical events, such as electrocoagulation, because the time it would take to produce an interpretable record would make it difficult to determine exactly what step in an operation caused a change in function of the auditory nerve.

Recording of the CAP from the auditory nerve has also shown that there are considerable differences in individual susceptibility to mechanical manipulation of the auditory nerve. In operations in the CPA when the retromastoid approach is used, such manipulations of the eighth nerve might occur, for instance, when the cerebellum is retracted. It has been indicated in earlier studies that medial-to-lateral retraction (106,107) places the eighth nerve at greater risk than does retraction in a caudal-to-rostral direction. This hypothesis has been confirmed by studies of CAP recordings from the

auditory nerve (71). Animal experiments have revealed that injuries are likely to occur where the auditory nerve passes through the cribriform plate (101,102,108).

Experience in intraoperative monitoring has also shown that the arachnoid membrane that covers CN VIII might be stretched by retracting the cerebellum and thereby stretching the eighth nerve. It was found that changes in auditory evoked potentials that occur during MVD operations can be reduced by opening the arachnoid membrane widely as soon as possible after it has been exposed (Jho and Møller, unpublished observation, 1990); this should be done even in operations in which only CN V must be exposed in order to carry out the operation. The reason that it is beneficial to make a large opening in the arachnoid membrane is probably that tensions along the edge of the opening then lessen or that the arachnoidal membrane that is connected to CN VIII can stretch the nerve when, for example, the cerebellum is retracted.

These are examples of how intraoperative neurophysiological monitoring can better promote the development of surgical methods that are more effective and have less risk.

ANESTHESIA REQUIREMENTS

Although slight changes in the ABR have been reported as a result of the administration of certain anesthetic agents (109,110), ABRs are remarkably insensitive to anesthesia. The type of anesthesia can therefore be chosen without any consideration as to whether or not ABR are to be monitored. However, it has been noted that the patient's body temperature has a significant effect on the latency of ABR. When the body temperature drops below 35.0°C, there is a noticeable increase in the latency of the peaks of the ABR (111). This should be remembered when interpreting slow changes in the ABR.

7

Monitoring of Somatosensory Evoked Potentials

Introduction
SSEP in Monitoring of the Spinal Cord
Recording SSEP for Monitoring Peripheral Nerves
Stimulation Technique and Parameters for SSEP Monitoring
Preoperative and Postoperative Tests
Interpretation of SSEP
Evoked Potentials From the Spinal Cord
SSEP as an Indicator of Ischemia From Reduced Cerebral Blood Perfusion
SSEP as an Indicator of Brainstem Manipulation
Trigeminal Evoked Potentials
Anesthesia Requirements for Monitoring Cortical Evoked Potentials

INTRODUCTION

Intraoperative recordings of somatosensory evoked potentials (SSEPs) were among the earliest used electrophysiological methods for monitoring function of the spinal cord and, for that matter of any neurological system. Orthopedics was the first specialty of surgery in which this method was used beginning in the 1970s in operations for scoliosis *(112–114)*. When SSEPs are monitored during operations involving the spinal cord, the responses are usually elicited by electrical stimulation of a peripheral nerve and recorded from electrodes placed on the scalp. The SSEPs obtained in that way are generated by successive excitation of neural structures of the ascending somatosensory pathway. These potentials thus consist of different components that appear with different latencies *(see* the description of the neural generators of the SSEP in Chap. 5).

From: *Intraoperative Neurophysiological Monitoring: Second Edition*
By A. R. Møller
© Humana Press Inc., Totowa, NJ.

The SSEPs elicited by electrical stimulation of areas of the skin (dermatomes) that are innervated by specific dorsal roots of the spinal cord were later introduced for more specific monitoring of the spinal cord segments and spinal nerve roots. Intraoperative recordings of SSEPs are also used for monitoring peripheral nerves *(see* Chap. 13). When used for monitoring of the function of the spinal cord, SSEPs only monitor the dorsal (sensory) portion of the spinal cord. When suitable methods were developed for monitoring the ventral (motor) portion of the spinal cord, such monitoring became an important part of intraoperative monitoring in operations where the spinal cord is at risk of being injured *(see* Chaps. 9 and 10).

The use of intraoperative monitoring of SSEPs as an indicator of brain ischemia is valuable during operations on aneurysms, during which the anterior circulation of the brain might be affected *(115)*. In such operations, upper limb SSEPs, elicited from the median nerve of the wrist, are used. The component of the recorded SSEP that is generated by in the primary somatosensory cortex (N_{20}) is used as an indicator of ischemia. In some cases, SSEP has also been used to monitor brainstem function, although auditory brainstem responses (ABRs) are usually found to be superior to SSEPs for this purpose (*see* Chap. 6) or might provide complimentary information. The ascending auditory pathway has several nuclei located in the brainstem, therefore providing rationale that ABR seems to be more sensitive to ischemia and surgical manipulations of the brainstem than SSEP, because the somatosensory system has basically only a fiber tract (the medial lemniscus) passing through the brainstem.

SSEP IN MONITORING OF THE SPINAL CORD

Intraoperative monitoring of spinal cord function is indicated in operations in which the blood supply to the spinal cord could be compromised, as well as in surgical procedures in which the spinal cord could be manipulated. Manipulations of the spinal cord and ischemia might occur in operations to remove spinal cord tumors, corrective surgery for scoliosis, spinal stenosis, and disc removal and in trauma surgery.

Beginning in the 1970s, orthopedic surgeons were the first surgical specialists to introduce intraoperative monitoring of the spinal cord using recordings of the SSEP (*112–114*), which was the only technique available at that time for monitoring spinal cord function. Intraoperative monitoring of SSEPs only monitors the sensory pathways of the spinal cord and thus, theoretically, the nonsensory pathways, such as the descending motor pathways, might therefore be injured without any noticeable change occurring in the recorded SSEP. This has been regarded to be a serious problem, especially because the blood supply to the part of the spinal cord where the ascending sensory pathways travel (the dorsal portion of the spinal cord) differs from the blood supply of the anterior (ventral) portion of the spinal cord where the descending motor pathways are located. Thus, a deficiency of blood supply or injury to

the ventral portion of the spinal cord could cause impairment of motor function (such as paraplegia) without any noticeable changes in the recorded SSEP. This matter has been discussed in much detail, and it is now possible to monitor the descending motor pathway intraoperatively (*116*) (*see* Chap. 10).

There are three limitations in this theoretical argument regarding the separation of the motor and sensory parts of the spinal cord that are important to understand. First, ischemic injury does not always exactly respect the division between the ventral and dorsal cord, so that vascular injuries to the ventral portion of the spinal cord can be reflected in changes in the SSEP (*117*). Second, mechanical injury to the cord outside of the anatomical location of intramedullary surgery will often affect both the ventral and dorsal portions of the spinal cord. Third, the pathways contributing to the SSEP are not purely limited to the dorsal column system (*118*), and pathways in the lateral cord such as the dorsal spinocerebellar tract might contribute to the conduction of the SSEP. Fourth, insults to the ventral portion of the spinal cord might cause a "spinal shock" and thereby affect the SSEP transiently. This might be because of the abundant connections in the spinal cord that connect different parts of the spinal cord.

Practical experience obtained from thousands of cases of spine operations in which SSEP were monitored intraoperatively has shown that monitoring of the SSEP in fact reduces the risk of paralysis and pareses in operations on the spine (119). *Of the 184 patients who suffered postoperative deficits in 51,263 operations in this study, injuries in 150 of these 184 patients were predicted on the basis of intraoperative SSEP monitoring, but detecting abnormalities intraoperatively was missed in 34 patients (false negatives). Although that represents a very small incidence of false-negative results of monitoring (34 of 51,263 operations, or 0.063%) the false-negative responses in the 184 who suffered postoperative deficits was high (34 in 184, 18.5%).*

Recordings of SSEPs are sensitive to changes in neural conduction, and small changes in the function of the dorsal column pathway in the spinal cord can be easily detected. However, changes in the waveform of such recordings might not only occur as a result of manipulations of the spinal cord that imply a risk of postoperative neurological deficits, but also harmless events such as changes in body temperature or changes in the anesthetic level might cause changes in the recorded potentials.

Stimulation

Electrical stimulation of peripheral nerves is used almost exclusively to elicit the SSEP used for intraoperative monitoring, but SSEPs elicited by electrical stimulation of specific areas of the skin (dermatome stimulation, **Fig. 6.1**) offer advantages in some operations. Monitoring the sensory part of the upper cervical portion of the spinal cord or the somatosensory pathways in the brainstem can be done by observing the SSEP elicited by electrical stimulation of the median nerve at the wrist. The median nerve contributes to dorsal roots of C_6, C_7, C_8, and T_1. The potentials that are evoked by stimulation of the ulnar nerve might be used as well. The ulnar nerve contributes to the dorsal roots of C_8 and T_1, whereas the radial nerve, which is rarely stimulated for evoking SSEPs, contributes to C_5, C_6, C_7, C_8, and somewhat to T_1.

For lower limb SSEP, it is common to stimulate the posterior tibial nerve at the ankle, but also the peroneal nerve at the knee is suitable for stimulation. For monitoring in operations where specific dorsal roots are at risk, stimulation of dermatomes is suitable (dermatomes are patches of skin that are innervated by specific dorsal roots) **(Fig. 7.1)**.

Because the median nerve at the wrist contributes to C_8 (and T_1) dorsal roots, the SSEP that is elicited by stimulation of the median nerve should be sensitive to injury of the spinal cord at and above the C_8 level. If the spinal cord below C_8 is at risk, the SSEP must be elicited by stimulation of a peripheral nerve on a lower limb (or an appropriate dermatome). Most often, the peroneal nerve at the knee or the posterior tibial nerve at the ankle is chosen to be stimulated.

It has also been shown that mechanical stimulation of the skin to activate receptors can be used to elicit SSEP responses *(121)*, but these methods of eliciting SSEP are not in general use in the operating room at present—mainly because the responses are of lower amplitude and have higher variability than those produced by electrical stimulation of a peripheral nerve.

Recording

When the SSEP is recorded in a clinical setting, several recording channels are used to differentiate between the different components of the response *(66)*; most of the current machines used in the operating room have 16 amplifiers and can thus record in up to 16 channels simultaneously.

The cortical (N_{20}) and midbrain (N_{18}) potentials evoked during stimulation of the upper limb SSEP could be recorded with the active electrode placed over the contralateral parietal cortex—2 cm behind C_3 or C_4 called C_3' or C_4' (10–20 system) *(53)* **(Fig. 7.2)**. The reference electrodes for such recordings are often placed on the forehead. Using a derivation involving an active electrode on the scalp and a noncephalic reference electrode placed on the shoulder or sternum *(55,56)* provides a better identification of early subcortical components of the SSEP in response to median nerve stimulation (P_9, P_{11}, P_{14}–P_{16}). The SSEPs have been effectively recorded with the reference electrode placed on the upper neck in the midline **(Fig. 7.3)**, and the active electrode placed on the contralateral parietal scalp about 7 cm lateral to the midline and 2–3 cm behind the plane of the C_z level (corresponding to C_3' or C_4') *(56)*. Recordings of lower limb SSEPs are usually done with the active electrode placed on C_z (or 2 cm behind) and the reference electrode either at a frontal scalp position or at a noncephalic location (shoulder or upper neck).

The most commonly monitored spinal/brainstem potentials are the P_9, P_{11}, and P_{14}–P_{16} and

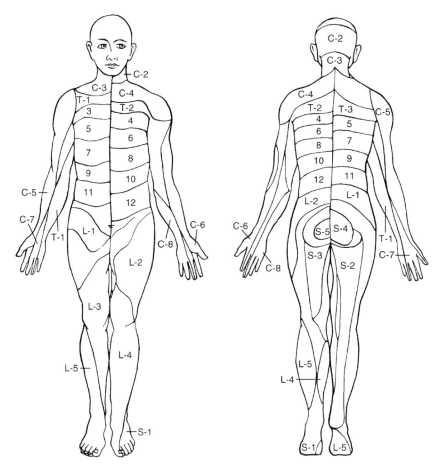

Figure 7.1: Dermatomes. (Reprinted from: Daube JR, Reagan TJ, Sandok BA, Westmoreland BF. *Medical Neurosciences*, 2nd ed. Rochester, MN: Mayo Foundation; 1986, with permission from the Mayo Foundation.)

N_{18}. The P_9 is generated where the nerves from the brachial plexus enter the spine; the P_{11} is generated internally in the dorsal horn of the spinal cord. The P_{14}–P_{16} are generated close to or in the dorsal column nuclei. Although the P_{14} is classically thought of as generated at the cervicomedullary junction, there is evidence that it has generators in many locations in the cord and hence, might not always change dramatically with injury to the cord *(122)*. The N_{18} of the upper limb SSEP that is generated by structures of the rostral brainstem can be recorded over a large part of the scalp. The N_{20} of the SSEP is generated in the primary somatosensory cortex and can (only) be recorded on the

side of the scalp that is contralateral to the stimulus site (median nerve at the wrist). Recordings from Erb's point reflect activity in the brachial plexus and, thus, is of value for ensuring effective stimulation of the median nerve **(Fig. 7.3)**.

There are cortical components (P_{40} or P_{37}) and subcortical components (N_{34} and N_{21}) of the lower limb SSEP that can have value for intraoperative monitoring (*see* **Fig. 5.17**). Recordings of the P_{40} or P_{37} components of the cortical components of the lower limb SSEP are usually made with the active electrode placed 2 cm posterior to the vertex (C_z') and the reference electrode placed at the forehead.

A

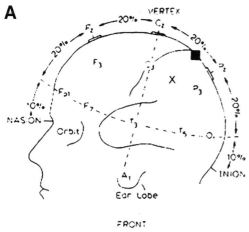

B

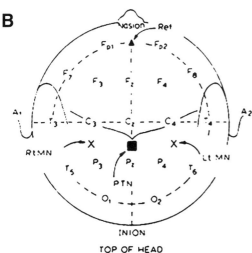

Figure 7.2: The 10–20 electrode system as described by the International Federation of Clinical Neurophysiology. (Reprinted from: Jasper HH. The ten twenty electrode system of the International Federation. *Electroenceph. Clin. Neurophysiol.* 1958;10:371–375, with permission from Elsevier.)

The N_{34} component of the subcortical responses originates in the brainstem. It is typically recorded using a F_{pz} to a cervical electrode. It is readily recorded in most patients but can be of low amplitude. The advantage of monitoring this potential during spine surgery is that it is much less sensitive to anesthetic effects than the cortical potentials. The N_{21} component of the SSEP is elicited by lower

limb stimulation and recorded from an electrode placed at T_{12} vertebra with the reference electrode on the iliac crest. Such early components have, however, not found wide use in intraoperative monitoring, and the electrode placement for recording these potentials usually causes unacceptable levels of electrical interference. Recordings from the popliteal fossa can be used to record the action potential volley traveling cranially in the peripheral nerve that is being stimulated at more distal locations, such as the posterior tibial nerve. This is of value for demonstrating that the stimulation produced an effective activation of the peripheral nerve.

Dermatomal Evoked SSEP

Monitoring of the spinal cord using recording of SSEPs that are elicited by stimulation of peripheral nerves as described earlier represents the sum of the neural conduction in many spinal nerve roots. Peripheral nerves receive input from large areas of the body and electrical stimulation of peripheral nerves therefore simulates the normal activation of sensory receptors (muscle receptors, joint receptors, and skin receptors) located in many different parts of the body. Such stimulation activates the spinal cord in a spatially unspecific manner because the peripheral nerve that is stimulated provides input to many segments of the spinal cord. Injury to a specific dorsal root or segment of the spinal cord might not affect the recorded SSEP to a great extent, because the contributions from intact dorsal roots mask the deficit in a single dorsal root or a single segment of the spinal cord.

The neural conduction in one or a few dorsal roots or spinal cord segments can be monitored by applying the stimulation to a well-defined small part (skin) of the body. Individual dorsal roots of the spinal cord carry the sensory nerve supply to patches of the skin, known as dermatomes, as illustrated in **Fig. 7.1**. The SSEPs obtained in response to electrical stimulation of individual dermatomes provide a way to monitor the function of specific dorsal roots and specific parts of the spinal cord **(Fig. 7.4)**.

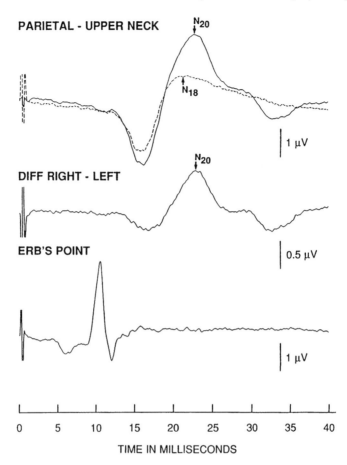

PARIETAL - UPPER NECK

N_{20}

N_{18}

1 μV

DIFF RIGHT - LEFT

N_{20}

ERB'S POINT

0.5 μV

1 μV

0   5   10   15   20   25   30   35   40

TIME IN MILLISECONDS

Figure 7.3: Typical SSEPs obtained by stimulating the median nerve at the wrist while recording on two channels from the two parietal positions 3 cm behind C_3 and C_4 (X in **Fig. 7.2**), with the reference electrode placed on the upper back, in a patient undergoing microvascular decompression to relieve spasmodic torticollis. Thus, the lower curve is the difference between the two recordings. Thus, the curve is similar to recording differentially between the two parietal locations and it shows mainly peak N_{20}. Also shown is the response from Erb's point (response from the brachial plexus).

Dermatomal SSEPs are much more sensitive to localized changes in neural conduction in dorsal roots and in a single spinal cord segment, than the SSEP that is elicited by stimulation of peripheral nerves although dermatomes overlap to some extend and more than one dorsal root may be activated when a dermatome is stimulated. However, the amplitude of dermatomal SSEP tend to be lower and the response exhibit a greater degree of variability than those obtained in response to stimulation of peripheral nerves **(Fig. 7.4)**.

RECORDING SSEP FOR MONITORING PERIPHERAL NERVES

Monitoring SSEPs can also serve to monitor neural conduction in peripheral sensory nerves. Vrahas et al. *(124)* described the technique of monitoring the sciatic nerve during operations for pelvic and acetabular fractures, during which surgical manipulations could injure the sciatic nerve. Any component of the SSEP can be used to detect changes in neural conduction in a peripheral nerve. The signs of injuries to a

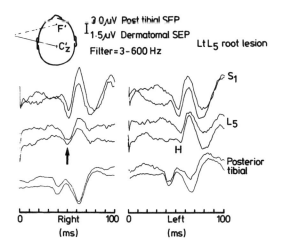

Figure 7.4: Comparison between responses elicited by stimulation of the S_1 and L_5 dermatome and the posterior tibial nerve. (Reprinted from: Katifi HA, Sedgwick EM. Evaluation of the dermatomal somatosensory evoked potential in the diagnosis of lumbosacral root compression. *J. Neurol. Psychol.* 1987;50:1204–1210, with permission from BMJ Publishing Group.)

peripheral nerve, like the sciatic nerve, are prolonged latency and reduction of the evoked potentials' amplitude. Prolongation of neural conduction in the peripheral nerve from which the SSEPs are elicited will affect the latencies of all peaks equally. The amplitude of the response recorded directly from a nerve in response to electrical stimulation (compound active potential [CAP]) decreases in direct proportion to the relative number of nerve fibers in which neural conduction is blocked, but the amplitude of the peaks of the SSEP decreases to a lesser degree. The amplitude of the components of the SSEP that are of cortical origin are likely to decrease less than those of earlier peaks. It is, therefore, appropriate to use components of the SSEP that are generated by more peripheral structures than the cortex for monitoring.

The response recorded from the T_{12} location is an example of a peripherally generated evoked potential that is assumed to originate in the dorsal column and, thus, represents neural activity that has not undergone any neural transformation in a nucleus. Therefore, the amplitude of this response accurately reflects the number of fibers of a nerve that is conducting, providing that supramaximal stimulation is used. A reduction in the amplitude of the T_{12} response by, for instance, 30% can be assumed to indicate that 30% of the nerve fibers are no longer active. However, far-field evoked potentials might be affected by changes in the course of the peripheral nerve that is being tested or changes in the geometry of the nerve, which, for example, might occur if the leg is abducted. Such manipulations could cause changes in the amplitude of the response *(125)* that should not be mistaken for signs of injuries to nervous tissue.

It might be practical to use sequential stimulation of the sciatic nerve on both sides so that the SSEP that is elicited by stimulation of the sciatic nerve on the operated side can be compared with that from the (assumed) unaffected side. Using the difference in the SSEP that is recorded from the two sides eliminates any influence caused from changes in the temperature of the limbs and other general changes such as in the level of anesthesia or blood pressure. Such changes would affect both sides equally.

Neural conduction in peripheral nerves of the arm and in the brachial plexus can be monitored by recording the SSEP using methods similar to those described earlier for the lower limb. In such cases, it is practical to use the P_{14}–P_{16} complex of the SSEP elicited by stimulation of the median nerve or the ulnar nerve, depending on which of these two nerves are at risk of being affected by the operation. The SSEP should be recorded as shown in **Fig. 7.3**—differentially from the contralateral parietal scalp at a position that is 3 cm behind C_3 or C_4 (C_3' and C_4'; marked by X in **Fig. 7.2**) and the upper neck.

If the operation is done distally on the arm or the leg, it is possible to record from the respective nerve proximal to the location of operation while stimulating the nerve electrically at a location that is distal to the site of the operation. This method is described in detail in Chap. 13.

Injuries to the brachial plexus could occur from positioning of the patient on the operating table. Such injuries might occur even in operations that are not affecting peripheral nerves on the arm or the brachial plexus at all. Injuries to the brachial plexus from positioning of the patient are rather common and it is justified to record SSEPs in response to median nerve stimulation during positioning of patients where the arm and shoulder are involved. Recording from Erb's point might also be useful, because such recordings yield responses from the brachial plexus and thus reflect changes in neural conduction of a peripheral nerve on the area that is proximal to the site of stimulation (**Fig. 7.3**).

Peripheral nerves on the arm and leg are mixed nerves in which the same nerve carries both sensory and motor fibers. When SSEPs are used to monitor neural conduction in such nerves, it is the sensory fibers that are tested. When direct recordings from nerves are used for monitoring, it is neural conduction in both sensory and motor fibers that is tested; when muscle responses are recorded in response to electrical stimulation of a mixed nerve, it is the motor portion of the nerve that is tested. It is useful to record responses from muscles that are innervated by nerves that are at risk of being injured during an operation; this might serve to monitor neural conduction in peripheral nerves as a supplement or replacement for recording the SSEPs.

The amplitudes of the responses that are obtained at the end of an operation could serve as a prognostic measure of the extent of an injury to a peripheral nerve, but such information should be treated cautiously because the responses obtained at the end of the operation cannot distinguish a temporary injury from a permanent injury.

For stimulation and recording, needle electrodes should be used; they should be placed percutaneously to reach the nerves in question, or within their close proximity. In operations to repair brachial plexus injuries, it might be of value to stimulate spinal roots electrical in the surgical field while recording cortical responses for the purpose of discriminating a root avulsion.

Pedicle Screws

Recording of SSEPs has been used for monitoring sensory nerve roots of the spinal cord during the placement of pedicle screws. Pedicle screws are used to hold spinal instrumentation in place, and when inserted, there is a risk that these screws will injure spinal nerve roots.

SSEP elicited by electrical stimulation of a peripheral nerve will enter activity into the spinal cord in several nerve roots; if one is damaged (e.g., by the pedicle screw), the input to the spinal cord will only decrease marginally and might not cause sufficient change in the SSEP to be detected. The specificity of such monitoring can be improved by using stimulation of dermatomes instead of peripheral nerves. However, both forms of monitoring of SSEP have shortcomings for monitoring insertion of pedicle screws, and is now largely replaced by recording of motor potentials EMG (either stimulated or free-running) *(126,127)* (discussed in Chap. 10).

STIMULATION TECHNIQUE AND PARAMETERS FOR SSEP MONITORING

Electrical stimulation of peripheral nerves can be applied using subdermal needle electrodes or surface electrodes. The electrodes should be placed close to the nerves that are to be stimulated. The distance between the two stimulating electrodes should be 1–2 cm. The negative electrode should be placed closest to the body (most proximal). For stimulation of specific dermatomes, surface electrodes (such as EKG pads) should be placed on the skin within the dermatome that is to be stimulated, 3–4 cm apart on one side of the body.

A constant-current stimulator is the best choice for stimulation of peripheral nerves and dermatomes because changes in the electrode impedance will not affect the current that is delivered to the nerve. When stimulating a peripheral and mixed nerve in an anesthetized patient who is not paralyzed, the stimulus current should be increased to a level at which a noticeable muscle twitch can be seen (twitch of the thumb when stimulating the median nerve, a twitch of the muscles on the leg when stimulating the peroneal nerve at the knee, or a twitch of the big toe when stimulating the posterior tibial nerves). If the anesthesia regime includes a muscle relaxant, a muscle response will not be detectable and the stimulus current level should be set to three to four times the threshold for a preoperative twitch. Muscle relaxants do not influence the effectiveness of stimulation because muscle relaxants do not affect neural conduction in peripheral nerves. If the optimal stimulus intensity cannot be determined in an individual patient, a setting of 20 mA has been recommended *(128)*, although others use current levels as high as 100 mA.

The number of nerve fibers that are activated by electrical stimulation increases with increasing stimulus strength up to the level at which the stimulation depolarizes all nerve fibers in the nerve that contribute to the SSEP. A strong stimulus will therefore produce a response with the highest possible amplitude. The optimal level of stimulation cannot be used in awake patients because it causes intolerable pain, but in anesthetized patients, it is possible to use optimal stimulus strength.

The stimulus rate should be set so that an interpretable record can be obtained in as short a time as possible. When the stimulus rate is increased above a certain value, the amplitude of the response decreases, but the number of responses that can be collected in a certain time increases with an increasing stimulus rate **(Fig. 7.5)**. Therefore, there is an optimal choice of the stimulus rate at which an interpretable record can be obtained within the shortest amount of time—namely the rate at which the product of the amplitude of the response and the stimulus rate has its maximal value *(128,129)*.

The stimulus strength used for stimulation of dermatomes should be adjusted so that it does not stimulate underlying structures (muscles). This can be done in patients who are not paralyzed by observing muscle contractions.

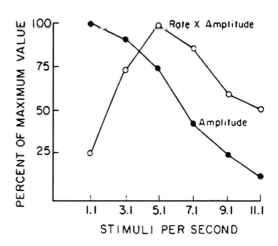

Figure 7.5: Effect of increasing the rate of the stimulus presentation (filled circles) on the amplitude of the SSEP in response to electrical stimulation of the posterior tibial nerve. Open circles show the product of the amplitude of the SSEP and the stimulus rate. (Reprinted from: Nuwer MR, Dawson EC. Intraoperative evoked potential monitoring of the spinal cord: enhanced stability of cortical recordings. *Electroenceph. Clin. Neurophysiol.* 1984;59:318–327, with permission from Elsevier.)

Stimulation of dermatomes could produce a response of a smaller amplitude; thus, more responses might need to be averaged to obtain an interpretable record **(Fig. 7.5)**. It might be practical to alternate between stimulating dermatomes that correspond to the level of the spinal cord that is being operated upon and stimulating a peripheral nerve that includes that same area of the spinal cord.

The stimulus rate affects various components of the SSEP differently and the optimal rates are therefore different for the different components. The optimal rate is lower when the evoked responses are elicited from the lower limbs than it is when elicited from the upper limbs. In most patients, the optimal stimulus rate for the SSEP is approx 10 pps when elicited by stimulation of a nerve on the upper limbs and approx 5 pps when elicited by stimulation of the lower limbs **(Fig. 7.5)** for the primary cortical components (N_{20} peak for upper limb SSEP and N_{45} peak for lower limb). In patients with peripheral neuropathy, such as might be caused by diabetes mellitus, a lower stimulus rate yields a better response (avoid selecting rates that are divisors of 60 Hz in North America and 50 Hz in Europe in order to reduce contamination of the recordings with line frequency signals *see* Chap. 18).

Each extremity should be stimulated, one at a time. Although some investigators have described the use of bilateral stimulation, this is not recommended because injury to one side only will cause a small change in such bilaterally elicited potentials because the response from the intact side will dominate and it might be impossible to detect even severe changes in the response from one side if the response from the other side was unchanged.

Recording SSEPs from the scalp can be done using needle electrodes as well as surface electrodes. Needle electrodes are easier to apply in the anesthetized patient but surface electrodes can be applied before the patient, is brought to sleep. Both types of electrode can provide stable recordings over many hours.

The response to stimulation of the median nerve (upper limb SSEP) is best recorded from electrodes placed over the contralateral parietal region of the scalp, 3–4 cm behind the central plane through C_3 and C_4 and 7 cm lateral from the midline (C_3' and C_4') (10–20 system). If recorded with the active electrode placed at C_z, the N_{20} peak is much attenuated and the N_{18} peak might dominate that region of the recording. If the active electrode is placed on the ipsilateral parietal region of the scalp, the N_{20} peak might not be noticeable at all, and only the N_{18} peak would be detectable in that range of latencies. Thus, recording from different locations on the scalp makes it possible to differentiate between the N_{18} and N_{20} peaks.

It is helpful in distinguishing between N_{18} and N_{20} to record two channels of SSEP—one channel differentially between an electrode on the right parietal scalp with a reference at the upper neck and the other channel from the left parietal scalp with the same reference (**Figs. 7.2** and **7.3**). (Most modern equipment offer as many as 16 channels for recordings; *see* Chap. 18).

A clear representation of the potentials generated in the dorsal column nuclei (P_{14}–P_{16}) can be obtained by placing the reference electrode at the inion or the upper neck. If the reference electrode is placed at the frontal portion of the scalp (F_z) or the forehead, these potentials are not prominent at all and the recorded potentials will be dominated by potentials of cortical origin (N_{20}) when the contralateral median nerve is stimulated. With the reference electrode placed at the neck, the recordings also yield earlier peaks such as P_9, which is generated by the activity entering the spinal cord, and P_{11}, which is generated internally in the spinal cord (*see* Chap. 5).

When recording the responses elicited by stimulation of the lower limbs, the active electrode should be placed in the midline, 3–4 cm posterior to the C_z, and the reference electrode placed either at a frontal location in the midline or on the upper neck. Because the potentials are recorded from the midline, the same electrode position can be used regardless of which side is being stimulated. To visualize early components of the lower limb SSEP, the reference electrode should be placed over the T_{12} vertebra. Recording differentially between C_z and T_{12} can be noisy because of the long distance between the two electrodes; therefore, more responses need to be averaged to get an interpretable record than when recording between C_z and a frontal location.

The responses to stimulation on both sides can be obtained on a single recording by stimulating left and right limbs in succession, with a sufficient delay to allow the entire response to stimulation of one side to be recorded before stimulating the other side. The use of such a "split screen" for display of the SSEP makes it possible to monitor the SSEP elicited from both sides simultaneously. The method can be used for both upper and lower limb SSEP. It is convenient to use a delay of 100 ms for both upper and lower limb SSEP (Fig. 7.6) (note

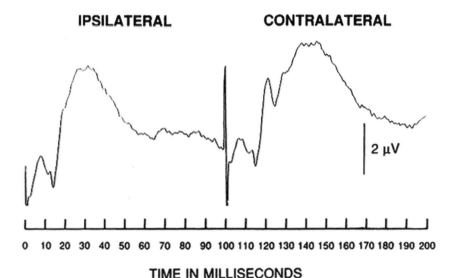

IPSILATERAL   **CONTRALATERAL**

2 µV

0 10 20 30 40 50 60 70 80 90 100 110 120 130 140 150 160 170 180 190 200

TIME IN MILLISECONDS

Figure 7.6: Examples of using a "split screen" to show upper limb SSEP from the left parietal side of the scalp (3 cm behind C_3), with a noncephalic reference at the upper dorsal neck, while stimulating the left median nerve at the wrist (left-hand record) and 100 ms later on the right median nerve (right-hand record). Note the prominent N_{20} peak from the contralateral side. The recordings were obtained in a patient undergoing MVD to relieve spasmodic torticollis.

the prominent N_{20} peak in the contralateral recording). The disadvantages of this method are that the time resolution on such records is less than when a single record is displayed. There might also be some form of interaction between the two responses from both sides. Modern equipment allows the display of the responses to stimulation of the two sides to be on two separate tracings, one positioned above the other, thus preserving the resolution of time the same way as when a single channel is displayed.

As has been mentioned previously, the two sides should never be stimulated simultaneously because that reduces the sensitivity of the SSEP in detecting changes in neural conduction on either side, and there would be a noticeable change in such SSEP only if neural conduction were affected on both sides at the same time.

The waveform of the SSEP is not only influenced by electrode positions, but it also depends on the recording parameters. The filter settings of the amplifiers affect the waveform of the recorded potentials considerably. Similar to what was discussed in the chapter on auditory brainstem responses (ABRs), it is important to use optimal filtering to minimize the number of responses that need to be averaged in order to obtain an interpretable record. Also, recordings of SSEP benefit from the use of zero-phase finite-impulse response digital filters (*see* Chap. 18). Similar filters as those described in the chapter on ABR can be used. If only electronic filters are used, the low cutoff should be set at 1–5 Hz (high-pass filter), and for the high cutoff (low-pass filter), a setting of 125 or 250 Hz will reproduce cortical responses faithfully. These filter settings might cause smoothing of early components such as the P_{14}–P_{16} peak of the SSEP elicited by stimulation of the median nerve. If these components are important for the interpretation of the SSEP, a higher low-pass cutoff setting should be chosen (e.g., 500 or 1000 Hz).

Responses elicited by median nerve stimulation should be viewed in a 40- or 50-ms-wide time window, whereas potentials that are elicited by lower limb stimulation should be viewed in an 80- to 100-ms-wide time window. The sampling rate for the analog-to-digital conversion should be at least 2000 Hz (0.5 ms sampling time) when a low-pass filter setting of 250 Hz is used, but it is more appropriate to use a 5- to 10-kHz sampling rate (*see* Chap. 18). Most modern equipment use a sampling rate that is assumed to be adequate and the user cannot normally alter the sampling rate.

When recording SSEPs, it is important to make a baseline recording for each individual patient before the operation (preferably after the patient has been anesthetized but before the operation is begun). The recordings made during the operation should be compared to that baseline. This baseline recording should be displayed superimposed on the current recordings. All modern equipment have the possibility for artifact rejection, which is based on the amplitude of the response. If the response includes an initial artifact from electrical stimulation, the first part of the recording should not be used for determining whether a record should be rejected or not (*see* Chap. 18).

It is imperative to be able to display the output of the amplifiers directly so that interference that might occur during an operation can be monitored and its waveform examined, which is a prerequisite for being able to eliminate such intermittent interference. That cannot be done on the basis of examination of the averaged waveform. If interference is so strong that it activates the artifact rejection all the time, then there is no way to know what the character of the interference is if the raw output from the amplifiers is not available.

PREOPERATIVE AND POSTOPERATIVE TESTS

Disorders that affect neural conduction in peripheral nerves might severely affect the outcome of intraoperative monitoring of SSEP, particularly lower limb SSEP. If the patient has a moderate-to-severe neuropathy, from, for example, diabetes mellitus, it might not be possible to elicit an interpretable response by electrical stimulation of a peripheral nerve or a dermatome. Older people even without definite symptoms normally have a lower amplitude of their SSEP because of (normal) age-related reduction of the number of active nerve fibers in peripheral nerves and larger variation of conduction velocities, which reduce the temporal coherence of the nerve activity that arrives at the dorsal column nuclei. These changes have a greater effect on lower limb SSEP than upper limb SSEP because of the longer nerve paths in the spinal cord and the longer peripheral nerves and spinal ascending sensory nerve tracts. The decreased temporal coherence results in a distorted pattern of the recorded SSEP and lower amplitude and longer latencies of all components. In mild cases of neuropathy, the amplitude of the recorded SSEP might be lower than normal and the latencies might differ only slightly from those of patients without such pathologies.

INTERPRETATION OF SSEP

In some operations, monitoring of the amplitude of any component is sufficient, whereas in other operations, it is of importance to be able to identify which structures are affected. Knowledge about the neural generators of the SSEP is essential in order to make correct interpretation of changes in the SSEP with regard to the anatomical location of the injury that has caused the observed changes in the SSEP. If peak N_{18} is mistaken for peak N_{20}, an error in interpretation of the anatomical location of the injury will occur because the neural generators of these two peaks are anatomically different (upper brainstem vs sensory cortex).

What Kind of Changes are Important?

Changes in the amplitude of specific peaks in the SSEP are important indicators of surgically induced injuries, but prolonged latencies are also important to consider *(130,131)*.

Some studies seem to indicate that changes (decreases) in the amplitude of the SSEP are more indicative of injury than are changes in the latencies *(130)*. The Jones et al. *(130)* study showed that if the amplitude of the earliest, and second, component of the lower limb SSEP decreased more than 40%, injuries that could cause permanent postoperative deficits were likely to have occurred. A 60% decrease was associated with a 50% risk of postoperative complications. Nuwer et al. *(131)* generally agreed with this evaluation. Studies have shown that the duration over which such changes occur is important, and if the duration of the disappearance of the recorded potentials is short, even a total disappearance of recordable potentials does not mean that (measurable) postoperative neurological deficits will occur *(131)*. What constitutes "a short time" is debated, and it has been indicated that even a 30-min disappearance of evoked potentials might not indicate that postoperative sensory deficits are likely to occur.

Large, but transient changes in the SSEP might be indications of spinal shock that could be caused by injury or ischemia of the ventral part of the spinal cord. Therefore, such changes in the SSEP should be considered a serious warning that requires immediate attention. Brown and Nash have emphasized the need to perform a wake-up test in cases where changes occur in the SSEP that cannot be regarded as being minimal *(132)* because such changes in the SSEP could indicate that descending motor pathways have become injured.

Effect of Temperature and Other Nonpathological Factors

Lowering the temperature of the limb on which a peripheral nerve is being stimulated electrically below that of normal body temperature causes a decrease in the neural conduction velocity of peripheral nerves and, thus, an increase in the latency of the SSEP. A decrease in the core temperature of the patient will cause decreased conduction velocity of the somatosensory pathway in the spinal cord. The latency of SSEP elicited by stimulation of

the median nerve also increases when the temperature of the limb that is stimulated decreases because it is often located outside the drape and thus exposed to the cold air of the operating room *(133)*. For SSEP elicited by stimulation of the posterior tibial nerve the prolongation of the latency has been estimated to be 1.15 ms/°C for the P_{40} peak *(134)*. Lower limb SSEP can usually be recorded at body temperatures as low as 25°C and SSEP elicited by stimulation of the median nerve could be recorded in patients with body temperatures as low as 20°C.

The amplitudes of the different components of evoked potentials is more susceptible to random changes than is the latency of specific peaks. However, better control of stimulation and recording has reduced such nonsurgically induced variations in the amplitude of the SSEP and, thus, made it possible to interpret changes in the SSEP with a higher degree of certainty.

EVOKED POTENTIALS FROM THE SPINAL CORD

Techniques have been described to record evoked potentials from electrodes placed close to the spinal cord *(29,135,136)*, and methods for direct electrical stimulation of the spinal cord have also been developed for intraoperative monitoring of the spinal cord *(137–141)*.

Spinal Evoked Potentials Elicited by Stimulation of Peripheral Nerves

Evoked potentials recorded directly from the exposed spinal cord or from locations close to the spinal cord in response to electrical stimulation of peripheral nerves have been utilized for many years to monitor the integrity of the spinal cord *(136,140–143)*. Such recordings are invasive and the electrodes are closer to the neural generators and, therefore, the recorded evoked potentials have much larger amplitudes than those recorded from the scalp.

Recording directly from the spinal cord while stimulating a peripheral nerve yields evoked potentials **(Fig. 7.7)** that are generated

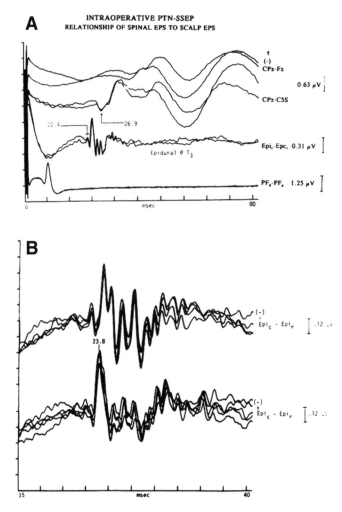

Figure 7.7: Examples of evoked potentials recorded directly from the spinal cord in response to stimulation of the posterior tibial nerve. (Reprinted from: Erwin CW, Erwin AC. Up and down the spinal cord: intraoperative monitoring of sensory and motor spinal cord pathways. *J. Clin. Neurophysiol.* 1993;10:425–436, with permission from Elsevier.)

in different parts of the spinal cord. The recorded potentials are largely unaffected by anesthesia, contrary to the case for the potentials that are generated in the cortex and recorded from the surface of the scalp. Because the recorded potentials have larger amplitudes than those recorded from the scalp, an interpretable record can be obtained much faster than when recording from scalp electrodes. The potentials that are recorded directly from the spinal cord have sharper peaks than the SSEP (Fig. 7.7) and, therefore, it is easier to detect smaller changes in the latencies of the potentials recorded from the spinal cord than it is for potentials recorded from the scalp. The technique of direct stimulation and recording from the spinal cord is more popular outside of United States (such as in Japan).

Two specific disadvantages of recording directly from the spinal cord exist; recording electrodes require placement on the surface of the spinal cord or near the spinal cord *(135)* and it is necessary to obtain a specific electrode position and maintain that position throughout the operation, as considerable changes could occur in the evoked potentials if the recording electrodes move only slightly during the operation.

Neurogenic Evoked Potentials. The responses that can be recorded at one location on the spinal cord to stimulation at another location of the spinal cord have been interpreted as being neurogenic motor evoked potentials (NMEP). The NMEP recordings were assumed to represent the motor (ventral) portion of the spinal cord, thus regarded to be a valuable substitution for recording motor evoked potentials *(141)*. However, later studies seem to show that the recordings (mainly) reflect activity in the dorsal column, thus sensory pathways *(144)*, but a small motor component can be detected *(145)*. These results were based on collision studies, in which stimulation of the spinal cord and that of a peripheral nerve are applied with appropriate time differences to determine which pathways (sensory or motor) such general electrical stimulation of the spinal cord activates *(see* Chap. 10).

Stimulation Technique and Parameters

The same stimulus parameters that are used when stimulating a peripheral nerve to elicit cortical SSEP can be used to elicit spinal cord potentials, but it is possible to use a more rapid stimulus rate when recording spinal cord potentials. This might not be so important because of the large amplitudes of the responses that are recorded directly from the spinal cord anyhow makes it possible to obtain an interpretable record in a short time. The electrodes used for stimulation and recording from the spinal cord are introduced using small catheters.

SSEP AS AN INDICATOR OF ISCHEMIA FROM REDUCED CEREBRAL BLOOD PERFUSION

Monitoring of SSEP is now in common use in operations where the frontal circulation might be compromises such as in aneurysm operations *(115)*. Monitoring of SSEP is superior to monitoring of visual evoked potentials (VEP) because changes in the VEP do not correlate well with ischemia of the occipital cortex or with insults to the visual pathways *(64)*. The use of monitoring of motor evoked potentials *(see* Chap. 10) is also valuable as indicator of ischemia and the use of that technique is increasing.

Basis for the Use of SSEP in Monitoring Ischemia

Prolongation of the interval between the P_{14} and the N_{20} peaks of the SSEP known as the central conduction time (CCT) **(Fig. 5.16)** *(51)* is used as an indicator to detect changes in the function of the central somatosensory nervous system structures. A prolongation of the CCT is taken as an indication of the beginning of ischemia; thus, it is a sign that the blood flow through the region of the brain that is involved in generating these potentials has decreased. (The conduction time of the median nerve often increase because the arm becomes cooler during long operations—but that does not affect the CCT.)

The animal experiments by Branston and co-workers *(146)* have shown that there is a direct relationship between the time it takes for the SSEP to disappear and the degree of ischemia. Experiments in baboons showed that the SSEP disappears when cerebral blood flow falls below 15–18 mL/100 g/min, but a more severe decrease (to about 10 mL/100 g/min) in blood flow is necessary to disturb ionic homeostasis to an extent that there is risk of permanent damage *(147)*. Studies in humans by Symon and co-workers *(148,149)* have shown that there is a relationship between the time it takes for the N_{20} peak of the SSEP to disappear after occlusion of an artery in aneurysm surgery and the risk of occurrence of permanent neurological deficit. The time it takes for the SSEP to no longer be detectable following occlusion (clamping) of a branch of the middle cerebral artery (MCA) was found to be crucial to the outcome of the operation. The shorter the time it takes, the higher the risk of permanent

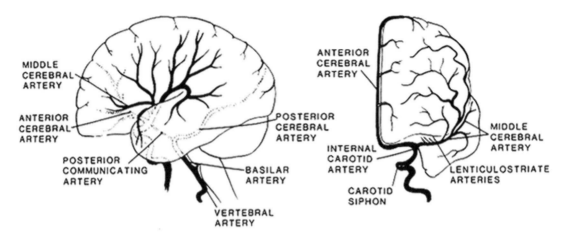

Figure 7.8: Blood supply by the middle and the anterior cerebral arteries.

deficits; if the time is less than 2 min, the risk is high for permanent deficits. Occlusion causes a lesser degree of ischemia when it takes a longer time for the SSEP to disappear. In patients in whom it took 4 min or more for the SSEP to disappear, 20 min of the absence of the N_{20} peak of the SSEP was tolerated when the carotid artery or the MCA was occluded. If the time it takes for the N_{20} peak to disappear is less than 4 min, the estimated time of tolerance is reduced to 10 min *(150)*. Studies in animal experiments and in humans *(151)* have shown that the SSEPs disappear more rapidly after repeated episodes of ischemia such as from repeated temporary clipping of an artery.

The use of SSEP in intraoperative monitoring of operations on aneurysms is not as effective when the anterior cerebral artery is affected. Symon and Murota *(149)* suggested that the use of SSEP elicited from the lower limbs (posterior tibial nerve stimulation) might be more effective in detecting ischemia caused by occlusion of the anterior cerebral artery than the use of SSEP elicited from the median nerve.

Symon and his group had also advocated the usefulness of SSEP monitoring as a predictor of outcome of basilar artery surgery, but Friedman et al. *(152)* pointed out that occlusion of the basilar artery might cause ischemia in areas of the brain other than those that affect the

SSEP, and the occurrence of such ischemia may therefore escape detection when monitoring SSEP **(Fig. 7.8)**.

Monitoring of SSEP can provide prediction of the outcome of operations on patients in whom intraoperative complications occur, such as bleeding of an aneurysm. Prolonged CCT at 5 d postoperative was found to indicate poor outcome *(149)*.

The same criteria for changes in CCT based on SSEP elicited from the median nerve has been used in other operations in which the blood flow might be altered intentionally to allow for surgical repair. Carotid endarterectomy, in which the carotid artery has to be clamped during removal of the atherosclerotic plague, is one example of an operation during which monitoring of SSEP is useful for evaluating whether the patient can tolerate an occlusion of the carotid artery. However, monitoring of EEG is now used more often for that purpose.

Practical Aspects of Recording SSEP for Detecting Ischemia

When monitoring of SSEP is used for detecting ischemia in the brain, it is assumed that neural transmission in the spinal cord is not at risk. SSEP elicited by stimulation of the median nerve is therefore as useful as SSEP elicited by stimulation of a nerve on the lower limbs. Because SSEP elicited by stimulation of the median nerve is more reliable than SSEP elicited by stimulation of the lower limbs, the median nerve SSEP is usually chosen for this purpose. The median nerves at the wrist should be stimulated one at a time. Stimulation of both median nerves at the same time should not be used for the reasons described earlier.

Determination of the CCT that is used as a measure of ischemia requires that P_{14} and N_{20} be reproduced well in the recordings of the SSEP. The P_{14} peak is best recorded from an electrode placed at the neck area, and the N_{20} peak is best recorded from an electrode placed over the contralateral parietal scalp **(Fig. 5.16)**. Therefore, it is appropriate to record differentially between electrodes placed on the contralateral scalp (3–4 cm behind C_3 or C_4) and the dorsal neck. It is practical to record from two channels, each one recording from either side of the scalp (3–4 cm behind C_3 or C_4) using the same reference at the neck for both channels. When operating on one side of the brain, principally the contralateral median nerve should be stimulated and recording obtained from the scalp on the side of the operations. Recording the SSEP from the opposite side in response to stimulation of the median nerve on the operated side to get the contralateral N_{20} might be useful.

When the SSEP is used as an indicator of ischemia, it must be remembered that there are other factors that could affect the CCT, such as the level of anesthesia, retraction of the brain, hypothermia, and hypotension. Whereas brain retraction might only affect one hemisphere, and thus SSEP recorded on one side only, general hypotension, hypothermia, and anesthesia will affect both sides essentially equally. That is one reason why it is valuable to record from both sides simultaneously. Lowering the blood pressure as is often done for facilitating aneurysm operations and other operations of the vascular system might affect the SSEP and the monitoring team should watch this closely.

If the blood flow in the MCA is affected, it can be expected to only cause changes in the response on one side, in which case, recordings from the other side can be used as a control to determine if changes are caused by general factors such as hypotension or the effect of anesthesia. In cases where the basilar circulation is manipulated, such as it might be in operations on basilar aneurysms, the SSEP recorded from both sides could be affected by a reduction in blood flow because of clipping of aneurysms or other interference with the circulation in the basilar system. Clamping of the anterior communicating artery sometimes affects the blood supply to both hemispheres, thus affecting the SSEP in response to stimulation of both sides' median nerves. Some monitoring equipment have the ability to alternately stimulate the two median nerves and to sort the recorded potentials so that they appear on two separate channels. Such a system is ideal for monitoring SSEP for the purpose of detecting cerebral ischemia.

Recording SSEP Compared With Direct Measurement of Blood Flow for Monitoring

Monitoring cerebral blood flow intraoperatively is valuable in some situations, but monitoring SSEP might be more suitable in many operations because it detects the effect of ischemia, whereas the amount of reduction in blood flow is not directly related to ischemia. Because SSEP measures changes in neuronal function (such as that caused by ischemia induced by reduced blood flow), it is probably a more reliable indicator of risk of permanent injury than measurements of blood flow, especially because ischemic tolerances vary from patient to patient and might be different under different circumstances.

Recordings of SSEP do not provide any information about how much oxygenation has decreased after it has reached the level at which the SSEP can no longer be recorded. After loss of SSEP, there is a "blind area" where no information about the progression of ischemia can be obtained. The rate of change in the SSEP, as mentioned earlier, indirectly (by extrapolation) renders information about how fast that critical level is reached. This extrapolation is based on the assumption that ischemia progresses at the same rate after the SSEP no longer can be recorded as it did before that occurred. Direct measurement of blood flow would cover such a "blind area" and would provide information all the way down to zero flow.

SSEP AS AN INDICATOR OF BRAINSTEM MANIPULATION

The value of intraoperative monitoring of SSEP in patients undergoing operations in which the brainstem might be manipulated is not as obvious as is the value of monitoring ABR, because there are no brainstem relay nuclei in the somatosensory system. The fiber tract of the medial lemniscus that passes through the brainstem might be affected by brainstem manipulation in a way that can be recorded as a change in the cortical SSEP, but presumably to a lesser degree than would nuclei.

TRIGEMINAL EVOKED POTENTIALS

Although trigeminal evoked potentials (TEPs) may be regarded as a "member" of the group of sensory evoked potentials known as SSEPs, TEPs are rarely used in intraoperative monitoring. When TEPs are elicited by electrical stimulation of branches of the trigeminal nerve, a response can be recorded from the scalp (C_z and O_z) (153,154) as well as from the exposed intracranial portion of the trigeminal nerve (155). The short-latency negative components with latencies of 0.9, 1.6, and 2.6 ms (155) were recorded from the trigeminal nerve where it enters the brainstem. These potentials represent neural activity in the trigeminal nerve—not in any more rostral structures—and such recordings can only be used to monitor the trigeminal (sensory) nerve. TEPs can also be elicited by tactile stimulation (air puffs) (156).

There are considerable differences in the results regarding the recording of TEP obtained in different laboratories and by different investigators, in particular regarding

long-latency (greater than 5 ms) components of the TEP elicited by electrical stimulation of a peripheral branch of the trigeminal nerve (154). At present, it does not seem that recording of TEPs is particularly useful in intraoperative monitoring, except possibly during trigeminal rhizotomy in patients with trigeminal neuralgia in whom it might be of value to monitor neural conduction in the trigeminal nerve (155).

ANESTHESIA REQUIREMENTS FOR MONITORING CORTICAL EVOKED POTENTIALS

The effect of anesthesia on SSEP is different for different components of the recorded SSEP. P_{14}–P_{16} components of the upper limb SSEP are little affected by any commonly used anesthetics (**Figs. 7.9** and **7.10**) (157). However, most intraoperative monitoring of SSEP is based on recording cortical evoked potentials from electrodes placed on the scalp. Halothane that was used earlier but rarely now causes increased CCT. This unfortunate effect is present even at low concentrations (158), but isoflurane seems to have less effect. Barbiturates that are often used in operations where the SSEP is to be monitored seem to have little effect on the SSEP (159).

Brown and Nash (132) presented an anesthesia protocol that can be used in connection with intraoperative monitoring of SSEP elicited by stimulation of the lower limbs. These investigators found that barbiturates (Secobarbital, 2 mg/kg intramuscularly), atropine (0.4 mg), and opioids (Fentanyl at the time of induction of anesthesia) can be used as premedications. For anesthesia, they recommend sodium thiopental for induction, followed by a bolus of narcotic (Fentanyl or Sufentanil) in addition to nitrous oxide, and a halogenated inhalation agent (132). There is doubt about how the different commonly used inhalation agents such as nitrous oxide interact with halogenated substances and/or whether they are equivalent on the basis of

ENFLURANE EFFECTS

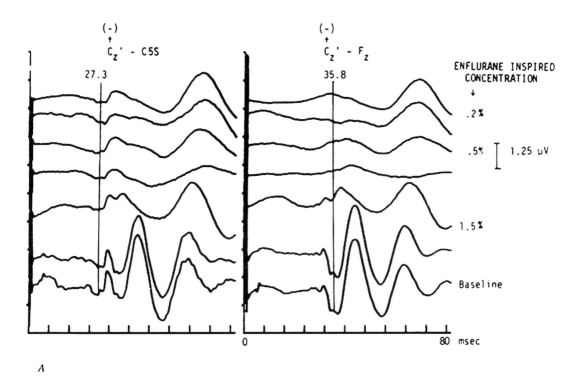

Λ

Figure 7.9: Effect of anesthesia (Enflurane) on the SSEP elicited by stimulating the posterior tibial nerve. (Reprinted from: Samra SK. Effect of isoflurane on human nerve evoked potentials. In: Ducker TB, Brown RH, eds. *Neurophysiology and Standards of Spinal Cord Monitoring.* New York, NY: Springer-Verlag; 1988:147–156, with permission from Springer.)

their MAC value[1] in their action to suppress cortical components of the SSEP *(160)*. (These agents, especially the halogenated agents, are constantly replaced with newer ones. The oldest, halothane, is rarely used. One of the newest Food and Drug Administration-approved halogenated inhalation agents is Sevoflurane but other similar agents are in use such as Desflurane. Other names of halogenated anesthetics are Isoflurane and Enflurane) (**Figs. 7.9** and **7.10**).

Total intravenous anesthesia (TIVA) techniques that are becoming into increasing use

can be designed so that its effect on the SSEP is less than that of inhalation anesthetics.

Brown and Nash *(132)* have noted that the administration of anesthetics by bolus injection have adverse effects on intraoperative monitoring such as recording of the SSEP and the effect on sensory evoked responses could be minimized by using a drug infusion to avoid transient effects of bolus administration. Anesthetic agents used to maintain anesthesia should therefore be administered by continuous infusion techniques.

Agents such as opioids (narcotics) that are used to achieve freedom of pain, β-adrenergic

---

[1]The effect of different anesthetic agents is often described by their "mean alveolar concentration" (MAC). 1MAC is the concentration that induces anesthesia in an average person (50% of the recipients move in response to incision).

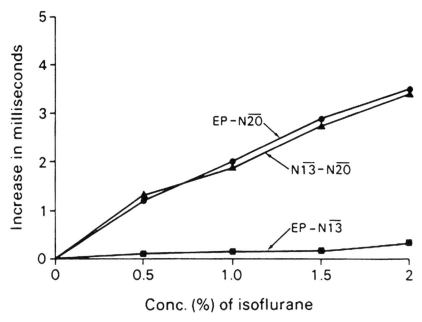

Figure 7.10: Effect of Isoflurane on the neural conduction times that are represented by the difference in the latencies of the different peaks in the SSEP elicited by stimulating the median nerve at the wrist. No effect is seen in the conduction from the brachial plexus (Erb's point; EP) to the dorsal column nuclei (EP-N_{13}), but there is a gradual increase in the central conduction time (CCT, N_{13}–N_{20}) with increasing concentration of Isoflurane. (Reprinted from: Samra SK. Effect of isoflurane on human nerve evoked potentials. In: Ducker TB, Brown RH, eds. *Neurophysiology and Standards of Spinal Cord Monitoring.* New York, NY: Springer-Verlag; 1988:147–156, with permission from Springer.)

blockers, nitroglycerine, and sodium Nitro Prusside, used to control blood pressure, do not affect monitoring of SSEP nor do other commonly used cardiovascular drugs, but vasodilators might cause shunting of blood flow away from the spinal cord and so their use should be discouraged during procedures where there is a risk of reduced blood flow to the spinal cord.

Some anesthetics, such as Etomidate, seem to enhance the cortical components of the SSEP rather than suppress them. Etomidate, for example, causes an increase in the amplitude of SSEP potentials of cortical origin *(162)*.

8

Monitoring of Visual Evoked Potentials

INTRODUCTION

Intraoperative monitoring of visual evoked potentials (VEPs) during neurosurgical operations has been described by several investigators *(63–65,68,83)* for the purpose of preserving vision in operations in which the optic nerve or optic tract is being manipulated or in operations that involved the occipital cerebral cortex *(163)*. It has been found difficult, however, to obtain reliable recordings of VEPs in anesthetized patients who did not undergo intracranial procedures *(164)*.

VEP AS AN INDICATOR OF MANIPULATION OF THE OPTIC NERVE AND OPTIC TRACT

Reports have, in general, been discouraging on the use of monitoring of VEPs for detecting injuries that could develop into postoperative visual deficits *(64,65)*. The results are much less clear than those obtained using other sensory modalities, and all investigators have reported both false-positive (intraoperative changes in the VEP but no postoperative deficits) and false-negative (no change in the VEP intraoperatively but postoperative deficits) results. One investigator *(83)* recorded several instances of convincing VEP changes during surgical manipulation of the optic chiasm and during episodes of hypotension, but without

From: *Intraoperative Neurophysiological Monitoring: Second Edition*
By A. R. Møller
© Humana Press Inc., Totowa, NJ.

any postoperative evidence of pathology. However, although the results were generally difficult to interpret, Raudzens *(83)* found that when VEPs remained unchanged throughout the operation, there was no deterioration of vision as a result of the operation. Nevertheless, he also reported that patients with visual defects preoperatively could have normal VEPs intraoperatively, so that the true value of monitoring VEPs to identify intraoperative damage remains questionable. These studies were done using light-emitting diodes (LEDs) mounted in an eye patch (goggles), with red light flashes reaching the patient's eyes through closed eyelids.

Another group of investigators *(65)* found that the value of intraoperative monitoring of VEPs for the purpose of preserving neural function of the visual system that is important to practical vision is small. This observation is in agreement with this author's own experience. The introduction of high-intensity flashes *(165)* as stimuli for monitoring VEPs intraoperatively seems to have increased the reproducibility of such evoked potentials. The use of high-intensity LEDs mounted in goggles that deliver flash stimuli for evoking visual evoked potentials *(165)* might solve the problem of adequate stimulation in anesthetized patients, but more studies are needed before a conclusion can be realized. More recently, monitoring of VEPs has been used in operations that involved the occipital cortex for treating epilepsy *(163)*. These investigators, using a strobe light to elicit the VEP found such monitoring useful in preserving central vision.

It has been difficult to determine whether recording of evoked potentials directly from the optic nerve *(68)* has any advantages over the use of VEPs recorded from the scalp, except for the probable lesser susceptibility of such subcortical responses to suppression from the use of inhalation anesthetics. This method of recording directly from the optic nerve or optic tract, however, does not seem to have advantages over recording of VEPs from electrodes placed on the scalp with regard to being able to signal when manipulations of the optic nerve or tract might be causing injuries that will result in a postoperative neurological deficit (impaired vision). Again, the reason for this does not seem to be the way the VEPs are recorded, but, rather, an inadequacy of the stimuli that is used. That a flash evoked VEP is poorly correlated with visual deficits is in agreement with experience in using VEPs in clinical diagnosis. Thus, it has been shown that flash evoked VEPs are much less specific in detecting neurological deficits of the visual system than are VEPs elicited by a reversing checkerboard pattern *(66)*. The reason for this is that the time pattern of light stimuli is not "important" to the visual system, which is more sensitive to changes in contrast; therefore, VEPs elicited by a reversing checkerboard pattern reveal more important deficits than do VEPs elicited by repetitive flashes. Clearly, techniques utilizing VEPs for preserving vision in operations near the optic nerve and the optic tract must be much more highly developed before they can be considered practical for clinical use. Additionally, it seems necessary to be able to focus some kind of a pattern on the retina of patients if intraoperative monitoring of VEPs is to be useful in detecting injuries that are important to vision. The introduction of high-intensity light flashes as stimuli might offer a solution to these problems *(165)*. Despite these shortcomings, VEPs are indeed used in intraoperative monitoring in some kinds of operation.

Techniques for Recording VEPs

The VEPs that are recorded intraoperatively are generally recorded using electrodes placed on the scalp at C_z and O_z locations. The electronic filters in the amplifiers are typically set to cutoff frequencies of 5 and 500 Hz for the high-pass and low-pass filters, respectively.

The flash stimuli can either be generated by a stroboscope type of flash generator or by LEDs that are bonded to a contact lens *(68)*.

Light-emitting diodes that are bonded to contact lenses and placed on the eye of the patient *(68,81)* have a low risk of injuring the cornea when contact lenses that are designed for protection of the eye are used, but great care must be taken to avoid injuring the cornea when the contact lenses are placed on the eye. Techniques of intraoperative monitoring using VEPs using LEDs that are placed in a goggle type of arrangement have also been described. The stimuli have red light transmitted through the closed eyelids. Although the intensity of the light that reaches the eye might be adequate to elicit an interpretable response, it might not be optimal to use red light for intraoperative monitoring during long operations because it is likely to be the only light that reaches the patient's eye during the operation and, therefore, the patient's eyes might become dark-adapted during the operation *(14)*. This will change the response gradually, which could be interpreted as a pathologic change. Thus, it might be better to use green light, which will not produce such an evident adaptation effect. Light stimulators that utilize high-intensity LEDs mounted in goggles *(165)* could avoid these problems.

ANESTHESIA REQUIREMENTS FOR VISUAL EVOKED POTENTIALS

Any recording of evoked potentials that relies on cortical responses is altered significantly by the use of inhalation anesthesia. This must be considered when using VEPs recorded from scalp electrodes for intraoperative monitoring and is similarly evidenced for other cortical responses such as somatosensory evoked potentials. In a recent study, the use of total intravenous anesthesia did not seem to increase the reliability of monitoring of VEPs *(164)* and stable recordings were difficult to obtain. It is not known to what extent short-latency VEPs, such as near-field potentials that can be recorded from the optic nerve or optic tract, are affected by inhalation anesthesia.

References to Section II

1. Brodel M. *Three Unpublished Drawings of the Anatomy of the Human Ear.* Philadelphia, PA: W.B. Saunders; 1946.
2. Møller AR. Noise as a health hazard. *Ambio* 1975;4:6–13.
3. Møller AR. *Hearing: Its Physiology and Pathophysiology.* San Diego, CA: Academic; 2000.
4. Pickles JO. *An Introduction to the Physiology of Hearing*, 2nd ed. London: Academic; 1988.
5. Zweig G, Lipes R, Pierce JR. The cochlear compromise. *J. Acoust. Soc. Am.* 1976;59:975–892.
6. Rhode WS. Observations of the Vibration of The Basilar Membrane in Squirrel Monkeys Using the Mossbauer Technique. *J. Acoust. Soc. Am.* 1971;49:1218–1231.
7. Sellick PM, Patuzzi R, Johnstone BM. Measurement of basilar membrane motion in the guinea pig using the Mossbauer technique. *J. Acoust. Soc. Am.* 1982;72:131–141.
8. Johnstone BM, Patuzzi R, Yates GK. Basilar membrane measurements and the traveling wave. *Hear Res.* 1986;22:147–153.
9. Spoendlin H. Structural basis of peripheral frequency analysis. In: Plomp R, Smoorenburg GF, eds. *Frequency Analysis and Periodicity Detection in Hearing.* Leiden: A. W. Sijthoff; 1970:2–36.
10. Flock A. Transducing mechanisms in lateral line canal organ. *Cold Spring Harbor Symp. Quant. Biol.* 1965;30:133–146.
11. Eggermont JJ, Odenthal DW, Schmidt DH, Spoor A. Electrocochleography: basic principles and clinical applications. *Acta Oto Laryng.* (Stockh) 1974;316:1–84.
12. Eggermont JJ, Spoor A, Odenthal DW. Frequency specificity of tone-bursts electrocochleography. In: Ruben RJ, Elberling C, Salomon G, eds. *Electrocochleography.* Baltimore, MD: University Park Press; 1976:215–246.
13. Møller AR. On the origin of the compound action potentials (N_1N_2) of the cochlea of the rat. *Exp. Neurol.* 1983;80: 633–644.
14. Møller AR. *Sensory Systems: Anatomy and Physiology.* Amsterdam: Academic Press; 2003.
15. Møller AR. *Evoked Potentials in Intraoperative Monitoring.* Baltimore, MD: Williams and Wilkins; 1988.
16. Lang J. Anatomy of the brainstem and the lower cranial nerves, vessels, and surrounding structures. *Am. J. Otol.* 1985;Suppl, Nov:1–19.
17. De Ridder D, De Mulder G, Walsh V, Muggleton N, Sunaert S, Møller A. Magnetic and electrical stimulation of the auditory cortex for intractable tinnitus. *J. Neurosurg.* 2004;100(3):560–564.
18. Jewett DL, Williston JS. Auditory evoked far fields averaged from scalp of humans. *Brain* 1971;94:681–696.
19. Møller AR, Jho HD, Yokota M, Jannetta PJ. Contribution from crossed and uncrossed brainstem structures to the brainstem auditory evoked potentials (BAEP): a study in human. *Laryngoscope* 1995;105:596–605.
20. Møller AR. Use of zero-phase digital filters to enhance brainstem auditory evoked potentials (BAEPs). *Electroenceph. Clin. Neurophysiol.* 1988;71:226–232.
21. Møller AR. *Neural Plasticity and Disorders of the Nervous System.* Cambridge: Cambridge University Press; 2005, in press.
22. Møller AR, Jannetta PJ. Compound action potentials recorded intracranially from the auditory nerve in man. *Exp. Neurol.* 1981;74: 862–874.
23. Hashimoto I, Ishiyama Y, Yoshimoto T, Nemoto S. Brainstem auditory evoked potentials recorded directly from human brain stem and thalamus. *Brain* 1981;104:841–859.
24. Spire JP, Dohrmann GJ, Prieto PS. *Correlation of Brainstem Evoked Response with Direct Acoustic Nerve Potential.* New York: Raven; 1982.
25. Scherg M, von Cramon D. A new interpretation of the generators of BAEP waves IV: results of a spatio temporal dipole. *Electroenceph. Clin. Neurophysiol.* 1985;62:290–299.
26. Møller AR, Jannetta PJ, Sekhar LN. Contributions from the auditory nerve to the brainstem auditory evoked potentials (BAEPs): results of intracranial recording in man. *Electroenceph. Clin. Neurophysiol.* 1988;71: 198–211.
27. Møller AR. Neural generators of auditory evoked potentials. In: Jacobson JT, ed. *Principles and Applications in Auditory Evoked Potentials.* Boston: Allyn & Bacon; 1994:23–46.
28. Kimura A, Mitsudome A, Beck DO, Yamada T, Dickens QS. Field distribution of antidromically activated digital nerve potentials: Models for far-field recordings. *Neurology* 1983;33: 1164–1169.

29. Lueders H, Lesser RP, Hahn JR, Little JT, Klein AW. Subcortical somatosensory evoked potentials to median nerve stimulation. *Brain* 1983;106:341–372.

30. Martin WH, Pratt H, Schwegler JW. The origin of the human auditory brainstem response wave II. *Electroenceph. Clin. Neurophysiol.* 1995; 96:357–370.

31. Buchwald JS, Huang CM. Far field acoustic response: origins in the cat. *Science* 1975;189: 382–384.

32. Achor L, Starr A. Auditory brain stem responses in the cat: I. Intracranial and extracranial recordings. *Electroenceph. Clin. Neurophysiol.* 1980;48:154–173.

33. Achor L, Starr A. Auditory brain stem responses in the cat: II. Effects of lesions. *Electroenceph. Clin. Neurophysiol.* 1980;48:174–190.

34. Møller AR, Burgess JE. Neural generators of the brain stem auditory evoked potentials (BAEPs) in the rhesus monkey. *Electroenceph. Clin. Neurophysiol.* 1986;65:361–372.

35. Lang J. Facial and vestibulocochlear nerve, topographic anatomy and variations. In: Samii M, Jannetta P, eds. *The Cranial Nerves.* New York: Springer-Verlag; 1981:363–377.

36. Fullerton BC, Levine RA, Hosford Dunn HL, Kiang NYS. Comparison of cat and human brain stem auditory evoked potentials. *Hear Res.* 1987;66:547–570.

37. Møller AR, Colletti V, Fiorino FG. Neural conduction velocity of the human auditory nerve: bipolar recordings from the exposed intracranial portion of the eighth nerve during vestibular nerve section. *Electroenceph. Clin. Neurophysiol.* 1994;92:316–320.

38. Spoendlin H, Schrott A. Analysis of the human auditory nerve. *Hear Res.* 1989;43:25–38.

39. Møller AR, Jannetta PJ. Auditory evoked potentials recorded from the cochlear nucleus and its vicinity in man. *J. Neurosurg.* 1983;59: 1013–1018.

40. Møller AR, Jho HD. Responses from the brainstem at the entrance of the eighth nerve in human to contralateral stimulation. *Hear Res.* 1988;37:47–52.

41. Møller AR, Jannetta PJ. Auditory evoked potentials recorded intracranially from the brainstem in man. *Exp. Neurol.* 1982;78: 144–157.

42. Møller AR, Jannetta PJ. Evoked potentials from the inferior colliculus in man. *Electroenceph. Clin. Neurophysiol.* 1982;53:612–620.

43. Lorente de No R. Action potentials of the motoneurons of the hypoglossus nucleus. *J. Cell Comp. Physiol.* 1947;29:207–287.

44. Davis H, Hirsh SK. A slow brain stem response for low-frequency audiometry. *Audiology* 1979;18:441–465.

45. Møller AR, Jannetta PJ, Jho HD. Click-evoked responses from the cochlear nucleus: A study in human. *Electroenceph. Clin. Neurophysiol.* 1994;92:215–224.

46. Møller AR, Jannetta PJ. Interpretation of brainstem auditory evoked potentials: Results from intracranial recordings in humans. *Scand. Audiol. (Stockh.)* 1983;12:125–133.

47. Landgren S, Silfvenius H. Nucleus Z, the medullary relay in the projection path to the cerebral cortex of group i muscle afferents from the cat's hind limb. *J. Physiol. (Lond.)* 1971;218: 551–571.

48. Penfield W, Rasmussen T. *The Cerebral Cortex of Man: A Clinical Study of Localization of Function.* New York, NY: Macmillan; 1950.

49. Møller AR, Jannetta PJ, Jho HD. Recordings from human dorsal column nuclei using stimulation of the lower limb. *Neurosurgery* 1990;26: 291–299.

50. Desmedt JE, Cheron G. Central somatosensory conduction in man: Neural generators and interpeak latencies of the far-field components recorded from neck and right or left scalp and earlobes. *Electroenceph. Clin. Neurophysiol.* 1980;50:382–403.

51. Hume AL, Cant BR. Conduction time in central somatosensory pathways in man. *Electroenceph. Clin. Neurophysiol.* 1978;45:361–375.

52. Desmedt JE. Somatosensory evoked potentials in neuromonitoring. In: Desmedt JE, ed. *Neuromonitoring in Surgery.* Amsterdam: Elsevier Science; 1989:1–21.

53. Jasper HH. The ten twenty electrode system of the International Federation. *Electroenceph. Clin. Neurophysiol.* 1958;10:371–375.

54. Gilmore R. Somatosensory evoked potential testing in infants and children. *J. Clin. Neurophysiol.* 1992;9:324–341.

55. Cracco RQ, Cracco JB. Somatosensory evoked potentials in man: farfield potentials. *Electroenceph. Clin. Neurophysiol.* 1976;41: 60–66.

56. Desmedt JE, Cheron G. Non-cephalic reference recording of early somatosensory potentials to finger stimulation in adult or aging normal man: differentiation of widespread N_{18} and contra-lateral N_{20} from the prerolandic P_{22}

and N$_{30}$ components. *Electroenceph. Clin. Neurophysiol.* 1981;52: 553–570.

57. Mauguiere F, Desmedt JE, Courjon J. Neural generators of N18 and P14 far-field somatosensory evoked potentials studied in patients with lesion of thalamus or thalamocortical radiations. *Electroenceph. Clin. Neurophysiol.* 1983;56:283–292.

58. Møller AR, Jannetta PJ, Burgess JE. Neural generators of the somatosensory evoked potentials: Recording from the cuneate nucleus in man and monkeys. *Electroenceph. Clin. Neurophysiol.* 1986;65:241–248.

59. Desmedt JE, Cheron G. Prevertebral (oesophageal) recording of subcortical somatosensory evoked potentials in man: the spinal P$_{13}$ component and the dual nature of the spinal generators. *Electroenceph. Clin. Neurophysiol.* 1981;52:257–275.

60. Allison T, Hume L. A comparative analysis of short-latency somatosensory evoked potentials in man, monkey, cat, and rat. *Exp. Neurol.* 1981;72:592–611.

61. Berkley KJ, Budell RJ, Blomqvist A, Bull M. Output systems of the dorsal column nuclei in the cat. *Brain Res. Rev.* 1986;396:199–226.

62. Erwin CW, Erwin AC. Up and down the spinal cord: Intraoperative monitoring of sensory and motor spinal cord pathways. *J. Clin. Neurophysiol.* 1993;10:425–436.

63. Wilson WB, Kirsch WM, Neville H, Stears J, Feinsod M, Lehman RAW. Monitoring of visual function during parasellar surger. *Surg. Neurol.* 1976;5:323–329.

64. Cedzich C, Schramm J, Fahlbusch R. Are flash-evoked visual potentials useful for intraoperative monitoring of visual pathway function? *Neurosurgery* 1987;21:709–715.

65. Cedzich C, Schramm J, Mengedoht CF, Fahlbusch R. Factors that limit the use of flash visual evoked potentials for surgical monitoring. *Electroenceph. Clin. Neurophysiol.* 1988;71:142–145.

66. Chiappa K. *Evoked Potentials in Clinical Medicine*, 3rd ed. Philadelphia: Lippincott–Raven; 1997.

67. Kraut MA, Arezzo JC, Vaughan HGJ. Intracortical generators of the flash VEP in monkeys. *Electroenceph. Clin. Neurophysiol.* 1985;62:300–312.

68. Møller AR. Electrophysiological monitoring of cranial nerves in operations in the skull base.

In: Sekhar LN, Schramm Jr VL, eds. *Tumors of the Cranial Base: Diagnosis and Treatment.* Mt. Kisco, New York: Futura; 1987:123–132.

69. Kimura J, Mitsudome A, Yamada T, Dickens QS. Stationary peaks from moving source in far-field recordings. *Electroenceph. Clin. Neurophys.* 1984;58:351–361.

70. Grundy B. Intraoperative monitoring of sensory evoked potentials. *Anesthesiology* 1983;58:72–87.

71. Møller AR, Jannetta PJ. Monitoring auditory functions during cranial nerve microvascular decompression operations by direct recording from the eighth nerve. *J. Neurosurg.* 1983;59:493–499.

72. Møller AR, Møller MB. Does intraoperative monitoring of auditory evoked potentials reduce incidence of hearing loss as a complication of microvascular decompression of cranial nerves? *Neurosurgery* 1989;24:257–263.

73. Colletti V, Bricolo A, Fiorino FG, Bruni L. Changes in directly recorded cochlear nerve compound action potentials during acoustic tumor surgery. *Skull Base Surg.* 1994;4:1–9.

74. Silverstein H, Norrell H, Hyman S. Simultaneous use of CO$_2$ laser with continuous monitoring of eighth cranial nerve action potential during acoustic neuroma surgery. *Otolaryngol. Head Neck Surg.* 1984;92:80–84.

75. Fischer C. Brainstem auditory evoked potential (BAEP) monitoring in posterior fossa surgery. In: Desmedt J, ed. *Neuromonitoring in Surgery.* Amsterdam: Elsevier Science;1989:191–218.

76. Linden R, Tator C, Benedict C, Mraz C, Bell I. Electro-physiological monitoring during acoutic neuroma and other posterior fossa surgery. *J. Sci. Neurol.* 1988;15:73–81.

77. Kuroki A, Møller AR. Microsurgical anatomy around the foramen of Luschka with reference to intraoperative recording of auditory evoked potentials from the cochlear nuclei. *J. Neurosurg.* 1995;82:933–939.

78. Møller AR, Jho HD, Jannetta PJ. Preservation of hearing in operations on acoustic tumors: an alternative to recording BAEP. *Neurosurgery* 1994;34:688–693.

79. Levine RA, Montgomery WW, Ojemann RG, Springer MFB. Evoked potential detection of hearing loss during acoustic neuroma surgery. *Neurology* 1978;28:339.

80. Levine RA, Ojemann RG, Montgomery WW, McGaffigan PM. Monitoring auditory evoked

potentials during acoustic neuroma surgery. *Ann. Otol. Rhinol. Laryngol.* 1984;93:116–123.

81. Sekhar LN, Møller AR. Operative management of tumors involving the cavernous sinus. *J. Neurosurg.* 1986;64:879–889.

82. Hatayama T, Møller AR. Correlation between latency and amplitude of peak V in brainstem auditory evoked potentials: intraoperative recordings in microvascular decompression operations. *Acta Neurochir. (Wien)* 1998;40: 681–687.

83. Raudzens RA. Intraoperative monitoring of evoked potentials. *Ann. NY Acad. Sci.* 1982;388: 308–326.

84. Chiappa K, Gladstone KG, Young RR. Brainstem evoked responses: Studies of waveform variations in 50 normal human subjects. *Arch. Neurol.* 1979;36:81–86.

85. Campbell KCM, Abbas PJ. The effect of stimulus repetition rate on the auditory brainstem response in tumor and non-tumor patients. *J. Speech Hear Res.* 1987;30:494–502.

86. Pratt H, Sohmer H. Intensity and rate functions of cochlear and brainstem evoked responses to click stimuli in man. *Arch. Otol. Rhinol. Laryngol.* 1976;212:85–92.

87. Jewett DL. The 3 channel Lissajous' trajectory of the auditory brain stem response. IX. Theoretical aspects. *Electroenceph. Clin. Neurophysiol.* 1987;68:386–408.

88. Gardi JN, Sininger YS, Martin WH, Jewett DL, Morledge DE. The 3-channel Lissajous' trajectory of the auditory brain-stem response. IV. Effect of lesions in the cat. *Electroenceph. Clin. Neurophysiol.* 1987;68:360–367.

89. Pratt H, Har'el Z, Golos E. Geometrical analysis of human three-channel Lissajous' trajectory of auditory brain stem evoked potentials. *Electroenceph. Clin. Neurophysiol.* 1984;58:83–88.

90. Hashimoto I. Auditory evoked potentials recorded directly from the human VIIIth nerve and brain stem: origins of their fast and slow components. *Kyoto Symp.* 1982;36(EEG Suppl.):305–314.

91. Hashimoto I. Auditory evoked potentials from the humans midbrain: slow brain stem responses. *Electroenceph. Clin. Neurophysiol.* 1982;53:652–657.

92. Møller AR, Jannetta PJ, Møller MB. Neural generators of brainstem evoked potentials. Results from human intracranial recordings. *Ann. Otol. Rhinol. Laryngol.* 1981;90:591–596.

93. Møller AR. Direct eighth nerve compound action potential measurements during cerebellopontine angle surgery. In: Höhmann D, ed. *Proceedings of the First International Conference on ECoG, OAE, and Intraoperative Monitoring.* Amsterdam: Kugler, 1993:275–280.

94. Silverstein H, Norrell H, Haberkamp T, McDaniel AB. The unrecognized rotation of the vestibular and cochlear nerves from the labyrinth to the brain stem: its implications to surgery of the eighth cranial nerve. *Otolaryngol. Head Neck Surg.* 1986;95:543–549.

95. Møller AR, Jho HD. Effect of high frequency hearing loss on compound action potentials recorded from the intracranial portion of the human eighth nerve. *Hear Res.* 1991;55:9–23.

96. Terr LI, Edgerton BJ. Surface topography of the cochlear nuclei in humans: Two and three-dimensional analysis. *Hear Res.* 1985;17:51–59.

97. Møller AR. Monitoring techniques in cavernous sinus surgery. In: Loftus CM, Traynelis VC, eds. *Monitoring Techniques in Neurosurgery.* New York, NY: McGraw-Hill: 1994:141–155.

98. Levine RA, Ojemann RG, Montgomery WW, McGaffigan PM. Monitoring auditory evoked potentials during acoustic neuroma surgery. Insights into the mechanism of the hearing loss. *Ann. Otol. Rhinol. Laryngol.* 1984;93:116–123.

99. Ojemann RG, Levine RA, Montgomery WM, McGaffigan PM. Use of intraoperative auditory evoked potentials to preserve hearing in unilateral acoustic neuroma removal. *J. Neurosurg.* 1984;61:938–948.

100. Winzenburg SM, Margolis RH, Levine SC, Haines SJ, Fournier EM. Tympanic and transtympanic electrocochleography in acoustic neuroma and vestibular nerve section surgery. *Am. J. Otol.* 1993;14:63–69.

101. Sekiya T, Møller AR. Avulsion rupture of the internal auditory artery during operations in the cerebellopontine angle: a study in monkeys. *Neurosurgery* 1987;21:631–637.

102. Sekiya T, Møller AR. Cochlear nerve injuries caused by cerebellopontine angle manipulations. An electrophysiological and morphological study in dogs. *J. Neurosurg.* 1987;67:244–249.

103. Møller AR. Late waves in the response recorded from the intracranial portion of the auditory nerve in humans. *Ann. Otol. Rhinol. Laryngol.* 1993;102:945–953.

104. Møller AR, Jho HD. Compound action potentials recorded from the intracranial portion of the

auditory nerve in man: effects of stimulus intensity and polarity. *Audiology* 1991;30:142–163.

105. Angelo R, Møller AR. Contralateral evoked brainstem auditory potentials as an indicator of intraoperative brainstem manipulation in cerebellopontine angle tumors. *Neurol Res* 1996;18:528–540.

106. Gardner WJ. Concerning the mechanism of trigeminal neuralgia and hemifacial spasm. *J. Neurosurg.* 1962;19:947–958.

107. Jannetta P. Hemifacial spasm. In: Samii M, Jannetta P, eds. *The Cranial Nerves.* Heidelberg: Springer-Verlag; 1981:484–493.

108. Møller AR, Sekiya T. Injuries to the auditory nerve: a study in monkeys. *Electroenceph. Clin. Neurophysiol.* 1988;70:248–255.

109. Cohen MS, Britt RH. Effects of sodium pentobarbital, ketamine, halothane, and chloralose on brain stem auditory evoked responses. *Anesth. Analg.* 1982;61:338–343.

110. Thornton C, Catley DM, Jorden C, Roystan D, Lehane JR, Jones JG. Enflurane increases the latency of early components of the auditory evoked response in man. *Br. J. Anesth.* 1981;53:1102–1103.

111. Stockard JJ, Sharbrough F, Tinker J. Effects of hypothermia on the human brain stem auditory response. *Ann. Neurol.* 1978;3:368–370.

112. Brown RH, Nash CL. Current status of spinal cord monitoring. *Spine* 1979;4:466–478.

113. Nash CL, Lorig RA, Schatzinger LA, Brown RH. Spinal cord monitoring during operative treatment of the spine. *Clin. Orthop.* 1977;126:100–105.

114. Engler GL, Spielholtz NI, Bernard WN, Danziger F, Merkin H, Wolff T. Somatosensory evoked potentials during Harrington instrumentation for scoliosis. *J. Bone Joint Surg.* 1978;60A:528–532.

115. Neuloh G, Schramm J. Monitoring of motor evoked potentials compared with somatosensory evoked potentials and microvascular Doppler ultrasonography in cerebral aneurysm surgery. *J. Neurosurg.* 2004;100:389–399.

116. Deletis V. Intraoperative neurophysiology and methodologies used to monitor the functional integrity of the motor system. In: Deletis V, Shils JL, eds. *Neurophysiology in Neurosurgery.* Amsterdam: Academic; 2002:25–51.

117. Robertazzi RR, Cunningham JNJ. Monitoring of somatosensory evoked potentials: a primer on the intraoperative detection of

spinal cord ischemia during aortic reconstructive surgery. *Semin. Thorac. Cardiovasc. Surg.* 1998;10:11–17.

118. York DH. Somatosensory evoked potentials in man: differentiation of spinal pathways responsible for conduction from the forelimb vs hindlimb. *Prog. Neurobiol.* 1985;25:1–25.

119. Nuwer MR, Dawson EG, Carlson LG, Kanim LE, Sherman JE. Somatosensory evoked potential spinal cord monitoring reduces neurologic deficits after scoliosis surgery: results of a large multicenter study. *Electroenceph. Clin. Neurophysiol.* 1995;96:6–11.

120. Daube JR, Reagan TJ, Sandok BA, Westmoreland BF. *Medical Neurosciences*, 2nd ed. Second Ed. Rochester, MN: Mayo Foundation; 1986.

121. Pratt H, Starr A. Somatosensory evoked potentials in natural forms of stimulation. In: Cracco RQ, Bodis-Wollner I, eds. New York, NY: Alan R. Liss; 1986:28–34.

122. Mauguiere F. Anatomic origin of the cervical N13 potential evoked by upper extremity stimulation. *J. Clin. Neurophysiol.* 2000;17:236–245.

123. Katifi HA, Sedgwick EM. Evaluation of the dermatomal somatosensory evoked potential in the diagnosis of lumbo-sacral root compression. *J. Neurol. Psychol.* 1987;50:1204–1210.

124. Vrahas M, Gordon RG, Mears DC, Krieger D, Sclabassi RJ. Intraoperative somatosensory evoked potential monitoring of pelvic and acetabular fractures. *J. Orthop. Trauma* 1992;6:505–508.

125. Desmedt JE, Nguyen TH, Carmeliet J. Unexpected latency shifts of the stationary P9 somatosensory evoked potential far field with changes in shoulder position. *Electroenceph. Clin. Neurophysiol.* 1983;56:628–634.

126. Maguire J, Wallace S, Madiga R, Leppanen R, Draper V. Evaluation of intrapedicular screw position using intraoperative evoked electromyography. *Spine* 1995;20:1068–1074.

127. Toleikis JR. Neurophysiological monitoring during pedicle screw placement. In: Deletis V, Shils JL, eds. *Neurophysiology in Neurosurgery.* Amsterdam: Elsevier; 2002:231–264.

128. Nuwer MR. *Evoked Potential Monitoring in the Operating Room.* New York, NY: Raven; 1986.

129. Nuwer MR, Dawson EC. Intraoperative evoked potential monitoring of the spinal cord: enhanced stability of cortical recordings.

Electroenceph. Clin. Neurophysiol. 1984;59: 318–327.

130. Jones SJ, Howard L, Shawkat F. Criteria for detection and pathological significance of response decrement during spinal cord monitoring. In: Ducker TB, Brown RH, eds. *Neurophysiology and Standards of Spinal Cord Monitoring.* New York: Springer-Verlag; 1988: 201–206.

131. Nuwer MR, Daube J, Fischer C, Schramm J, Yingling CD. Neuromonitroing during surgery. Report of an IFCN committee. *Electroenceph. Clin. Neurophysiol.* 1993;87:263–276.

132. Brown RH, Nash CLJ. Standardization of evoked potential recording. In: Ducker TB, Brown RH, eds. *Neurophysiology and Standards of Spinal Cord Monitoring.* New York: Springer-Verlag; 1988:1–10.

133. Coles JG, Taylor MJ, Pearce JM, et al. Cerebral monitoring of somatosensory evoked potentials during profoundly hypothermic circulatory arrest. *Circulation* 1984;70:1096–1102.

134. Rheineck Van Leyssius AT, Kalkman CJ, Bovill JG. Influence of moderate hypothermia on posterior tibial nerve somatosensory evoked potentials. *Anesth. Analg.* 1986;5:475–480.

135. Lueders H, Gurd A, Hahn J, Andrish J, Weiker G, Klem G. A new technique for intraoperative monitoring of spinal cord function: multichannel recording of spinal cord and subcortical evoked potentials. *Spine* 1982;7:110–115.

136. Maccabee PJ, Levine DB, Pinkhasov EI, Cracco RQ, Tsairis P. Evoked potentials recorded from scalp and spinous processes during spinal column surgery. *Electroenceph. Clin. Neurophysiol.* 1983;56:569–582.

137. Tamaki T, Takano H, Takakuwa K. Spinal cord monitoring: basic principles and experimental aspects. *Central Nervous Syst. Trauma* 1985;2: 137–149.

138. Tsuyama N, Tsuzuki N, Kurokawa T, Imai T. Clinical application of spinal cord action potential measurement. *Int. Orthoped.* (SICOT) 1978;2:39–46.

139. Tamaki T, Tsuji H, Inoue S, Kobayashi H. The prevention of iatrogenic spinal cord injury utilizing the evoked potential. *Int. Orthoped.* (SICOT) 1981;4:313–317.

140. Owen JH. Intraoperative stimulation of the spinal cord for prevention of spinal cord injury. *Adv. Neurol.* 1993;63:271–288.

141. Owen JH, Bridwell KH, Grubb R, et al. The clinical application of neurogenic motor evoked potentials to monitor spinal cord function during surgery. *Spine* 1991;16:S385–S390.

142. Cohen AR, Young W, Ransohoff J. Intraspinal localization of the somatosensory evoked potential. *Neurosurgery* 1981;9:157–162.

143. Jones SJ, Edgar MA, Ransford AO. Sensory nerve conduction in the human spinal cord: Epidural recordings made during scoliosis surgery. *J. Neurol. Neurosurg. Psychiatry.* 1982;45:446–451.

144. Toleikis JR, Skelly JP, Carlvin AO, Burkus JK. Spinally elicited peripheral nerve responses are sensory rather than motor. *Clin. Neurophysiol.* 2000;111:736–742.

145. Pereon Y, Nguyen ST, Delecrin J, et al. Combined spinal cord monitoring using mixed evoked potentials and collision techniques. *Spine* 2002;27:1571–1576.

146. Branston NM, Symon L, Crockard HA, Pasztor E. Relationship between the cortical evoked potential and local cortical blood flow following acute middle cerebral artery occlusion in the baboon. *Exp. Neurol.* 1974;45:195–208.

147. Astrup J, Symon L, Branston NM, Lassen NA. Cortical evoked potentials and extracellular K+ and H+ at critical levels of brain ischemia. *Stroke* 1977;8:51–57.

148. Symon L, Hargadine J, Zawirski M, Branston N. Central conduction time as an index of ischemia in subarachnoid haemorrhage. *J. Neurol. Sci.* 1979;44:95–103.

149. Symon L, Murota T. Intraoperative monitoring of somatosensory evoked potentials during intracranial vascular surgery. In: Desmedt JE, ed. *Neuromonitoring in Surgery.* Amsterdam: Elsevier Science; 1989:263–274.

150. Momma F, Wang AD, Symon L. Effects of temporary arterial occlusion on somatosensory evoked responses in aneurysm surgery. *Surg. Neurol.* 1987;27:343–352.

151. Spetzler RF, Selman WR, Nash CL, Brown, RH. Transoral microsurgical odontoid resection and spinal cord monitoring. *Spine* 1979;4:506–510.

152. Friedman WA, Kaplan BJ, Day AL, Sypert GW, Curran MT. Evoked potential monitoring during aneurysm operation: observations after fifty cases. *Neurosurgery* 1987;20:678–687.

153. Bennett MH, Jannetta PJ. Trigeminal evoked potentials in human. *Electroenceph. Clin. Neurophysiol.* 1980;48:517–526.

154. Stechison MT, Kralick FJ. The trigeminal evoked potential: Part I. Long-latency

responses in awake or anesthetized subjects. *Neurosurgery* 1993;33:633–638.

155. Stechison MT, Møller AR, Lovely TJ. Intraoperative mapping of the trigeminal nerve root: technique and application in the surgical management of facial pain. *Neurosurgery* 1996;38:76–82.

156. Hashimoto I. Trigeminal evoked potentials following brief air puff: enhanced signal-to-noise ratio. *Ann. Neurol.* 1988;23:332–338.

157. Sloan TB, Heyer EJ. Anesthesia for intraoperative neurophsysiologic monitoring of the spinal cord. *J. Clin. Neurophysiol.* 2002;19:430–443.

158. Wang AD, Costa e Silva IE, Symon L, Jewkes D. The effect of halothane on somatosensory and flash evoked potentials during operations. *Neurol. Res.* 1985;7:58–62.

159. Drummond JC, Todd MM. The effect of high dose sodium thiopental on brainstem auditory and median nerve somatosensory evoked responses in humans. *Anesthesiology* 1985;63:249–254.

160. Frazier WT. Effects on anesthetic drugs on spinal cord monitoring: an update. In: Ducker TB, Brown RH, eds. *Neurophysiology and Standards of Spinal Cord Monitoring.* New York, NY: Springer-Verlag; 1988:125–139.

161. Samra SK. Effect of isoflurane on human nerve evoked potentials. In: Ducker TB, Brown RH, eds. *Neurophysiology and Standards of Spinal Cord Monitoring.* New York, NY: Springer-Verlag; 1988:147–156.

162. McPherson RW, Bell S, Traystman RJ. Effects of thiopental, fentanyl, and etomidate on upper extremity somatosensory evoked potentials in humans. *Anesthesiology* 1986;65:584–589.

163. Curatolo JM, Macdonell RA, Berkovic SF, Fabinyi GC. Intraoperative monitoring to preserve central visual fields during occipital corticectomy for epilepsy. *J. Clin. Neurosci.* 2000; 7:234–237.

164. Wiedemayer H, Fauser B, Armbruster W, Gasser T, Stolke D. Visual evoked potentials for intraoperative neurophysiologic monitoring using total intravenous anesthesia. *J. Neurosurg. Anesthesiol.* 2003;15:19–24.

165. Pratt H, Martin WH, Bleich N, Zaaroor M, Schacham SE. A high-intensity, goggle-mounted flash stimulator for short-latency visual evoked potentials. *Electroenceph. Clin. Neurophysiol.* 1994;92:469–472.

SECTION III

MOTOR SYSTEMS

Chapter 9
 Anatomy and Physiology of Motor Systems
Chapter 10
 Practical Aspects of Monitoring Spinal Motor Systems
Chapter 11
 Practical Aspects of Monitoring Cranial Motor Nerves

Loss of spinal motor function, either total or partial, always has severe consequences, as does loss or impairments of the function of the cranial motor systems. Loss of neural function can be devastating, but with the use of intraoperative monitoring and development of better surgical methods, such as microneurosurgery, such risks have been significantly reduced. Therefore, monitoring of spinal and cranial motor systems is an important part of intraoperative neurophysiological monitoring. In order to fully utilize the possibilities that such monitoring offers in reducing the risks of postoperative motor deficits, it is important to understand the basic anatomy and function of the motor systems. The cranial motor systems differ in many ways from the spinal motor system. This section describes the anatomy and the physiology of both systems, beginning with the spinal motor system.

The use of intraoperative neurophysiological recordings is not limited to detecting intraoperative neural injury, but it is also gaining greater importance in guiding the surgical procedure itself especially during "functional neurosurgery." This will be discussed in more detail in Chap. 15. Movement disorder such as Parkinson's disease, essential tremor, dystonia, and possibly Gilles de la Tourette syndrome can be successfully treated by placing lesions or stimulating electrodes in specific functional parts of the basal ganglia and thalamus. This implies that the neurophysiologist must understand both the pyramidal and extrapyramidal motor systems in detail. Therefore, this section includes a detailed description of the anatomy and physiology of the basal ganglia and the thalamus (Chap. 9), and a discussion of some of the disorders that are treatable by interventions aimed at these structures. The practical aspects of monitoring of the spinal motor system and cranial motor nerves are covered in Chaps. 10 and 11. The practical aspects of identifying specific tissue (such as parts of the basal ganglia) is covered in Chap. 15 (Section V), which also covers mapping of the spinal cord, brainstem, and nerve roots.

9

Anatomy and Physiology of Motor Systems

INTRODUCTION

The anatomy and the physiology of motor systems have been studied extensively in animal experiments. However, the animals used in the 1970s were mainly cats, the motor systems of which have considerable differences from that of humans. Even when monkeys were used for such studies, it became evident that their motor systems were different from that of humans. The limited possibilities of studying especially the neurophysiology of the human motor systems has caused knowledge about the human motor system to be limited. Studies in the operating room have contributed valuable information about the human motor system. This chapter will provide a basic description of the anatomy and functional organization of the motor system. When the information stems from studies in animals, it will be pointed out that the description might have discrepancies regarding the situations in humans. We will describe the spinal motor system and cranial nerve motor system separately in this section.

From: *Intraoperative Neurophysiological Monitoring: Second Edition*
By A. R. Møller
© Humana Press Inc., Totowa, NJ.

GENERAL ORGANIZATION OF THE SPINAL MOTOR SYSTEMS

The spinal motor system can be divided in upper and lower parts. The upper part consists of the cerebral cortex, basal ganglia, and cerebellum, and the lower part consists of the spinal cord, including the alpha motoneurons (the "common final pathway"). The descending pathways from the motor cortex and from motor nuclei in the brainstem and cerebellum terminate on neurons in the spinal cord. Here, they not only control alpha motoneurons but also spinal interneurons, and descending pathways can control the excitability of alpha motoneurons, spinal reflexes, and other complex neural circuits in the spinal cord, such as the central pattern generator (CPG) for walking.

The descending motor pathways have traditionally been divided into extrapyramidal and pyramidal pathways, but as the understanding of the interplay between the basal ganglia and the motor cortex has increased, that separation has been less important. The separation is still referred to clinically by neurologists because it characterizes two different groups of symptoms from the motor system.

For many purposes, it is appropriate to divide the motor system into the lateral and the medial systems *(1)*. The lateral system comprises the corticospinal and rubrospinal system, and activity

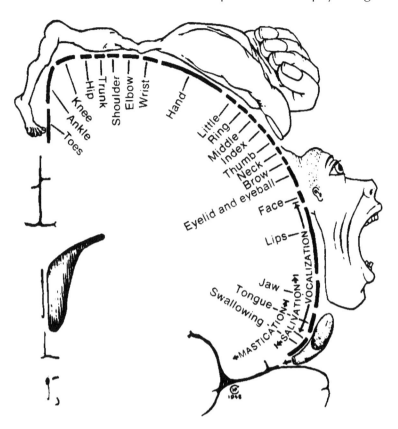

Figure 9.1: Illustration of the somatotopic organization of the motor cortex. (Reprinted from: Brodal P. *The Central Nervous System.* New York: Oxford University Press; 1998, with permission from Oxford University Press.)

in these systems controls muscles in distal limbs. The medial system comprising the reticulospinal, tectospinal, and vestibulospinal descending pathways controls proximal limb muscles and trunk muscles.

Upper Motoneuron

The motor cortex generates motor commands. The primary motor cortex is somatotopically organized in a way similar to the somatosensory cortex **(Fig. 9.1)**. The hands and the face comprise the largest parts of the motor cortex, and they are located on the lateral and dorsal surfaces of the brain. The trunk occupies a small part of the motor cortex, and the distal legs are represented by a region that is hidden between the two hemispheres. The primary cortex receives input from higher order cortical motor regions such as premotor cortical (PMC) areas **(Fig. 9.2)** and the supplementary motor area (SMA). The motor cortex also receives input from the somatosensory cortical areas. The motor cortex sends information to the basal ganglia and brainstem structures, and it receives input from the brainstem, cerebellum, and the basal ganglia via the thalamus **(Fig. 9.3)**. The main descending pathways from the motor cortex terminate in interneurons in different segments of the spinal cord and in nuclei of cranial motor nerves.

Considerable neural processing occurs in the motor cortex itself, and that is reflected in the descending activity. The organization of the motor cortex is dynamic and its processing might change with time or as a result of input from other parts of the brain as expression of

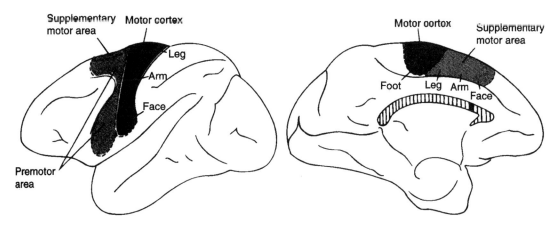

Figure 9.2: Motor, premotor, and supplementary motor cortical areas. The illustration refers to the monkey. (Reprinted from: Brodal P. *The Central Nervous System.* New York: Oxford University Press; 1998, with permission from Oxford University Press.)

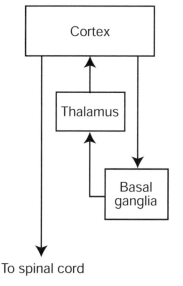

To spinal cord

Figure 9.3: Connections between the basal ganglia and the primary motor cortex. (Reprinted from: Møller AR. *Neural Plasticity and Disorders of the Nervous System.* Cambridge: Cambridge University Press; 2005, with permission from Cambridge University Press.)

neural plasticity. Drugs such as those used in anesthesia can affect cortical processing and excitability of cortical neurons.

Basal Ganglia

Traditionally, the term "basal ganglia" is used to collectively describe the caudate nucleus, the

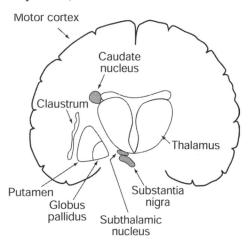

Figure 9.4: Anatomical organization of the basal ganglia and the motor thalamus. (Reprinted from: Møller AR. *Neural Plasticity and Disorders of the Nervous System.* Cambridge: Cambridge University Press; 2005, with permission from Cambridge University Press.)

putamen, and the globus pallidus. However, various investigators have included different nuclei under the term "basal ganglia," including the substantia nigra, the subthalamic nucleus (STN), and the claustrum **(Fig. 9.4)** because they are related functionally to the other parts of the basal ganglia *(2)*. The caudate nucleus and the putamen, as the primary inputs to the basal ganglia, possess many similarities and are often

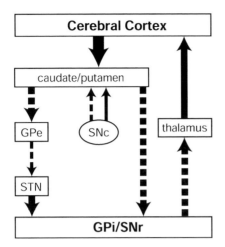

Figure 9.5: Simplified scheme of the connections between the cerebral cortex and some of the nuclei of the basal ganglia and the thalamus. Solid arrows show excitation and interrupted arrows show inhibition. (Reprinted from: Møller AR. *Neural Plasticity and Disorders of the Nervous System.* Cambridge: Cambridge University Press; 2005, with permission from Cambridge University Press.)

referred to as the striatum or neostriatum. The putamen and the globus pallidus are known as the lentiform nucleus. Several previously unrecognized subdivisions of these nuclei are now known and their function begins to be understood. For example, the globus pallidus consists of an external segment (globus pallidus external part [GPe]) and an internal segment (globus pallidus internal part [GPi]). A part of the substantia nigra is the pars reticulata (SNr) and another part is known as the substantia nigra pars compacta (SNc) (**Fig. 9.5**). These nuclei are of special interest in connection with movement disorders.

The basal ganglia process information from all parts of the cerebral cortex, including the motor cortex, and relay information to other subcortical structures and the thalamus. Reciprocal connections to the motor cortex are via the motor portion of the thalamus (**Fig. 9.3**).

It should be noted that all connections between the components of the basal ganglia are inhibitory, with one exception, namely the connections between the STN and the Gpi/SNr,

which are excitatory. The output of GPi and SNr provides tonic inhibition on thalamocortical neurons *(4)*, but the direct dopaminergic nigrostriatal pathway from SNc might also modulate the activity in the two striato-pallidal pathways in two different ways, one of which facilitates transmission in the "direct" pathway, whereas the other is inhibiting transmission in the "indirect" pathway *(5)*.

The basal ganglia are associated with movement disorders such as Parkinson's disease (PD), Huntington's disease (HD), and Gilles de la Tourette syndrome *(6)*. The possibility of successfully treating some of these disorders by making lesions or by electrical simulation of specific structures of the basal ganglia has led to the development of surgical methods that require electrophysiological guidance in their application. This increased interest in treatments that involves surgical interventions of specific parts of nuclei of the basal ganglia and the thalamus has resulted in a need for a better understanding of the function of the basal ganglia and their anatomy. Much of the research on the normal and pathological function of the basal ganglia, has been done in the operating room and it has resulted in a more differentiated view of the role of these ganglia in movement control and movement disorders.

The input to the basal ganglia from the primary motor cortex converges on the striatum, which consists of the caudate nucleus and the putamen, the centromedian nucleus (CM) of the thalamus, and the substantia nigra (**Fig. 9.5**). The putamen receives input both from the primary motor cortex (MI) and primary somatosensory cortex (SI), whereas the caudate nucleus mostly receives input from association cortices *(2)* (**Fig. 9.6**). The STN connects to the globus pallidus and the substantia nigra, in a reciprocal way, and to a lesser degree, the STN receives input from the motor cortex (**Fig. 9.7**). The output from the basal ganglia mainly originates from the GPi and the substantia nigra. The nuclei of the striatum send "direct" inhibitory input to the GPi and SNr. What is known as the "indirect" route projects to the GPi/SNr via the GPe and the STN. This means that the GPi and

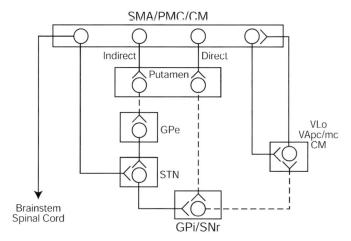

Figure 9.6: Schematic of direct and indirect pathways of the basal ganglia *(8)*. SMA: supplementary motor area; PMC: premotor cortex; CM: centromedian nucleus of thalamus. (Reprinted from: Møller AR. *Neural Plasticity and Disorders of the Nervous System.* Cambridge: Cambridge University Press; 2005, with permission from Cambridge University Press.)

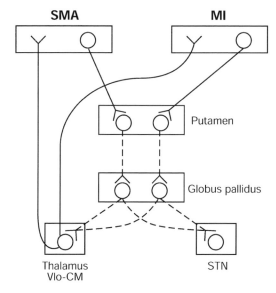

Figure 9.7: Connections between the basal ganglia and motor cortex and supplementary motor cortex. (Reprinted from: Møller AR. *Neural Plasticity and Disorders of the Nervous System.* Cambridge: Cambridge University Press; 2005, with permission from Cambridge University Press.)

SNr nuclei receive input from the striatum that is interrupted in the GPe and STN, as well as input that is not interrupted in these structures *(7)*.

The fact that the basal ganglia receive input from the motor cortex and deliver its output back to the motor cortex makes descending pathways from the motor cortex (corticospinal tract) contain information from the basal ganglia. This is why the distinction between pyramidal and extrapyramidal tracts has become invalid from an anatomical and physiological point of view, although that old distinction could have some relevance regarding the collection of symptoms in disorders of the motor system.

The role of the basal ganglia in control of motor activity is complex and several hypotheses about the role of these nuclei have been presented. It has been suggested that the basal ganglia are involved in the planning of movements *(8)* and this hypothesis is supported by the existence of connections to premotor areas, (SMAs) **(Fig 9.7)**, and the prefrontal motor cortex (PMC) **(Fig. 9.6)**.

Disorders Related to the Basal Ganglia. Much of our understanding of the role of the basal ganglia in motor control has been gained from studies done in patients with PD and other motor disorders who were treated either using lesions in the basal ganglia or by implantation of electrodes in specific parts of these nuclei for deep brain stimulation (DBS).

Degeneration of dopamine-producing cells in the SNc has for a long time been assumed to play the major role in producing the typical symptoms of PD. The subsequent rerouting of information in the basal ganglia is assumed to cause the bradykinesia (slow movements), tremor, and postural instability that are the classical signs of PD. PD has also other more complex symptoms, such as "freezing."

There is evidence that many factors are involved in the pathogenesis of PD. Hereditary factors and oxidative stress are probably implicated. Neurotoxicity by the neurotransmitter glutamate also likely contributes to the development of the disease (9). Age is the major risk factor for PD, and patients with PD often have other typical age- related neurological disorders (10). The involvement of neural plasticity (3) has, however, been mostly ignored in forming hypotheses about the pathologies of PD, but the fact that training of various kinds is beneficial in reducing the symptoms and signs of PD supports the hypothesis that expression of neural plasticity is involved in creating the symptoms and signs of PD.

HD is a progressive neurodegenerative disorder clinically characterized by chorea and cognitive decline. Anatomically, the abnormalities primarily affect the caudate nucleus and the putamen. Although patients with HD have massive degeneration in these nuclei, the substantia nigra does not seem to be affected, and so the clinical manifestations of these two disorders (HD and PD) of the basal ganglia are expected to be substantially different. The excitatory input from the thalamus to the cortex, which is decreased in PD, is increased in HD (9). Globus pallidus is often affected in HD but not PD.

Studies have shown that the input to the striatum from the SNc is unaffected in HD but that inhibition from the striatum onto the LGP is decreased and inhibition on the STN from LGP is increased. The excitation from both the STN to SNr and to the medial segment of globus pallidus (MGP) is decreased, whereas

it is increased in PD. In HD, inhibition on the thalamus from the MGP and SNr is decreased, whereas it is increased in PD. Other areas of the central nervous system (CNS) become affected as the disease progresses and neuronal loss occurs in the cerebral cortex, mainly affecting layers III, V, and VI. Increase in thalamic excitation of the cortex is assumed to be the cause of the increased, and often inappropriate, motor activity that is characteristic of patients with HD (11).

Much less is known about the pathophysiology of Gilles de la Tourette syndrome (6), which is a movement disorder that is characterized by sudden, rapid, recurrent movements (tics). Individuals with this disorder also have other symptoms such as uttering of odd and inappropriate sounds (coprolalia). It is believed that abnormalities within the cortico-striato-palido-thalamic circuit contribute to these symptoms. Recently, some patients with Tourette's syndrome have been treated successfully using DBS (bilateral thalamic stimulation), which reversed the symptoms (12).

Thalamus

The motor portion of the thalamus is involved in processing of movement information and it links the basal ganglia to the motor cortex. Lesions made in specific nuclei of the thalamus have been shown effective in treating movement disorders, as they have been in the treatment of sensory disorders and pain (see Chap. 15). Surgical lesions have now largely been replaced by implantation of electrodes for chronic electrical stimulation of specific nuclei (DBS).

Cerebellum

The cerebellum is of less interest from an intraoperative monitoring perspective than the basal ganglia and the thalamus. However, increasing understanding of the many functions of the cerebellum might in the future make it a target of similar interventions in treatment of movement disorders, as we have seen develop for the basal ganglia during the past two or three decades.

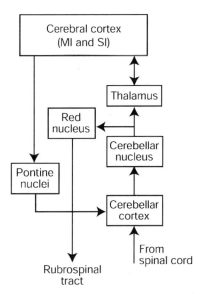

Figure 9.8: Schematic of the connections of the intermediate zone of the cerebellum. (Reprinted from: Møller AR. *Neural Plasticity and Disorders of the Nervous System.* Cambridge: Cambridge University Press; 2005, with permission from Cambridge University Press.)

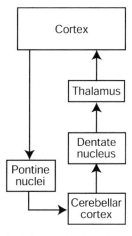

Figure 9.9: Schematic showing some important connections from the cortex to the cerebellum. (Reprinted from: Møller AR. *Neural Plasticity and Disorders of the Nervous System.* Cambridge: Cambridge University Press; 2005, with permission from Cambridge University Press.)

The cerebellum processes information from other CNS structures, but the cerebellum does not initiate movements. The cerebellum receives extensive input from sensory and proprioceptive sources such as the skin, joints, and muscle spindles through the spinocerebellar tract and from the vestibular system. The cerebellum connects to the basal ganglia, the spinal cord, and neurons in the primary motor cortex **(Fig. 9.8)**. Many of these connections are reciprocal **(Fig. 9.9)**. The dentate nucleus of the cerebellum connects to the thalamus and thereby communicates with the primary motor cortex.

Nuclei in the pons of the brainstem receive information from the primary motor and sensory cortices, which, in turn, provides input to the cerebral cortex via the nuclei in the cerebellum and the thalamus **(Fig. 9.10)**. For example, the red nucleus receives some of its input from the dentate nucleus of the cerebellum. The cerebellar hemispheres receive input from many sources such as the superior colliculus, pretectal nuclei, and the red nucleus

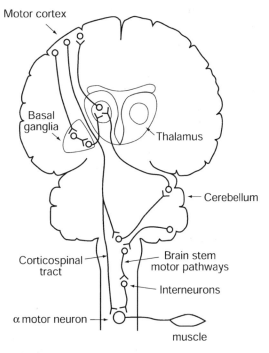

Figure 9.10: Anatomical location of major motor pathways. (Reprinted from: Møller AR. *Neural Plasticity and Disorders of the Nervous System.* Cambridge: Cambridge University Press; 2005, with permission from Cambridge University Press.)

through the inferior olive in the medulla *(2)* (**Fig. 9.10**). Finally, it has become evident that the cerebellum has many other functions than motor functions, including cognitive and memory functions.

DESCENDING SPINAL PATHWAYS

The descending pathways of the spinal cord are organized anatomically together with ascending sensory pathways (**Fig. 9.11**).

The descending pathways are of two main groups: the medial and the lateral systems *(1)*. The (dorso) lateral pathways include the corticospinal and rubrospinal tracts (**Fig. 9.12**), whereas the vestibulospinal, reticulospinal, and tectospinal tracts comprise the medial system (**Fig. 9.14**). The fibers of the descending motor pathways terminate on cells in the ventral horn of the spinal cord (**Fig. 9.13**).

The pathways of the lateral system provide voluntary, sophisticated motor control for fine movements, mainly controlling muscles of distal limbs, especially the hands. It is almost exclusively the lateral tracts that are monitored in operations where the spinal cord is at risk of being injured. The pathways of the medial system have general functions such as control of posture and control of basic function like walking. The medial group of pathways controls mainly trunk and proximal limb muscles. The medial system activates extensors more than flexors.

Lateral Pathways

The lateral system (also known as the dorso-lateral system) comprises two pathways: the corticospinal and the rubrospinal pathways (**Fig. 9.12**). The corticospinal system is most developed in primates, which makes studies of the motor system in other mammals less representative for humans. Many aspects of the corticospinal system in humans is incompletely known because of the limited number of studies of primates and the differences between humans and other primates.

Corticospinal (Pyramidal) Tract. The corticospinal tract connects cortical motor neurons with alpha motoneurons in the spinal cord, either directly or via one synapse in propriospinal interneurons. Most of the approx 2 million fibers of the corticospinal tract are fast conducting fibers, but only a small percentage of which connect directly (monosynaptically) to alpha motoneurons, whereas the remaining fibers terminate on propriospinal interneurons that connect directly to alpha motoneurons (**Fig. 9.12**).

The corticospinal tract alone passes through the pyramids, whereas other descending pathways pass through other parts of the medulla. This is why the corticospinal tract has been known as the pyramidal tract and the other tracts were known as the extrapyramidal tracts—a distinction that is no longer valid.

The main parts of the lateral pathways cross the midline at the level of the lower medulla, but it has been stated that 15% of the corticospinal fibers in humans do not cross the midline; there are large individual variations *(2)*. The corticospinal tract is asymmetric in about 75% of the population *(2)*, the right side often being larger than the left side *(2)*.

Some of the corticospinal fibers originate in the somatosensory cortex (**Fig. 9.13**), which explains why motor responses can be obtained by stimulating the somatosensory cortex.

Rubrospinal Tract. The rubrospinal tract originates in the nucleus ruber, which receives indirect input from the motor cortex. This pathway has very few fibers in humans (estimated to be 1% of those of the corticospinal tract in monkey and man *[2]*) and the functional importance of the rubrospinal tract in humans has been questioned. It is probably of little importance for monitoring purposes.

Medial Pathways

The pathways of the medial system consist of the reticulospinal, tectospinal, and vestibular spinal pathways (**Fig. 9.14**). The tracts of the medial system are less direct motor pathways than those of the lateral system, and the medial system comprises pathways with different

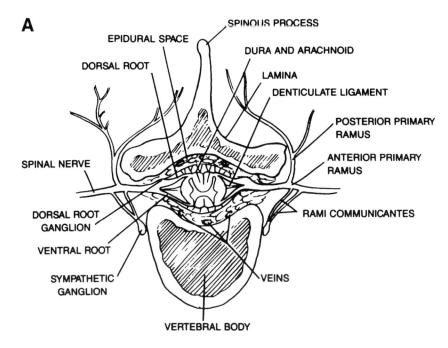

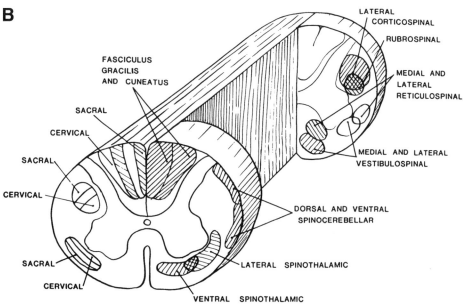

Figure 9.11: Spinal motor systems: **(A)** schematic of the anatomy of the spinal cord; **(B)** schematic of the anatomical location of ascending and descending sensory and motor pathways in the spinal cord. (Reprinted from: Daube JR, Reagan TJ, Sandok BA, Westmoreland BF. *Medical Neurosciences,* 2nd ed. Rochester, MN: Mayo Foundation; 1986, with permission from the Mayo Foundation.)

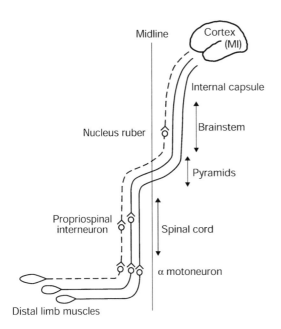

Figure 9.12: Simplified schematic of the lateral descending motor pathways from the motor cortex, showing the corticospinal and rubrospinal pathways. (Reprinted from: Møller AR. *Neural Plasticity and Disorders of the Nervous System.* Cambridge: Cambridge University Press; 2005, with permission from Cambridge University Press.)

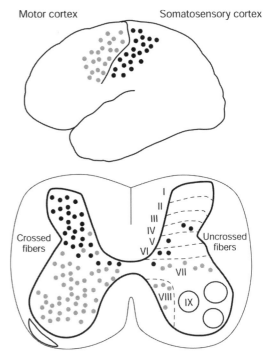

Figure 9.13: Termination of the corticospinal tract in the spinal cord. (Reprinted from: Møller AR. *Neural Plasticity and Disorders of the Nervous System.* Cambridge: Cambridge University Press; 2005, with permission from Cambridge University Press; after Brodal P. *The Central Nervous System.* New York: Oxford University Press; 1998.)

origins. The tracts of the medial system are, phylogentically, the oldest motor pathways.

The motor tracts that belong to the medial system have both crossed and uncrossed tracts **(Fig. 9.14)**, and their fibers terminate on neurons in the ventromedial zone of the spinal gray. These pathways mostly control propriospinal interneurons, the axons of which terminate on the motoneurons that control muscles on the trunk and girdle and proximal limb muscles. The fibers of these tracts terminate predominantly on propriospinal neurons and other interneurons in the spinal cord. The medial motor system mostly controls extensor muscles and muscles that are involved in posture ("antigravity" muscles).

Reticulospinal, Tectospinal, and Vestibular Spinal Pathways. The tectospinal and vestibulospinal fibers are mainly crossed *(14)* **(Fig. 9.14)** but have small, uncrossed parts.

The reticulospinal pathway originates in cells in the reticular formation of the brainstem; there, neurons receive input from many other nuclei and from the cerebral cortex. The colliculi (tectum) and the cerebellum also contribute. The fibers of the reticulospinal tract that originate in the pontine reticular formation travel in the ventral funiculus, whereas fibers from the medullary portion travel in the ventral part of the lateral funiculus **(Fig. 9.11)** *(2)*. The fibers of the reticulospinal tract form collaterals that terminate on both sides of the spinal cord **(Fig. 9.14)**. Activity in the reticulospinal fibers can have both inhibitory and excitatory influence on spinal motoneurons *(2)*, and reticulospinal fibers can influence both alpha and gamma motoneurons. The

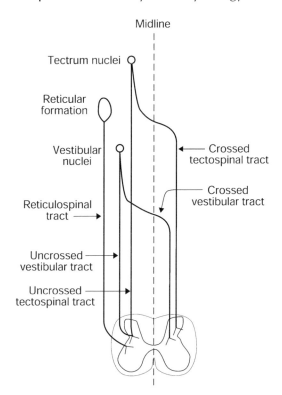

Figure 9.14: Simplified schematic of medial descending motor pathways showing the vestibular, tectospinal, and reticulospinal tracts. (Reprinted from: Møller AR. *Neural Plasticity and Disorders of the Nervous System.* Cambridge: Cambridge University Press; 2005, with permission from Cambridge University Press.)

reticulospinal tract contributes to maintaining posture and can orient the body in crude stereotyped movements *(2)*.

The importance in intraoperative monitoring of the reticulospinal tract is probably mostly related to its role of facilitating the alpha motoneuron. The reticulospinal tracts are suppressed by many forms of anesthesia. (For more details about the anatomy of motor tracts, *see* ref. *3*.)

Nonspecific Descending Systems

The noradrenalin (NA)–serotonin pathways belong to a nonspecific system originating in the raphe nuclei *(2) (see* ref. *3)* and they project to the spinal cord. Neurons in the locus coeruleus

also project to the spinal cord where they can affect the excitability of spinal neurons that are part of the motor system. In addition, the neurons of these nuclei connect to many regions of the brain *(2)*.

The fibers of the NA–serotonin pathways terminate throughout the gray matter in the spinal cord, where they can modulate neural activity in neurons that are part of the motor system, including alpha motoneurons. The NA–serotonin system generally increases the excitability of alpha motoneurons *(15,16)*. One important function of these descending pathways is adjusting muscle tone, such as suppressing skeletal muscle activity, which occurs, for example, during rapid eye movement sleep *(2)*. These facilitatory systems are sensitive to anesthetic agents; the reduction in the activity of these systems, caused by anesthetics, is likely to contribute to the decreased excitability of motor systems that is observed during surgical operations.

LOWER SPINAL MOTONEURON

Lower motor neurons consist of interneurons in the spinal cord and the alpha motoneuron from which the motor nerves emerge and through which all spinal motor activity must pass (the "common final pathway").

Segmental Pathways

At a first glance, the corticospinal tract appears as a rather simple pathway that connects neurons in the primary motor cortex to alpha motoneurons in the spinal cord— a pathway that activates complex circuitry in the spinal cord. The processing of motor commands in the spinal cord, however, is extensive. In fact, most input to cells in the spinal horns originates in other cells in the gray matter of the spinal cord, and there is a complex network of connections between neurons in the spinal cord that provides extensive intrasegmental and intersegmental processing. This processing is important for the normal function of the motor system and it is also important for assessing changes in function, such as in diagnosis of movement disorders and in intraoperative monitoring of motor systems.

The lateral system of descending pathways (corticospinal and rubrospinal systems) provides disynaptic and polysynaptic input to the spinal motoneuron from different parts of the cerebral motor areas and from other supraspinal sources. Corticospinal fibers make complex collateral connections with neurons in many subcortical centers (1,14,17). Some of these collaterals connect with neurons in several different areas of the spinal cord and extend over many spinal cord segments.

The neural networks in the spinal cord perform extensive integration of somatosensory and proprioceptive information with supraspinal motor commands occurring in the spinal cord. Spinal cord processing involves multiple feedback loops (including reflexes), the gain of which is affected by several sources of supraspinal input and by proprioceptor input. This means that the spinal cord has wide ranges of computational capabilities.

The interneurons in the spinal cord provide local processing of the input from supraspinal sources, which can be extensive, before the motor commands reach the alpha motoneurons. These local spinal circuits can generate complex commands on their own without supraspinal input, such as with walking (CPG).

Spinal proprioceptive interneurons that receive their input from corticospinal neurons also receive excitatory and inhibitory input from many segmental sources, and thereby, descending input to alpha motoneurons can be modulated (2,18–20).

Studies in which microstimulation of a specific site on the cortex were done showed that activity in small groups of cortical neurons can cause descending activity in many different tracts and evoke contraction of many different muscles (14).

Alpha Motoneurons

Alpha motoneurons that are located in layer IX of the ventral horn of the spinal cord are, as mentioned earlier, the targets of the descending motor tracts. These neurons are the "final common pathway" for motor control. Their axons form the ventral spinal roots and the motor portions of spinal nerves that innervate skeletal (extrafusal) muscles. The motor portion of peripheral nerves also contains the axons of gamma neurons that innervate the (intrafusal) muscles of muscle spindles.

Alpha motoneurons have many synapses (estimated to be approx 10,000–50,000 on a single motoneuron) that connect input from different sources. The input to alpha motoneurons comes from corticospinal fibers, but most corticospinal fibers activate alpha motoneurons through propriospinal interneurons and other local (excitatory and inhibitory) segmental interneurons. These spinal interneurons receive their input from supraspinal sources through long descending pathways (corticospinal, rubrospinal, vestibulospinal, and reticulospinal tracts), but most of the input to neurons in the spinal cord comes from other neurons in the spinal cord, thus originating in local spinal circuits (14,21).

Spinal Reflexes

The fibers of all descending pathways give off many collateral fibers, some of which connect to neurons that are involved in spinal reflexes. This is one way in which descending motor pathways control movement. Spinal reflexes are important for many types of movement and some functions such as walking. Neural circuits in the spinal cord without supraspinal input can perform breathing, but descending activity from supraspinal structures can modulate these functions. Some reflexes are relatively simple, such as the monosynaptic stretch reflex and other reflexes involving supraspinal circuits are complex. Typically, spinal reflexes are modulated by supraspinal input and input from neurons in the same and other spinal segments. The input to spinal reflexes from descending pathways such as the corticospinal tract and those of the medial system play an important role in processing of information from the motor cortex, as well as execution of motor commands. One of the simplest of spinal reflexes is the Renshaw reflex,

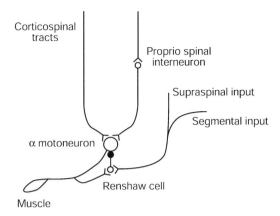

Figure 9.15: Input from corticospinal tracts to alpha motoneurons, showing Renshaw inhibition and modulation of that. (Reprinted from: Møller AR. *Neural Plasticity and Disorders of the Nervous System.* Cambridge: Cambridge University Press; 2005, with permission from Cambridge University Press.)

which feeds information that travels in the motor nerves back to the alpha motoneuron. Even though this reflex appears as a simple one-synapse feedback system, its action can be modulated by input from neurons in the spinal cord and from supraspinal sources **(Fig. 9.15)**. The same is the case for other spinal reflexes. Thus, also the "simple" monosynaptic stretch reflex can be modulated by supraspinal input and input from other segments of the spinal cord.

Dormant and Active Connections

Morphological studies show connections from the motor cortex to the striatum, several groups of thalamic nuclei, the red nucleus, pontine nuclei, the mesencephalic, pontine and medullary parts of the reticular formation, dorsal column and trigeminal sensory nuclei, and the lateral reticular nucleus *(22)*. It must, however, be pointed out that these connections that are often shown in diagrams in textbooks are mostly based on morphological studies, and much less is known about which of these connections are active at any given time and what their functional roles are. There is no doubt that activity in many of the fibers in these fiber tracts terminate in synapses that do not normally conduct. The

existence of such dormant connections represents redundancy that might be activated through expression of neural plasticity. Many phenomena can cause expression of neural plasticity, such as injuries or changes in demand. More important for intraoperative monitoring is perhaps the fact that connections that normally are conducting nerve impulses might cease that performance because of the effect of anesthesia. The adverse effect of that is probably most apparent when it results in reduced facilitatory input to motoneurons.

Value of Animal Studies

A large part of our knowledge about the function of the corticospinal system and the processing that occurs in the spinal cord is based on studies in animals such as the cat, which has only a few corticospinal fibers in the neck that terminate monosynaptically on alpha motoneurons (lamina IX; **Fig. 9.13**); therefore, the results of some of these studies are not representative for humans. Intraoperative recordings that can be done together with monitoring are important for increasing our understanding of the function of these systems in humans. Early work by Penfield *(23,24)* has paved the way for such studies.

Blood Supply to the Spinal Cord

Recording of somatosensory evoked potentials (SSEPs) was the earliest method used to intraoperatively monitor the function of the spinal cord, as described in Chap. 7. Monitoring of the SSEPs, however, only test the function of the sensory parts of the spinal cord. The sensory pathways that are monitored by recording SSEPs occupy the dorsal and lateral portions of the spinal cord, whereas the motor pathways occupy the ventral portion **(Fig. 9.11B)**. The effect of ischemia and other insults to the ventral portion of the spinal cord, therefore, does not cause direct changes in the SSEP.

The motor (ventral) portion of the spinal cord has a different blood supply than the dorsal portion of the spinal cord, where the sensory portion of the spinal cord is located **(Fig. 9.16)**. Compromises of the blood supply

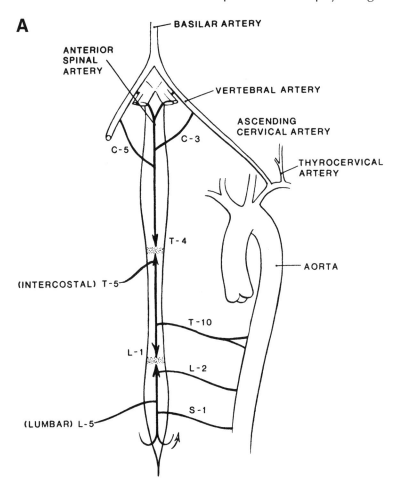

Figure 9.16: Blood supply to the spinal cord: **(A)** Schematic of the spinal cord with indications of areas supplied by the posterior and the anterior spinal arteries, and the area that is supplied by the circumferential vessels; **(B)** anterior spinal artery: radicular arteries are variable in location, shown here as C-3, C-5, T-4, T-10, L-1, L-2, and S-1; stippled areas indicate zones of marginal blood supply; **(C)** schematic of the blood supply to the spinal cord; **(D)** drawing showing how the posterior spinal arteries supply the spinal cord. (Reprinted from: Daube JR, Reagan TJ, Sandok BA, Westmoreland BF. *Medical Neurosciences*, 2nd ed. Rochester, MN: Mayo Foundation; 1986, with permission from the Mayo Foundation.)

to the ventral portion of the spinal cord might therefore occur without the dorsal part of the spinal cord being affected and thus go unnoticed if only the SSEP is monitored. Monitoring of the function of the ventral portion of the spinal cord is important during operations in which there is risk of ischemia of the spinal cord. Technical difficulties, mainly related to producing a satisfactory activation of the motor systems of the

spinal cord in an anesthetized patient, delayed the introduction of such monitoring for general use. Techniques for extracranial stimulation of the motor cortex for activating descending motor tracts in the spinal cord are now available, and the use of such techniques is increasing. Development of suitable anesthesia regimen has contributed to the success of monitoring of motor systems (*see* Chaps. 10, 16).

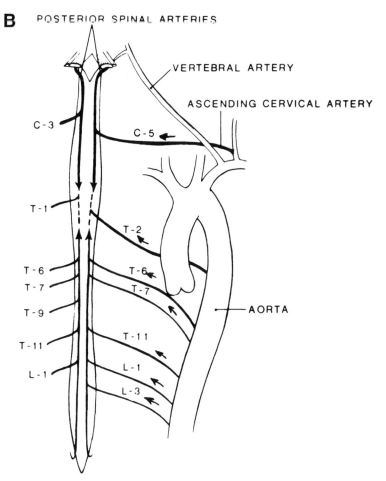

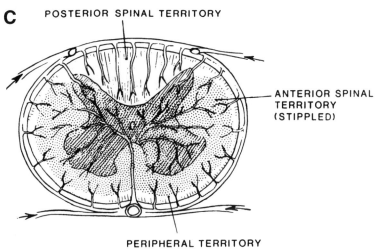

Figure 9.16: *(Continued)*

D

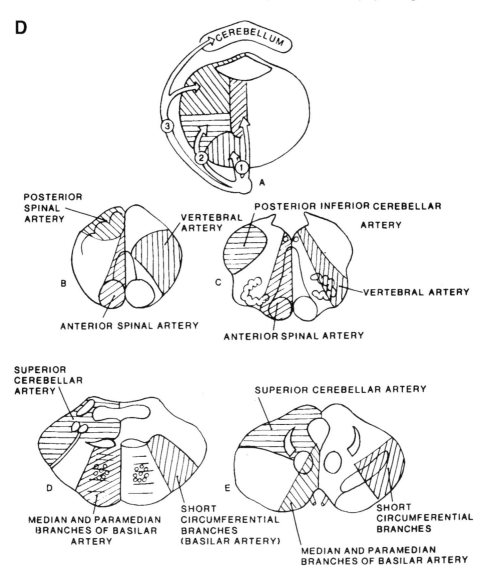

Figure 9.16: *(Continued)*

PHYSIOLOGY OF THE SPINAL MOTOR SYSTEM

The physiology of the lateral system is better known than that of the medial system. However, it is an obstacle to understanding the physiology of the lateral system that this system is different in the animal species from which our knowledge originates. Studies in humans done during surgical operations have contributed to our understanding of the physiology of these systems. The increasing use of neurophysiological methods in connections with operations on the spinal cord opens possibilities for many future studies.

Descending Activity (D and I Waves) of the Corticospinal System

Transcranial magnetic and electrical stimulation of the motor cortex can elicit responses in descending motor tracts that are useful for

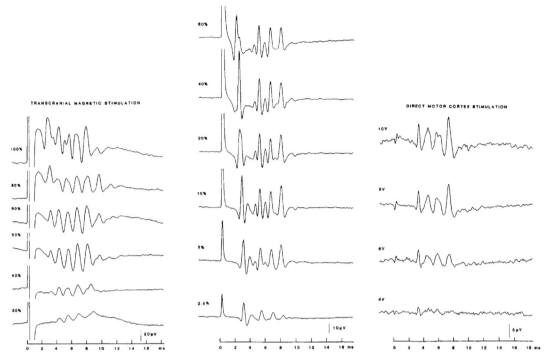

Figure 9.17: Effect of stimulus intensity on the response from the surface of the exposed spinal cord in a monkey to different forms of cortical stimulation: **left column:** transcranial magnetic stimulation; **middle column:** transcranial electrical stimulation; **right column:** direct electrical stimulation of the exposed cortex. The responses were recorded from the spinal epidural space by a monopolar electrode placed on the dorsal surface of the dura at the T_{11} level. Negativity is shown as an upward deflection. (Reprinted from: Kitagawa H, Møller AR. Conduction pathways and generators of magnetic evoked spinal cord potentials: a study in monkeys. *Electroenceph. Clin. Neurophysiol.* 1994;93:57–67, with permission from Elsevier.)

intraoperative monitoring of the spinal cord. The responses to direct or transcranial electrical and magnetic stimulation of the primary motor cortex consist of a series of distinct (negative) waves *(25–28)* that are often labeled D and I waves **(Fig. 9.17)**. The D wave (direct wave) is generated by direct activation of descending pathways from the primary motor cortex. The I waves, or indirect waves, are assumed to be generated by successive activation of cortical neurons in deeper and deeper layers of the primary motor cortex.

The recordings shown in **(Fig. 9.17)** reveal descending activity. The initial negative wave (D wave) is seen to be followed by a series of negative waves (I waves). The I waves are most

likely generated by activity in the same tracts, and elicited by activation of other cells in the motor cortex.

It has been hypothesized that (transcranially applied) electrical current in the unanesthetized individual activates nerve cells in the cortex by stimulating vertical fibers that then activate cells transsynaptically in succession, producing the I waves. The interval between I waves of approx 1.5 ms can be explained by synaptic delay and conduction delay in the associated axons. The fact that frontally oriented electrode placement **(Fig. 9.18**; anode at C_z, cathode 6 cm frontal to C_z) favors generation of I waves has been explained by assuming that such orientation of the stimulating

electrical field activates cortico-cortical projections of vertically oriented interneurons
(29) **(Fig. 9.18)**.

Some investigators have reported that D
waves are affected by anesthesia in a similar
way, as a decrease in stimulus intensity *(31)*.
This effect of anesthesia on the D waves has
been explained to be the effect of change in the
fluid space in the cortex rather than a change in
synaptic efficacy. Thus, Deletis *(32)* has presented evidence that the effect on D waves from
anesthesia is caused by vasodilatation that
changes the electrical properties of the surrounding area of the cerebral cortex, the stimulation of
which causes the D waves.

When the electrical stimulation is applied to
the exposed surface of the cortex, there is no
noticeable effect of anesthesia on the D waves,
which is in good agreement with the assumption
that the D waves that are elicited by electrical
stimulation of the motor cortex is, in fact, a
result of stimulation of the axons that leave the
cerebral cortex, thus the beginning of the corticospinal tract. Electrical stimulation of axons are
normally unaffected by anesthesia.

The I waves are affected more by anesthesia
than the D waves, and anesthesia decreases the
number of I waves that can be identified. The
effect is different from that of a decrease in
stimulus intensity *(31)*, supporting the hypothesis that the I waves depend on synaptic transmission in cortical interneurons and these
components of the response to cortical stimulation are therefore affected by anesthesia. The
effect of anesthesia on the I waves can thus be
explained by the change in synaptic efficacy.
In the deeply anesthetized animals or humans,
the synaptic transmission in these vertically
oriented axons to the cell bodies is abolished
and, therefore, only the D waves become present in recordings from the spinal cord (*see
also*, ref. *3*).

Responses recorded in awake humans who
had epidural electrodes placed at the C_1–C_2
spinal levels *(33)* or in operations for scoliosis
(Fig. 9.19) *(28)* in response to transcranial
magnetic and electrical stimulation, are similar
(28). The direction (and thus the position of the

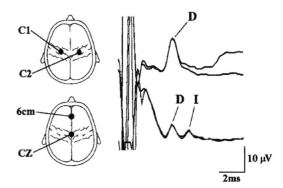

Figure 9.18: Effect of orientation of transcranial electrical stimulation on D and I waves
recorded from the upper thoracic spinal cord in
an operation for a spinal tumor. C_1 and C_z were
anodes. (Reprinted from: Deletis V. Intraoperative neurophysiology and methodologies used to
monitor the functional integrity of the motor system. In: Deletis V, Shils JL, eds. *Neurophysiology
in Neurosurgery.* Amsterdam: Academic Press;
2002:25–51, with permission from Elsevier, after
ref. *30*.)

stimulating coil) affects the waveform of the
recorded potentials *(29)*.

Although single-pulse transcranial stimulation can elicit contractions of skeletal muscles in
awake individuals, its effectiveness is diminished in patients under general (surgical) anesthesia *(34)*. Reduced facilitatory input to the
spinal cord from supraspinal sources is one of
the reasons why it is necessary to use trains of
impulses to elicit muscle responses from cortical
stimulation in anesthetized individuals (*see
ref. 3*). Stimulating the primary motor cortex
with a single impulse in the awake individual
cvoke activity in descending motor pathways
that generate excitatory postsynaptic potentials
(EPSPs) that are sufficient to reach the threshold
of alpha motoneurons. In the awake individual,
facilitation of the motoneuron is provided by
descending pathways such as the reticulospinal
tract that originates in the reticular formation of
the brainstem and influences the excitability of
spinal interneurons. In the anesthetized individual, the EPSPs elicited by a single impulse are
not sufficient to reach the threshold of the alpha
motoneuron because of a lack of such facilitation

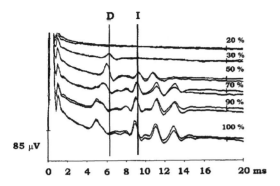

Figure 9.19: Similar recordings as in **Fig. 9.17**, done in a patient undergoing a scoliosis operation. D and I waves are shown from a 14-yr-old child with idiopathic scoliosis. The stimuli were applied through electrodes placed at Cz and 6 cm anterior. 100% = 750 V. (Reprinted from: Deletis V. Intraoperative neurophysiology and methodologies used to monitor the functional integrity of the motor system. In: Deletis V, Shils JL, eds. *Neurophysiology in Neurosurgery.* Amsterdam: Academic Press; 2002:25–51, with permission from Elsevier, after ref. *32*.)

and, therefore, temporal summation of EPSPs elicited by several successive stimuli is necessary to exceed the threshold of alpha motoneurons. Such trains of stimuli are easier to generate by electrical transcranial stimulation than by magnetic stimulation (*see* Chap. 10).

Stimulation of the somatosensory cortex (SI) can also activate descending motor pathways and elicit muscle contractions, but it requires a higher intensity than stimulation of the primary motor cortex. The descending activity gives rise to distinct potentials that can be recorded from the exposed spinal cord.

MEDIAL SYSTEM

The medial system innervates muscles in the proximal limbs and the trunk. This system has so far received little interest from a monitoring point of view, although it is known that spinal cord injuries can cause deficits of the medial system and subsequent pareses or paralysis of the muscles that are innervated by that system (innervating the trunk and proximal limb muscles; *see* p. 167). Such deficits manifest by difficulties in walking and maintaining posture and deficits in the use of proximal limb muscles. Further development of neurophysiological monitoring is needed for reducing the risk of iatrogenic injuries to the medial motor system.

Brainstem Control of Motor Activity

The brainstem reticular formation plays an important role in controlling muscle tone and on the excitability of spinal motoneurons, including the alpha motoneurons. This influence is mainly mediated to the spinal cord through the reticulospinal tract originating in the brainstem. This system enables brainstem structure to control the excitability of spinal motoneurons and interneurons. Whereas too much activity from the reticular activating system in the awake individual causes hyperexcitability and hyperactivity, too little activation results in difficulties in eliciting muscle responses from stimulation of the cerebral motor cortex.

The primary response recorded from the corticospinal tract of the spinal cord (the D wave) in response to transcranial electrical or magnetic stimulation *(35)* is insensitive to anesthesia, whereas electromyographic (EMG) responses are suppressed by general anesthesia. This shows that the suppressive effect of anesthesia on descending activity in the corticospinal system elicited by stimulation of the motor cortex is small. This means that even in an anesthetized patient, information from the motor cortex (if stimulated electrically) arrives at the propriospinal neurons and the alpha motoneurons with little noticeable effect from anesthesia. It seems unlikely that anesthesia should have an effect on this chain of two neurons (propriospinal interneuron and alpha motoneuron) in the direct corticospinal system. Therefore, there must be other reasons for difficulties in eliciting motor response (and EMG responses) in the anesthetized patient by cortical stimulation (*see also*, ref. *3*).

The generation of motor activity requires one more step than the generation of neural activity in the corticospinal tract, as reflected by D and I waves—namely that of excitation of alpha motoneurons. There are at least two reasons for the decreased excitability at the spinal cord level from anesthesia: It can be caused by a local effect on synaptic excitability of alpha motoneurons and propriospinal neurons (the only two neurons involved in the activation of muscles from the corticospinal pathways, *see* **Fig. 9.12**) or it can be caused by reduced facilitatory input to the alpha motoneurons from spinal or supraspinal sources. Reduced supraspinal facilitatory input to motoneurons is probably the main cause of the reduced excitability of alpha motoneurons. The sources of such facilitatory effect are the activity that is descending in the tracts of the medial system (primarily the reticulospinal tract). It is also known that the activity in the corticospinal tract that is reflected in the I waves is facilitatory to motoneurons. The I waves are suppressed by anesthesia; this means that the facilitatory effect of the activity that is reflected in the I waves is lost in the anesthetized patient.

The reticular formation also influences the excitability of spinal reflexes such as the stretch reflex. This means that input from the reticular activating system has an effect on the motor system similar to the effect of input from the reticular system on sensory systems (36); normal excitability of both the sensory and motor systems thus depend on the degree of wakefulness and through the activity of the brainstem reticular system. This is important for intraoperative monitoring of the motor systems because anesthesia that decreases wakefulness by reducing the output of the reticular formation reduces the facilitatory input to motor systems, inducing paralysis, and that is one of the factors that causes the well-known difficulties in evoking motor responses by cortical stimulation in the anesthetized individual (37,38).

Thus, activity in the corticospinal tract alone cannot elicit muscle contractions, and facilitation from other sources are necessary in addition to motor commands or artificial stimulation of the motor cortex to elicit muscle contractions. This means that the difficulties in obtaining muscle responses to stimulation of the cerebral cortex with single impulses in the anesthetized individual is caused by an elevated threshold of the alpha motoneurons (and propriospinal neurons) as a result of reduced facilitatory input from high supraspinal structures and, consequently, the requirement for temporal summation.

The EMG response naturally also depends on the function of the muscle endplates, but these are less sensitive to anesthesia, as is evident from the ability to elicit muscle contractions by electrical stimulation of motor nerves in surgically anesthetized (but not paralyzed) patients.

Central Control of Muscle Tone and Excitability. The effect of facilitation from high supraspinal centers on the excitability of motor systems can be demonstrated in the awake individual by changing the attention to the body part where muscle contractions are elicited by magnetic stimulation of the motor cortex **(Fig. 9.20)**. The response to a single impulse can be modulated by the individual's attention to the muscles that are activated (39). The amplitude of the recorded EMG response increases when the subject "thinks of the hand," whereas the amplitude decreases when "thinking of something else" (39).

Spinal Control of Muscle Excitability. The observed effect that changing the attention can change the muscle response elicited by cortical stimulation demonstrates clearly how activity from high CNS structures (including mental activity) can modulate the excitability of motor systems. Voluntary contraction of the muscles in question can also facilitate the response to magnetic stimulation of the cortex. A somewhat different example of facilitation of spinal motor activity is the familiar "Jendrassik maneuver"[1];

---

[1]The Jendrassik maneuver is used clinically to increase the excitability of lower extremity stretch reflexes. Practically, the patient is asked to hook the hands together by the flexed fingers and strongly pull against them, while the monosynaptic stretch reflex is activated by tapping on the patella tendon.

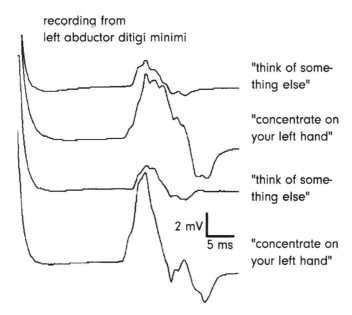

Figure 9.20: Illustration of facilitatory and inhibitory influence from high CNS levels on the response of a muscle in the hand of an awake human subject in response to transcranial magnetic stimulation of the motor cortex. (Reprinted from: Rösler KM. Transcranial magnetic brain stimulation: a tool to investigate central motor pathways. *News Physiol. Sci.* 2001;16:297–302, with permission from the American Physiological Society.)

where a spinal reflex (monosynaptic stretch reflex) is modulated (enhanced) by voluntary contraction of muscles that are innervated from different spinal segments. This is an example of how activity in one segment of the spinal cord can affect the function of different and distant spinal segments.

It has thus been clearly demonstrated in different kinds of experiment that a multitude of factors can influence the excitability of alpha motoneurons *(18,40,41)*.

ORGANIZATION OF CRANIAL MOTOR NERVE SYSTEM

Cranial motor nerves originate in motonuclei that correspond to the ventral horn of the spinal cord. The motor nuclei receive their input from the motor cortex or from subcortical sources. Some cranial nerves are purely motor nerves and some are purely sensory nerves, whereas others are mixed sensory and motor nerves. These mixed cranial nerves are not clearly separated in motor and sensory roots as are spinal nerves. Three cranial motor nerves innervate the extraocular muscles: the oculomotor nerve (CN III), the trochlear nerve (CN IV), and the abducens nerve (CN VI). CN IV and CN VI are pure somatic motor nerves, whereas CN III is a mixed nerve, the motor portion of which controls three of the five extraocular muscles. CN III also contains autonomic fibers that control the size of the pupil and accommodation. Loss of function of CN III essentially renders the eye useless. CN V, although mainly sensory (portio major), also has a motor portion (portio minor) that innervates the muscles of mastication. The tensor tympani muscle of the middle ear and some muscles of the pharynges that control the opening of the eustachian tube (velo palatine and others) are also innervated by the portio minor of CN V. The facial nerve (CN VII) is mainly a motor nerve that innervates the facial muscles as well as the stapedius muscle and the stylohyoid and digastric muscles, but it also contains sensory (taste) fibers. The taste fibers in CN VII originate in the anterior two-thirds of the tongue. CN VII also contains autonomic motor fibers that innervate the salivary glands as well as those glands that secrete tears (lacrimatory glands).

The lower cranial motor nerves — the glossopharyngeal nerve (CN IX), the vagus nerve (CN X), the spinal accessory nerve (CN XI), and the hypoglossal nerve (CN XII) — are mixed nerves that contain sensory, motor, and autonomic fibers. Practical aspects on monitoring of cranial motor nerves is discussed in Chap. 11.

10

Practical Aspects of Monitoring Spinal Motor Systems

Introduction
Monitoring During Specific Surgical Procedures
Stimulation of Cervical Motor Roots
Effects of Anesthesia on Monitoring Spinal Motor System

INTRODUCTION

This chapter concerns practical aspects on monitoring spinal motor systems. (Monitoring of cranial motor nerves is discussed in Chap. 11.) It discusses techniques for stimulation of the motor cortex and the spinal cord and for recording the responses.

The traditional method for intraoperative monitoring of the function of the spinal cord has been to record somatosensory evoked potentials (SSEPs), as described in Chap. 5. The sensory pathways that are monitored by recording SSEPs occupy the dorsal and lateral portions of the spinal cord, whereas the motor pathways occupy the ventral portion (*see* Chap. 9, **Fig. 9.16**). The ventral portion of the spinal cord has a different blood supply than the dorsal portion of the spinal cord (**Fig. 9.16**). The motor tracts can therefore be injured without the sensory pathways being affected. This means that monitoring of the SSEP does not detect changes in the function of the ventral (motor) part of the spinal cord and the descending motor tracts can be injured without causing any changes in the SSEP. Therefore, it is important to monitor spinal motor systems during operations in which the spinal cord is at risk of being manipulated.

From: *Intraoperative Neurophysiological Monitoring: Second Edition*
By A. R. Møller
© Humana Press Inc., Totowa, NJ.

Technical difficulties, mainly related to producing a satisfactory activation of the motor tracts of the spinal cord in an anesthetized patient, have delayed the general use of monitoring of spinal motor systems. Recent developments of techniques for transcranial electrical and magnetic stimulation of the motor cortex and of anesthetic techniques that allow activating spinal motor systems have provided the basis for general and practical use of intraoperative monitoring of spinal motor systems. Monitoring of SSEPs is, however, still used and it is valuable in reducing the risks of injury to the spinal cord.

Before monitoring of the motor pathways became technically possible and only SSEP was monitored, it was reported that the risk of injury to the motor portion of the spinal cord was low if SSEP monitoring was combined with selective wake-up tests *(42)*. The reason for the success of SSEP monitoring in reducing the risk of motor deficits might be that these investigators were observant of small reversible changes in the SSEP that occur when the motor pathways are injured. Such functional changes that occur in the sensory part of the spinal cord when the motor parts are injured might be explained by the fact that changes in function of one part of the spinal cord can spread throughout the spinal cord as a "spinal shock."

Monitoring the Corticospinal System

Transcranial magnetic or electrical stimulation of the motor cortex is now the most common method used for activating the motor cortex for monitoring the motor portion of the spinal cord *(28)*. It must, however, be kept in mind that the anatomic pathways involved during monitoring of transcranial motor evoked potentials (TC-MEPs) are the lateral motor system *(1)* (*see* Chap. 9) consisting of the corticospinal system and possibly including the rubrospinal system. This means that monitoring using transcranial electrical or magnetic stimulation exclusively monitors the system that innervate muscles of distal limbs, leaving the muscles of the proximal limbs and muscles of the trunk essentially unmonitored. Injuries to the parts of the spinal cord that control these muscles can therefore occur without any changes in the response of the corticospinal system; as of yet, the clinical significance of this fact has not been explored.

Electrical stimulation of the spinal cord is also used for monitoring motor systems. Such stimulation might activate descending motor systems other than the lateral system, such as the medial system *(1)* and sensory systems (*see* Chap. 9), and it is therefore not a monitor of motor systems alone.

Transcranial Stimulation of the Motor Pathways

Monitoring of TC-MEPs are noninvasive methods that make use of either electrical impulses applied through electrodes placed on the scalp or by strong magnetic impulses. These methods were described many years ago *(34,43,44)*, but the use of these methods in the operating room is complicated by several factors, one of which is the effect of anesthesia *(45)*; the results obtained show considerable variation among patients *(46)*. To date, it has mainly been electrical transcranial stimulation that has been used for routine intraoperative monitoring of operations where the spinal cord is at risk *(28,47–49)*, but the practical use of magnetic stimulation has also been described *(50)*. However, technical obstacles using magnetic stimulation still exist, and it is presently transcranial electrical stimulation of the cortex that is the preferred method for activating the motor system intraoperatively *(28,49)*.

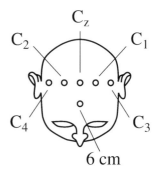

Figure 10.1: Electrode placement for electrical stimulation of the cerebral motor cortex. (Based on ref. *28.*)

Transcranial Electrical Stimulation of the Motor Cortex. It is generally assumed that anodal (positive) current applied to the surface of the cortex is more effective than cathodal (negative) current for activating descending motor tracts *(26)*. (For a theoretical analysis of transcranial electrical stimulation of the motor cortex, *see* ref. *51.*) Cathodal current elicits a more variable response with a higher threshold.

Transcranial electrical stimulation of the motor cortex requires that a large voltage be applied to the stimulating electrodes. Depending on the type of electrode used, several hundred volts might be necessary to obtain a response the intensity of which is painful in the awake patient. This limits the possibility of obtaining preoperative and postoperative recordings using techniques similar to those being used intraoperatively.

Although gold cup EEG electrodes can be used, corkscrew electrodes are most commonly used for transcranial electrical stimulation *(28)*. For stimulation of upper extremities the electrodes should be placed at C_3–C_4 locations (10–20 system, **Fig. 7.2A**, Chap. 7) and at C_1–C_2 for lower extremities. Becuase the anode is the effective stimulating electrode, at least for weaker stimulation, it should be placed on C_1 or C_3 to elicit a response in the right limbs, and C_2 or C_4 for activating muscles on left limbs. Electrode placement with the anode at the vertex (C_z), and the cathode at a location that is 6 cm anterior to that also provides efficient stimulation. Stimulation (**Fig. 10.1**) at

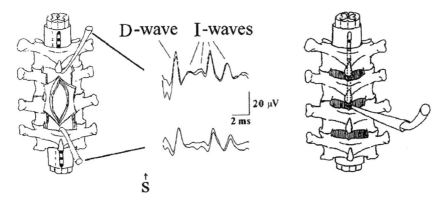

Figure 10.2: Recording of the response from the spinal cord in an operation for a spinal cord tumor, using two catheter electrodes each with three cylinder electrodes, one placed caudal and one placed rostral (for control purposes) to the surgical field. The top recording shows the response that approaches the tumor region and the lower recordings show the response having passed the tumor region. The right illustration shows placement of an epidural electrode in an operation where the spinal cord was not exposed. (Adapted from: Deletis V, Shils JL, eds. *Neurophysiology in Neurosurgery.* Amsterdam: Academic Press; 2002, and ref. *52.*)

these locations elicit clear D and I waves from the corticospinal tract as seen when recorded from the spinal cord **(Fig. 10.2)**.

Stimulators used for activating neural tissue (peripheral nerves and cells or fiber tracts in the central nervous system [CNS]) *(53–55)* might be either constant-current or constant-voltage generators (for a theoretical treatment of constant current stimulation, *see* ref. *51*). Constant-current stimulators for TC-MEPs have the advantage that the current delivered to the head is independent of the electrode impedance and the impedance of the electrode–tissue interface. This is important for two reasons: First, the probability of injury to tissue depends on current density and so will not suddenly change during a surgical procedure if the electrode impedance changes; second, the degree of activation of a cablelike axon is proportional to the gradient of the current traveling *(56)* along the axon. Because this is proportional to the total current produced by the stimulator, the neurophysiological effects of constant-current stimulation will be independent of the electrode impedance and the impedance of the electrode–tissue interface. Of course, this does not guarantee that the current delivered to neural structures is independent of changes in the impedance of

other structures such as the scalp and brain, which might cause shunting of electrical current. Changes in the geometry of the skull or presence of air inside the skull, replacing some of the cerebrospinal fluid (CSF) can also affect the current flow through the cortical tissue that is to be activated. When a constant-current stimulator is used and the electrode impedance increases, the stimulator must deliver a higher voltage in order to deliver the same current. Therefore, a stimulator has certain limitations for how high a voltage it can produce and that limitation might be different for different models of stimulators. If the resistance becomes larger than a certain value, the voltage limit of the stimulator will restrict the current and the stimulator will deliver a smaller current than that to which it is set. Many standard constant-current stimulators that are designed for clinical use have a current limit of 100 mA. Connecting two stimulators in parallel can double that limit, but this is still an order of magnitude lower than the 1.5-A current limit of a transcranial voltage stimulator (*see also* Chap. 18).

If constant-voltage stimulation is employed, it is important to take into account that the impedance of the tissue of corkscrew electrodes

placed at C_3–C_4 and F_p–C_z' might be 100–200 Ω
and the electrode impedance for large-surface
electrodes might be 120–220 Ω *(57)*. However,
these impedance values vary from electrode to
electrode and are dependent on the frequency
of the stimulus and the stimulus voltage
because the electrode–tissue system is nonlin-
ear. The total impedance also includes an
internal impedance in the stimulator, which is
120 Ω for a common type of stimulator
designed for TC-MEP monitoring (Digitimer
type D 185).

Using short pulse widths of typically
50–100 µs favors fast D wave recovery times
and enables interpulse intervals below 2 ms
(58). Used for eliciting MEPs through transcranial stimulation, fast and slow charges provide
similar intraindividual variability but fast-
charge stimulation seems to be more efficient
and requires approx 35% less total charge for
the same response as stimulation with a slow
charge. The latency of the response is not different for the two kinds of stimulation *(59)*.

Electrical impulses activate fibers in the
cerebral cortex rather than cell bodies *(60)*.
The efficacy of stimulation depends on the orientation of the generated current vector,
which, in turn, depends on the electrode montage. Electrode placements at C_3–C_4 for upper
extremity stimulation or C_z'–F_z for lower
extremities produce vertically oriented current
vectors that are ideal for stimulation of the
descending axons of the motor cortex that
become the corticospinal tract. Placing the
stimulating electrodes closer together creates
more horizontally oriented current vectors,
thus activating cortical fibers that generate I
waves in the corticospinal tract. Increasing the
stimulus strength deepens the penetration of
the electrical current in the brain, stimulating
cells at deeper layers of the motor cortex and
therefore activating different parts of the corticospinal tract. In operations where the motor
cortex is exposed, it is possible to stimulate the
cortex directly by placing grid electrodes on
the surface of the cortex or by using a small
bipolar stimulator (**Fig. 10.3**). Such direct
electrical stimulation can elicit responses in

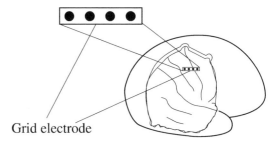

Grid electrode

Figure 10.3: Placement of electrodes over
the exposed cerebral motor cortex. (Based on
ref. *28.*)

descending motor pathways in a way similar to
transcranial stimulation *(27)*.

When stimulating the motor cortex directly,
the use of short pulse trains typically employed
in transcranial stimulation is preferred to the
long-duration 60-Hz stimulation used in the
traditional Penfield technique, because of the
lower risk of seizures. The Penfield technique,
however, must be used when cognitive testing
is performed *(61)*.

Transcranial Magnetic Stimulation. Transcranial magnetic stimulation of the motor cortex makes use of strong impulses of magnetic
fields to induce electrical current in the motor
cortex. Magnetic stimulation of the nervous
system is an attractive method for eliciting neural activity in descending motor tracts of the
spinal cord. It can activate structures deep
within the brain in awake humans without
causing any noticeable discomfort or risks.
Magnetic stimulation *(26,34)* can activate the
motor cortex and elicit volleys of neural activity in the corticospinal tract in a way similar to
those elicited by electrical stimulation of the
motor cortex *(25,27)*. Thus, magnetic stimulation evokes potentials that can be recorded
from the spinal cord as D and I waves similar
to those seen in the response to electrical stimulation of the motor cortex *(27)*.

The orientation of the magnetic field affects
its effectiveness in stimulating different populations of cells in the motor cortex *(62)*. The
site of activation might be at the spike trigger

zone of these neurons, or the fibers of the deep layers of the cortex might be activated, depending on the orientation of the magnetic field.

Practical Use of Magnetic Stimulation of the Motor Cortex. Magnetic stimulation is accomplished by passing a strong electrical impulse of current through a coil. Many different designs of such coils have been described, and several of these are now commercially available. Because stimulation of the motor cortex for eliciting activity in the descending motor tracts depends on the orientation of the magnetic field, it is important to position the coil correctly *(63)*.

The strong magnetic field that is generated can cause large stimulus artifacts that could interfere with the recorded responses. In the laboratory, it is possible to eliminate stimulus artifacts by injecting an appropriate amount of current (in opposite phase) into the recording circuit *(26)*, but such methods are usually too elaborate to be used in the operating room. We have shown that it is possible to record adequately clean responses from face muscles even though the recording site is close to the location of the stimulating coil, provided that appropriate precautions are taken *(64)*. Leads from the recording electrodes should be straight and pointing away from the patient. Artifacts should be prevented from overloading the amplifiers by keeping the amplification very low (*see* Chap. 18). It is also important to use electronic filters that are set wide and to use computer programs to remove the artifacts before the recorded potentials are subjected to further (digital) filtering. That, together with the use of finite-impulse response digital filters, reduces the time smearing of the artifacts so that the artifact does not overlap in time with the response.

Unfortunately, transcranial magnetic stimulation has several other drawbacks that have limited its use in the operating room for transcranial cortical stimulation. One such disadvantage is the bulkiness of the equipment; another is related to the difficulties in generating a rapid succession of magnetic impulses, as is required to overcome the effect of anesthesia

(38,65) when recording electromyogenic (EMG) potentials. Other deterrents in the use of magnetic stimulation in the operating room include the fear that magnetic stimulation might activate vast regions of the brain at the same time and thereby possibly leading to epileptic seizures or other adverse effects. These worries, however, seem to have been exaggerated, although in rare cases, epileptic seizures might indeed have been induced by magnetic stimulation in patients with a history of epilepsy. Additionally, there has been concern that the generated magnetic fields could cause metallic instruments to move or affect other electronic devices in the operating room.

Recording of the Response to Electrical or Magnetic Stimulation

The response from the descending motor tracts (corticospinal tract) can be recorded from the spinal cord using epidural electrodes. The subsequent muscle responses can be recorded as EMG potentials.

Recording From the Spinal Cord. Transcranial electrical stimulation of the motor pathways in humans generates D and I waves in the descending tracts. These waves can be recorded from electrodes placed in the epidural space of the spinal cord. D waves are so named because they are assumed to be elicited by direct activation of corticospinal fibers, whereas I waves are the result of indirect activation of corticospinal fibers through transsynaptic activation *(66)*. The I waves consist of a volley of waves that were first identified in animal experiments and later in humans *(67)*. Contributions to these I waves could also come from the ventral corticospinal tract that is located in the anterior funiculus. This latter tract has bilateral contributions.

The D waves are negative peaks that are assumed to be generated by activity in the dorsal corticospinal tract *(68)*. Similar waves are observed in response to transcranial magnetic stimulation and in response to direct electrical stimulation of the exposed cortical surface *(69)*.

Katayama et al. *(69)* described a method that utilized recordings of spinal potentials from electrodes placed on the spinal cord in response to electrically stimulation of the cortical surface of the brain in order to identify the motor cortex. Recording electrodes were placed in the epidural space of the cervical spinal cord to record evoked potentials from the descending (motor) pathways while probing the surface of the cortex with an electrical stimulating electrode *(69)*. When a D wave was recorded from the spinal cord, it was taken as an indication of activation of the motor cortex. These investigators also found that this response was not affected by surgical anesthesia or muscle relaxants.

The presence of the D and I waves in response to transcranial stimulation in humans indicates that the applied stimulation indeed activates the motor pathways. The latency of the D wave increases when the recording site in the epidural space in the spinal cord is moved caudally, which is in good agreement with the assumption that the D wave is generated by traveling impulses in descending motor tracts, as has been shown in animal experiments *(27,70)*.

The I waves are later components in the response from descending motor tracts in the spinal cord that are evoked by stimulation of the primary motor cortex through cortical–cortical connections. The initial component in responses to magnetic or electrical stimulation of the motor cortex is a negative peak that corresponds to the D wave, and it is generated in the dorsal corticospinal tract; 4 negative peaks (N_2, N_3, N_4, and N_5) are the I waves. The D and I waves recorded in humans are similar to those described animals *(27,69)*. The presence of the D waves is an indication that the descending corticospinal tract is intact proximally (centrally) to the site where they are recorded.

For recording D and I waves, epidural electrodes can be type JX-300 (Arrow International, Reading, PA). This electrode has three platinum–iridium recording cylinders placed 18 mm apart. The electrode has a double lumen that allows flushing the recording area with saline *(28)*. Such an epidural catheter electrode can be placed percutaneously, which is favored in procedures performed in Japan *(71)*. Other centers (in the United States) place the

recording electrode after laminectomy and so forth *(28)*. It is also possible to use a standard four-contact depth electrode (AD-TECH Medical Instrument Corp., Racine, WI).

The D and I waves are not affected by muscle relaxants, but their latency will increase after cooling of the spinal cord, with minimal effect on the amplitude of the recorded potentials *(32)*. This is in accordance with the fact that these responses are the result of propagated activity in fiber tracts.

Interpretation of Recorded Responses

Electrical and magnetic stimulation tend to activate the descending anterior corticospinal tract, but they also activate other descending tracts that might contribute to the recorded D waves, such as the lateral tracts. Furthermore, stimulation of the motor cortex might activate the corticospinal tract bilaterally. If the D waves recorded from the spinal cord become decreased to 50% of their original amplitude, it might mean that 50% of the total number of fibers are rendered nonconducting; however, if only one side is affected, that might mean that 100% of the corticospinal tract on the side has completely ceased to conduct nerve impulses. Therefore, the generally accepted limit of 50% decrease in the amplitude of the D wave is ambiguous. Although it might be true that 50% loss of conduction of corticospinal fibers might limit the successful outcome (without paralysis) if it occurs evenly on both sides tracts, but if it is caused by 100% loss of fibers on one side, it is a sign that predicts poor outcome.

In operations for intramedullary spinal cord tumors, the disappearance of the motor potentials is regarded as a temporary phenomenon that does not affect outcome if the amplitude of the D wave remains above 50% of its baseline. It has been assumed that if the amplitude of the D wave declines greater than 50%, it indicates a high risk of paralysis (paraplegia for the lower spinal cord and quadriplegia for cervical tumors) *(72)*.

Because it is often attempted to stimulate only one side of the brain, namely the side to which the anode of the stimulating electrodes is applied, it is expected that the D wave will be from only one side; however, it is not known how much of the D wave is from the anterior corticospinal tract and whether other tracts also contribute to the response.

It is important to consider that such monitoring concerns the corticospinal tract (lateral system) only and thus acts to protect only control of those muscles that are innervated by the corticospinal tract from paralysis or paresis. The other descending tract (medial system) that innervate proximal limb muscles and the trunk (*see* Chap. 9) have, so far, not been monitored practically. Loss of distal limb mobility is the most obvious postoperative deficit observed, because the examination is commonly done with the patient in bed, and because of that, deficits of the trunk muscles are not as readily observed. However, neurologists who allow a longer postoperative interval before examining patients (when they are ambulatory) often find that patients have problems walking and keeping posture after spinal cord operations although they have little abnormalities in their use of distal limbs. The observed deficits of truck muscles must then be caused by injuries to the medial motor system of descending motor tracts in the spinal cord (*see* Chap. 9), which are not normally monitored during spinal cord operations.

The importance of the corticospinal and rubrospinal system (lateral spinal motor system) has increased during evolution and is probably greater in humans than even in monkeys (*see* Chap. 9). However, the importance of one of the tracts of the medial system, the vestibulospinal tract, is obvious from experience with patients who have lost their vestibular function because of conditions such as vestibular neuronitis or from ototoxic antibiotics. Such patients experience severe deficits that can be related to motor function arbitrated by the medial system, affecting posture and other functions of trunk muscles. Although these symptoms decrease with time and might totally disappear in young individuals, the deficits that are caused by loss of function related to the vestibulospinal tract indicate that

at least one part of the medial descending system is essential. Although little is known about the functional importance of the other tracts of the medial motor system, the experience from loss of function of the vestibulospinal system indicates that there is a need to specifically monitor the medial system in addition to monitoring the corticospinal system.

Recording of Muscle Evoked Potentials

Monitoring spinal cord function on the basis of recordings of muscle activity that is elicited by transcranial stimulation is an effective method for detecting injury to the spinal cord provided that appropriate stimulus and recording parameters are used. It is, however, a disadvantage that muscle relaxants cannot be used. It is also more difficult to obtain EMG responses than response from the spinal cord because recordings of EMG potentials depend on the excitability of alpha motoneurons, which is decreased by anesthetics (because of reduced facilitatory input from high CNS centers; *see* Chap. 9). It is also important that the recording be made from appropriate muscles and attention must be paid to the patient's preoperative condition regarding paresis or paralysis of specific muscle groups.

The stimulation of the motor cortex that is normally used in such forms of monitoring causes activation of mainly the corticospinal tract that mostly innervates distal muscles of the extremities. Therefore, recordings of EMG potentials should be made from muscles on the distal extremities such as the hand **(Fig. 10.4)**. Small hand muscles are most appropriate to record from because many corticospinal fibers converge on their motoneurons. For the lower extremities, the abductor hallucis brevis is the optimal muscle from which EMG potentials can to be recorded because its motoneurons have a rich innervation by corticospinal fibers *(28)*. The tibialis anterior is an alternative muscle to use. Recordings are typically performed with needle electrodes in specific muscles; although advantages of this method vs surface electrodes for recording TC-MEPs have not been evaluated.

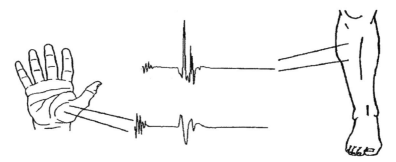

Figure 10.4: Recording of motor evoked potentials from muscles (EMG potentials) elicited by trains of electrical impulses applied to the motor cortex. (Adapted from: Deletis V. Intraoperative neurophysiology and methodologies used to monitor the functional integrity of the motor system. In: Deletis V, Shils JL, eds. *Neurophysiology in Neurosurgery.* Amsterdam: Academic Press; 2002:25–51, with permission from Elsevier, and ref. *52.*)

Interpretation of EMG Potentials. One of the major problems with the use of TC-MEPs is determining criteria for providing warnings on the basis of changes in the EMG responses. One problem lies in the fact that there is some inherent variability in the amplitude of the muscle responses. Another problem lies in the fact that muscle responses are often polyphasic and extended over time so that it is difficult to quantify them. Most practitioners now use one of two methods to avoid this latter problem. One approach, the threshold method *(73)*, involves measuring the lowest level of stimulation for which MEPs can be obtained. An increase in threshold by more than, for example, 100 V for transcranial electrical stimulation can be regarded as significant. One considerable problem with this approach is determining how much the stimulus intensity can be increased to obtain a response before it is a sign of a significant change in function. When using constant-voltage stimulation, changes in the electrode impedance or the accumulation of intracranial air could cause changes in the threshold that are not related to pathological changes in neural tissue. Another approach assumes that a significant change has occurred only if the MEPs disappear entirely. The lack of good solutions to these problems has been an obstacle to the acceptance of the use of EMG recordings together with transcranial stimulation of the spinal motor system.

Stimulation of the Spinal Cord

Several kinds of intraoperative electrical stimulation of the spinal cord have been described. One method makes use of electrical stimulation of the spinal cord and recording of the responses from a different location of the spinal cord. This method, promoted by Japanese neurosurgeons *(71)*, makes use of recordings of stimulus-elicited potentials from the spinal cord, independent of the anatomical location of their sources. This means that any fiber tract, descending or ascending, will be represented in such recordings, but to an extent that depends on the exact placement of the stimulating and recording electrodes. Both the dorsal column and the corticospinal tracts have been suggested as contributing to such responses. These responses are thus nonspecific and their value for intraoperative monitoring of the spinal cord has been questioned *(74)*.

Stimulation of the spinal cord by needles placed percutaneously, in decorticated spinous processes, or by epidural placed electrodes, can activate the entire spinal cord in a nonspecific way. Both motor and sensory pathways can be activated in that way. Collision studies have shown that neurogenic MEPs (NMEPs) that were elicited by such stimulation of the spinal cord could be recorded from peripheral nerves. The recorded potentials consist of large-amplitude motor components, which had shorter latencies than the longer latency and small-amplitude polyphasic sensory potentials *(75)*. Such reports promoted the usefulness of these responses.

In recent years, questions have arisen as to the accuracy or the interpretation of recordings of the response to direct stimulation of the spinal cord. More detailed studies of the recorded potentials elicited by stimulation of the spinal cord using collision techniques have shown that the responses to spinal cord stimulation mainly reflect transmission in the dorsal column, thus testing the sensory pathway and not the motor pathways. A polyphasic component in the response that might be caused by transmission in motor pathways sometimes could be seen. Collision studies have shown that sensory pathways generate the main components of the responses. These studies suggest that the descending volleys of activity, known as NMEPs, that result from percutaneous spinal stimulation are primarily, but not totally, composed of descending antidromic sensory components *(76,77)*. The source of these potentials is the dorsal column pathways that generate components of the SSEPs, rather than motor components. These results are supported by clinical studies *(78)*.

Recording Muscle Responses. Recording of the neural activity in descending motor pathways from electrodes placed in the epidural space of the spinal cord is an invasive method that cannot always be applied. Another technique makes use of electrical stimulation of the spinal cord while recording the responses from specific muscles (EMG) *(79)* or from peripheral nerves *(80)*.

Recording of muscle responses (EMG responses) from distal limb muscles elicited by cortical stimulation can also be used to monitor the corticospinal tract. However, whereas the D waves are little affected by anesthesia, the EMG responses are attenuated or abolished by many anesthetics and are, of course, reduced in amplitude by partial neuromuscular blockade *(38)*.

Methods using direct recordings from the spinal cord have been used for identification of the anatomical location of the motor cortex. It seems that the degree of invasiveness that is necessary for placing a recording electrode in the epidural space of the spinal cord is greater than what could normally be considered acceptable for that purpose. Other methods are available for identifying the anatomical location of the primary motor cortex. Thus, methods that can determine the anatomical localization of the central sulcus (*see* Chap. 14) provide information on the anatomical location of the motor cortex and are just as effective without requiring the placement of electrodes in the epidural space of the spinal cord. Perhaps of greater concern in using such methods for identifying the primary motor cortex is that stimulation of areas of the cerebral cortex other than the primary motor areas, might give rise to muscle contractions; even electrical stimulation of the sensory cortex might produce muscle contractions. Therefore it is now preferred to use recordings of SSEPs directly from the surface of the exposed cortex for the purpose of localizing the sensory and motor cortical areas (*see* Chap. 14).

Monitoring F and H Responses

Yet another method of monitoring the function of the spinal cord makes use of the stimulation of a peripheral mixed nerve and recording EMG responses from muscles innervated by the nerve (*see* p. 229). The antidromic volley elicited in the motor fibers by electrical stimulation of a mixed nerve can elicit an F response, which is caused by backfiring of motoneurons. Stimulating the sensory part of a mixed nerve might also elicit an H response because stimulation of proprioceptive fibers activates the monosynaptic stretch reflex activating the alpha motoneurons (*see* Chap. 9). (Naturally, stimulation of the motor part of a mixed nerve can also elicit a direct motor response by orthodromic activation of motor fibers.)

MONITORING DURING SPECIFIC SURGICAL PROCEDURES

The previously described methods for monitoring the motor system are suitable for many different kinds of operation that affect the spinal cord. When monitoring specific kinds of operations, slightly different variations of these methods are often used.

Scoliosis Operations and Removal of Spinal Cord Tumors

Transcranial electrical stimulation is now in common use for monitoring of operations on the spinal cord such as during tumor removal, trauma, and correcting spinal deformities such as scoliosis. D waves can be recorded from the spinal cord, and EMG responses from muscles that are innervated by ventral roots that leave the spinal cord at levels below the location at which the operation is done. EMG potentials are usually recorded from muscles on distal limbs such as hands or feet, depending on the location on the spinal cord where the operation is done. It has been a rule that preservation of the D wave to at least 50% of its preoperative amplitude is important, but loss of the EMG potentials has been regarded to be less serious and not a reason to abort the operation or change its course, as was discussed earlier.

Placement of Pedicle Screws

Placement of pedicle screws implies a risk of injuring spinal roots. Therfore, it is important to be able to determine the location of the tip of a pedicle screw while it is being inserted. Without monitoring, the risk of neurological deficits from pedicle screw placement procedures is rather high *(81)*. Imaging techniques have been shown less effective than electrophysiological methods for such monitoring.

There are two ways in which the proximity of a pedicle screw to a spinal root can be determined using intraoperative neurophysiological monitoring techniques. One method makes use of recording EMG potentials from a muscle that is innervated by the motor root that is at risk of being damaged *(82,83)* and electrical stimulation is applied to the pedicle screw (which is supposed to be electrically conducting) **(Fig. 10.5)**. Another method is based on monitoring spontaneous motor activity.

The use of recording of spontaneous (free-running) EMG potentials assumes that the

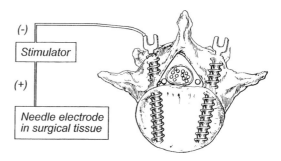

Figure 10.5: Principles of stimulation of a pedicle screw with electrical impulses. (Reprinted from: Toleikis JR. Neurophysiological monitoring during pedicle screw placement. In: Deletis V, Shils JL, eds. *Neurophysiology in Neurosurgery*. Amsterdam: Elsevier; 2002:231–264, with permission from Elsevier.)

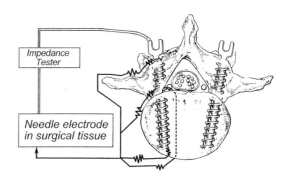

Figure 10.6: Illustration of different current paths that will "steel" stimulus current from the nerve root. (Reprinted from: Toleikis JR. Neurophysiological monitoring during pedicle screw placement. In: Deletis V, Shils JL, eds. *Neurophysiology in Neurosurgery*. Amsterdam: Elsevier; 2002:231–264, with permission from Elsevier.)

nerve root is sensitive to mechanical stimulation. Using electrical stimulation of the pedicle screw is probably better because it can test the closeness of the pedicle screw by determining the threshold of the electrical stimulation.

Some investigators have used constant-current stimulation for that purpose *(84,85)*. However, the applied current can take many paths other than the one through the nerve root **(Fig. 10.6)**, and, worse, the electrical conductivity in these

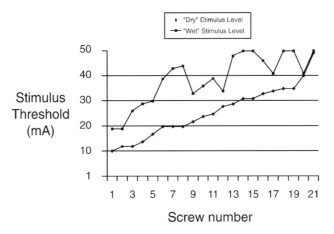

Figure 10.7: Illustration of how the threshold of EMG responses depends on how wet the surgical field is. (Reprinted from: Toleikis JR. Neurophysiological monitoring during pedicle screw placement. In: Deletis V, Shils JL, eds. *Neurophysiology in Neurosurgery.* Amsterdam: Elsevier; 2002:231–264, with permission from Elsevier.)

paths are likely to vary during an operation in accordance with how wet the environment is. Different degrees of wetness of the surrounding can affect the results because of shunting **(Fig. 10.7)** *(84)*.

When variable-current shunting occurs, it changes the stimulation of the nerve root if a constant-current stimulator is used. This is similar to that experienced when stimulating intracranial structures such as the facial nerve in operations for vestibular schwannoma, as is discussed in Chap. 11. The remedy for the problem is to use a constant-voltage stimulator rather than a constant-current source *(54,86)*. Using a constant-voltage source will make the electrical current that is delivered to the nerve root independent of the shunting from variable wetness of the surgical field where the stimulation is done.

STIMULATION OF CERVICAL MOTOR ROOTS

Magnetic stimulation of cervical motor roots is a practical way to elicit neural activity in motor nerves *(87)*. This method is used for diagnostic purposes and is beginning to find practical use in

intraoperative monitoring. When interpreting the results of such stimulation, it must be remembered that nerves have sensitive regions affected by magnetic stimulation. One of the most important such sensitive areas is where a nerve is bent *(88,89)*. Nerves from the lower spine form the cauda equine and these nerves have a sharp bend when they exit the spine. Magnetic stimulation will therefore activate that part preferentially *(62,64,90)* and, consequently, moving the stimulating coil along the nerve and its root will yield a response with the same latency.

EFFECTS OF ANESTHESIA ON MONITORING SPINAL MOTOR SYSTEM

Anesthesia has a profound effect on motor evoked potentials *(37,38,45,65)*. The effect is greatest on muscle responses (EMG), and it is least on early epidural responses (D waves). There is some effect on I waves from anesthesia.

Effects on Epidural Responses to Stimulation of the Motor Cortex

The epidural response in a baboon under isoflurane anesthesia show that the D waves are

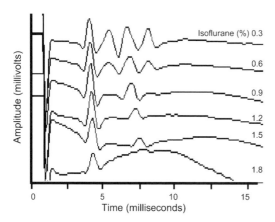

Figure 10.8: The effect of increasing isoflurane concentrations on the epidural response to transcranial electrical motor cortex stimulation in a ketamine-anesthetized baboon. (Reprinted from: Sloan T. Anesthesia and motor evoked potential monitoring. In: Deletis V, Shils JL, eds. *Neurophysiology in Neurosurgery.* Amsterdam: Elsevier Science; 2002, with permission from Elsevier.)

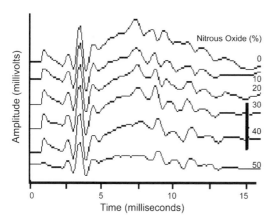

Figure 10.9: The effect of increasing nitrous oxide concentrations on the epidural response to transcranial electrical motor cortex stimulation in a ketamine-anesthetized baboon. Note that although the D wave is maintained, the I waves are lost, similar to isoflurane. (Reprinted from: Sloan T. Anesthesia and motor evoked potential monitoring. In: Deletis V, Shils JL, eds. *Neurophysiology in Neurosurgery.* Amsterdam: Elsevier Science; 2002, with permission from Elsevier.)

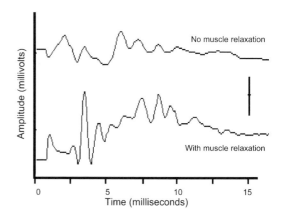

Figure 10.10: Recording from the epidural space from transcranial electrical motor stimulation with (**bottom**) and without (**top**) muscle relaxation. Note that the muscle artifact obscures the identification of I waves. (Reprinted from: Sloan T. Anesthesia and motor evoked potential monitoring. In: Deletis V, Shils JL, eds. *Neurophysiology in Neurosurgery.* Amsterdam: Elsevier Science; 2002, with permission from Elsevier.)

little affected by anesthesia, but the amplitude of the I waves decreases when the concentration is increased from 0.3 to 2.1%, with less effect seen on the D wave (**Fig. 10.8**). The I waves are lost at higher concentrations of the anesthetics used. Nitrous oxide also attenuate I waves in the epidural responses in a way similar to isoflurane *(38)* (**Fig. 10.9**).

Muscle relaxants, having their major site of action at the neuromuscular junction, attenuate or abolish muscle response, but have little effect on other electrophysiological recordings such as epidural recordings of D and I waves. Epidural recordings of the response to transcranial or spinal stimulation are often contaminated by activity in overlying muscle. Because muscle relaxants abolish such unwanted noise (**Fig. 10.10**), muscle relaxants might in fact improve the quality of recordings of D and I waves by eliminating the interference from the muscle activity on the recorded responses.

Effects on EMG Activity

The choice of anesthesia is probably more important for recordings of cortically evoked

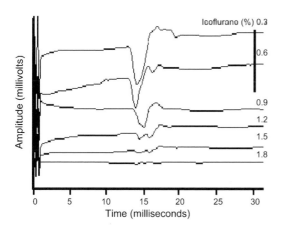

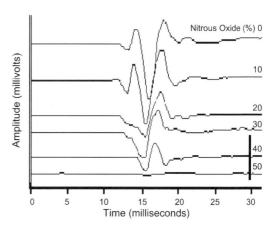

Figure 10.11: The effect of increasing isoflurane concentrations on the compound muscle action potential (CMAP) response to transcranial electrical motor cortex stimulation in a ketamine-anesthetized baboon. (Reprinted from: Sloan T. Anesthesia and motor evoked potential monitoring. In: Deletis V, Shils JL, eds. *Neurophysiology in Neurosurgery.* Amsterdam: Elsevier Science; 2002, with permission from Elsevier.)

Figure 10.12: The effect of increasing nitrous oxide concentrations on the CMAP response to transcranial electrical motor cortex stimulation in a ketamine-anesthetized baboon. As can be seen, the amplitude is progressively decreased with increasing concentrations, similar to isoflurane. (Reprinted from: Sloan T. Anesthesia and motor evoked potential monitoring. In: Deletis V, Shils JL, eds. *Neurophysiology in Neurosurgery.* Amsterdam: Elsevier Science; 2002, with permission from Elsevier.)

muscle responses (EMG potentials) than for any other modality of intraoperative monitoring. The level and the kind of anesthesia that is used affect the ability of cortical stimulation to elicit motor responses in different ways, but there might also be individual variations regarding the excitability of the motor system that should not be overlooked. The focus has been on the excitability of the motor cortex, but it seems more likely that the problems are related to the effect of anesthetics on the excitability of spinal cord neurons, including the alpha motoneurons, that depends on many factors, including internal spinal cord neural circuits and descending facilitatory input to the spinal cord (*see* Chap. 9).

Inhalation agents affect muscle MEPs elicited by a single impulse to an extent that the response cannot be recorded *(38,91)*. The effect of inhalation agents increases with the concentration, and even low concentrations (e.g., less than 0.2–0.5% isoflurane) affect the MEP *(38)* **(Fig. 10.11)**.

Nitrous oxide is a common component of general anesthesia. Nitrous oxide has been used combined with opioids ("nitrous-narcotic" anesthetic technique) in operations where cortically evoked muscle responses are recorded, and it has been used to supplement intravenous-based anesthetics such as propofol or etomidate *(38,92)*. Nitrous oxide depresses transcranial evoked muscle responses and it produces more profound changes in myogenic TC-MEP than any other inhalation anesthetic agent when compared at equipotent anesthetic concentrations *(92)*. The effect of nitrous oxide increases with its concentration **(Fig. 10.12)**, mimicking the effects of isoflurane (i.e., loss of compound muscle response **[Fig. 10.11]** and I waves at higher concentrations **[Fig. 10.8]**).

Studies have suggested that etomidate is an excellent agent for induction of anesthesia and its use during monitoring TC-MEPs *(38)*. Etomidate has the least degree of amplitude depression of muscle evoked potentials *(93)*.

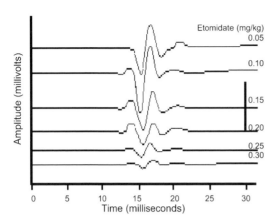

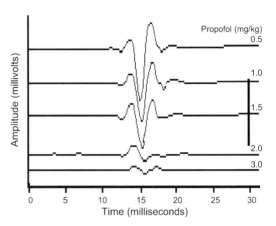

Figure 10.13: The effect of increasing doses of etomidate on the CMAP response to transcranial electrical motor cortex stimulation in a ketamine-anesthetized baboon. As can be seen, the amplitude is progressively decreased with increasing concentrations, similar to isoflurane. Note an initial increase in CMAP amplitude at low doses. (Reprinted from: Sloan T. Anesthesia and motor evoked potential monitoring. In: Deletis V, Shils JL, eds. *Neurophysiology in Neurosurgery*. Amsterdam: Elsevier Science; 2002, with permission from Elsevier.)

Figure 10.14: Effect of increasing doses of propofol on the CMAP response to transcranial electrical motor cortex stimulation in a ketamine-anesthetized baboon. (Reprinted from: Sloan T. Anesthesia and motor evoked potential monitoring. In: Deletis V, Shils JL, eds. *Neurophysiology in Neurosurgery*. Amsterdam: Elsevier Science; 2002, with permission from Elsevier.)

Clearly, the choice of anesthesia makes a marked difference in the ability to record MEP following transcranial stimulation of the motor tracts. Studies have suggested that the muscle response to transcranial magnetic stimulation can be more sensitive to the inhalation agents than electrical stimulation *(37)*. It appears that the best technique for monitoring of MEP is a total intravenous anesthesia technique (TIVA). Current drug combinations usually include opioids with ketamine, etomidate, or closely titrated propofol infusions *(38)* (*see* Chap. 16).

Like other anesthetics, its effect on motor evoked potentials increases with increasing concentration **(Fig. 10.13)**, but at low doses, it causes an initial increase of the amplitude of the motor responses and that effect is more prominent for transcranial magnetic evoked responses than transcranial electrical evoked responses. Etomidate has little effect on epidural-recorded D and I waves.

Propofol is a sedative–hypnotic intravenous agent that is rapidly metabolized. Propofol has gained extensive use and it is often combined with other agents such as opioids. It has an effect on the EEG similar to barbiturates and it has a depressant effect on motor response amplitude. Increasing concentrations of propofol have an effect on TC-MEPs similar to inhalation agents, with loss of CMAPs **(Fig. 10.14)** and I waves at higher concentrations *(38)*.

Mechanisms of Suppression of Motor Responses by Anesthetics

It has been hypothesized that the suppression of motor responses by anesthetics is caused by depression of the alphamotoneuron synapses. The fact that the D wave is resistant to anesthetic depression shows that the descending activity in the corticospinal tract is unaffected by anesthesia and that means that the excitatory synaptic input to the alpha motoneurons are probably also intact. The propriospinal interneurons that relay most of the descending activity in the corticospinal tracts to the alpha motoneurons (*see* Chap. 9, **Fig. 9.12**) are unlikely to be so sensitive to anesthesia that transmission of motor activity to the alpha motoneurons would be interrupted *(91)*. That has been taken to support the hypothesis that the effect of anesthetics on the MEP is on the alpha motoneuron cell level *(94)* and this hypothesis is further supported by the fact that the H reflex is also suppressed by halogenated inhalation anesthetics *(95)*. However, the effect on the alpha motoneuron might be a result of reduced excitatory input to alpha motoneurons rather than a direct effect on synaptic transmission to motoneurons. Suppression of alpha motoneurons could be caused by loss of I waves that provide a facilitatory influence on the alpha motoneurons and other facilitatory supraspinal and spinal input. Repetitive I waves appear to be necessary for producing myogenic responses in the unanesthetized state *(96)*.

The effect of anesthesia on the recorded EMG potentials is likely caused by reduced facilitatory influence from central structures on spinal motoneurons and local spinal circuits that normally enhance the excitability of the motoneuron.

The facilitatory inputs from supraspinal sources and from local spinal circuits are generated by long chains of neurons and are thus sensitive to anesthesia *(3)*.

The reduced facilitatory input to alpha motoneurons decreases their sensitivity in such a way that a larger excitatory postsynaptic potential (EPSP) is required to activate these motoneurons. That is most likely the main reason why a single impulse to the cerebral cortex cannot generate an EPSP of sufficient amplitude to reach this higher firing threshold in the anesthetized patient. The suppression of motor activity can be overcome by applying multiple impulses in rapid succession to the motor cortex. Such stimulation elicits multiple D waves (and possibly I waves), and temporal summation of this activity at the alpha motoneuron causes an EPSP of sufficient amplitude to reach

the threshold of alpha motoneurons, resulting in a peripheral nerve and motor response *(98)* **(Fig. 10.15)**. Such repeated stimulation can cause (temporal) summation of EPSPs at the alpha motoneurons to an extent that makes the membrane potential exceed the threshold even with the lack of facilitatory input. Technically, it is easy to generate a suitable train of electrical impulses for stimulating the motor cortex, but it is difficult to generate trains of magnetic impulses in a rapid succession.

The effect of temporal integration decreases with an increasing interval between the successive stimuli, and an optimal effect is achieved when intervals of 1–2 ms are used, but it can be effective for intervals up to 10 ms *(98)* (*see* **Fig. 10.15**). The optimal interstimulus interval can vary with the anesthetic effect *(65)*. If inhalation agents are used with the multipulse technique, a "tuning" of the stimulation interstimulus interval might improve the effectiveness of the monitoring.

The first time that a train of impulses is applied might not elicit a response, but repeated stimulation might lead to a muscle response **(Fig. 10.16)**. This effect is different from simple temporal summation of the EPSP and it might involve complex neural circuits. The facilitatory effect of activation of the monosynaptic stretch reflex (H reflex) can also help to overcome the anesthetic effect *(100)*.

There is no doubt that eliciting a motor response is complex, with the interaction between excitatory and inhibitory inputs to alpha motoneurons arriving from many different parts of the CNS, some naturally being from motor centers but other input arriving from, for example, the reticular formation and also from sensory systems, including the somatosensory cortex. This means that spinal stimulation techniques could monitor a mixture of sensory and motor pathways that might change with the type and dosage of the anesthetic agent used.

Muscle Relaxants

Any form of muscle relaxation brought about by a muscle endplate blocker (such as

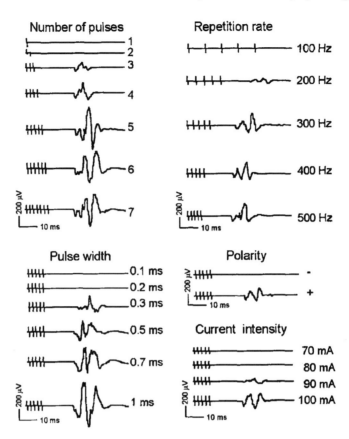

Figure 10.15: Influence of varying stimulation parameters on MEPs recorded from the thenar muscle and elicited by transcranial electrical stimulation with stimulating electrodes placed at $C_3 + 2$ cm or $C_4 + 2$ cm). The interstimulus interval was 2 ms, and a constant current of 100 mA was used. (Reprinted from: Neuloh G, Schramm J. Intraoperative neurophysiological mapping and monioring for supratentorial procedures. In: Delecrin J, Shils JL, eds. *Neurophysiology in Neurosurgery.* Amsterdam: Elsevier; 2002:339–401, with permission from Elsevier.)

curarelike agents) or by depolarizing agents (succinylcholine) affects the stimulus-elicited EMG potentials. Partial muscle blockade accomplished by muscle endplate-blocking drugs have a greater effect on responses that follow the initial response: the more so the shorter the time between stimuli. Continuous activity, such as mechanically elicited or injury-elicited (spontaneous) EMG activity, is attenuated more than single responses. If a short-acting endplate-blocking agent is used, it is important to be aware that the paralyzing

action disappears gradually and at a rate that differs from patient to patient and muscle group to muscle group. The rate at which muscle function is regained depends on the age, weight, and so forth of the patient, what other diseases might be present, and what other medications have been administered. During the time that the muscle-relaxing effect is decreasing, stimulation of a motor nerve with a train of electrical shocks will give rise to a relatively normal muscle contraction in response to the initial electrical stimulus, but the response to

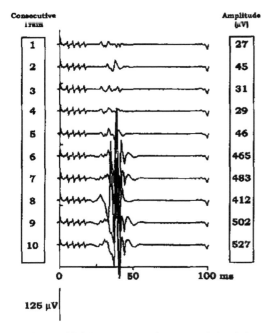

Figure 10.16: Response from the right abductor hallucis brevis muscle in response to repeated presentations of trains consisting of five stimuli; duration = 0.1 ms, intensity = 288 mA repeated at a rate of one per second, anode over C_3 and cathode over C_4. (Reprinted from: Sloan T. Anesthesia and motor evoked potential monitoring. In: Deletis V, Shils JL, eds. *Neurophysiology in Neurosurgery*. Amsterdam: Elsevier Science; 2002, with permission from Elsevier.)

subsequent impulses decreases and will be less than normal. The effect of muscle relaxants of the endplate-blocking type can be shortened ("reversed") by agents such as neostigmine that inhibit the breakdown of acetylcholine and thereby make better use of the acetylcholine receptor sites that are not blocked by the muscle relaxant used. However, a prerequisite for the use of such "reversing" agents is that a fair amount of muscle response (10–20%) has returned before reversing is attempted. It is important to note that such reversing does not immediately return the muscle function to normal, as the effect of the muscle relaxant will last for some time.

Some investigators have advocated the use of partial neuromuscular blockade that reduces the amplitude of the muscle response (a controlled degree of blockade [10–20% of single twitch remaining, or two of four twitches remaining in a "train of four" response]), whereas others have been reluctant to advocate such procedures and have recommended total absence of muscle-relaxing agents in the anesthesia regimen. This reluctance to use partial neuromuscular blockade comes from experience with monitoring of the facial nerve in operations for vestibular schwannoma. This is an area of anesthesia and monitoring that awaits the results of further studies.

11

Practical Aspects of Monitoring Cranial Motor Nerves

Introduction
Monitoring of the Facial Nerve
Monitoring the Motor Portion of CN V
Monitoring of Cranial Nerves III, IV, and VI
Monitoring Lower Cranial Motor Nerves
Transcranial Magnetic or Electric Stimulation

INTRODUCTION

Cranial motor nerves are at risk of being injured during many neurosurgical operations of the skull base, such as operations to remove different kinds of tumor. Cranial motor nerves can also be at risk during operations on the vascular system of the brain. The risk of loss of function of cranial motor nerves during surgical procedures can be reduced by appropriate use of intraoperative neurophysiological monitoring, thus decreasing the risk of postoperative deficits that have more or less severe consequences. Methods are available that can monitor the motor function of cranial nerves CN III, CN IV, CN V, CN VI, CN IX, CN X, CN XI, and CN XII.

When any one of these nerves are involved in tumors or when regions of the brain that are close to these nerves are manipulated or dissected, proper identification of the nerves intracranially is a prerequisite for preserving their functions.

Operations involving the face might place the branches of the facial nerve at risk for sustaining injury. The peripheral (extracranial) course of the facial nerve might also be at

risk of being injured during operations, such as those that involve the parotid gland. During operations in the chest and on the thyroid gland, the recurrence nerve (a branch of the vagal nerve, CN X) could sustain injury. CN IX, CN X, and CN XI might be at risk of being injured during operations around the jugular foramen, such as to remove tumors in that region. Carotid endarterectomy might also involve some of these lower cranial nerves. Some cranial motor nerves might sustain injuries along their extracranial course during operations in the upper neck.

This chapter describes how state-of-the-art electrophysiological methods can be used for intraoperative monitoring of cranial motor systems in different operations. Methods to monitor cranial motor nerves are described and discussions are presented on the benefits of such monitoring during neurosurgical operations in these particular nerves are at risk of being injured. We will begin with discussing monitoring of the facial nerve because the techniques used for that are applicable to monitoring of other cranial motor nerves.

MONITORING OF THE FACIAL NERVE

The facial nerve could be injured in a variety of operations, but most frequently it occurs

From: *Intraoperative Neurophysiological Monitoring: Second Edition*
By A. R. Møller
© Humana Press Inc., Totowa, NJ.

during operations to remove vestibular schwannoma.[1] Loss of facial function is a major handicap. Cosmetically, it is disastrous and, practically, a total loss of facial nerve function makes it difficult to eat. Additionally, eye problems are likely to develop because of the lack of tears produced; also, not being able to close the eyelid properly could result in injury to the cornea. Artificial tear solutions can be used to avoid drying of the cornea, which would result in eye pain and the risk of impaired vision resulting from corneal bruises. Implanting a (gold) spring in the eyelid that facilitates automatic closing of the eyelid by using gravitational force is helpful, but there is no doubt that loss of facial nerve function dramatically influences the life of anyone, and even a moderate impairment of facial function can be a severe handicap. Therefore, no effort should be spared to preserve the function of the facial nerve during operations in which it is being manipulated. Intraoperative neurophysiological monitoring of the function of the facial nerve is rewarding in that it can make a major difference in the outcome of an operation in which the facial nerve is involved or is being manipulated.

Facial Nerve Monitoring in Removal of Vestibular Schwannoma

Intraoperative monitoring of facial nerve function during operations to remove vestibular schwannoma is now officially recognized as a valuable adjunct to such operations. Thus, it was stated in a "Consensus Statement" of the National Institutes of Health Consensus Development Conference (held December 11–13, 1991) that

There is a consensus that intraoperative real-time neurologic monitoring improves the surgical management of vestibular schwannoma, including the preservation of facial nerve function and possibly improves hearing preservation by the use of intraoperative auditory brainstem response monitoring. New approaches to monitoring acoustic nerve function may provide more rapid feedback to the surgeon, thus enhancing their usefulness.

Intraoperative monitoring of cranial nerves V, VI, IX, X, and XI also has been described, but the full benefits of this monitoring remains to be determined. In the "Conclusion and Recommendation" of this report, it is stated: *"The benefit of routine intraoperative monitoring of the facial nerve has been clearly established. This technique should be included in surgical therapy of vestibular schwannoma. Routine monitoring of other cranial nerves should be considered," (Consensus Statement 1991, p. 19).* The benefit of intraoperative monitoring of the facial nerve has been confirmed in many subsequent studies.

Vestibular schwannoma comprise the great majority of the tumors in the cerebellopontine angle (CPA). The proximity between the facial nerve (CN VII) and the eighth cranial nerve (CN VIII), from which these tumors originate, places the facial nerve at risk when a vestibular schwannoma is being removed. Additionally, the anatomical proximity of the facial nerve to the eighth cranial nerve causes the tumor to "engulf" the facial nerve. Often, the tumor might have caused injury to the facial nerve prior to surgical intervention; therefore, some patients with vestibular schwannoma might have slight facial weakness before the operation. Even in cases in which the facial nerve is not directly involved in the vestibular schwannoma, there is a risk of injuring the facial nerve resulting from surgical manipulations in connection with removal of the tumor.

The facial nerve is more likely to become involved as a tumor increases in size. When a tumor is larger than 2.5 cm in diameter, there is a substantial possibility that the facial nerve has been displaced and often divided by the tumor. The facial nerve might be involved in the tumor capsule or it might be damaged by the tumor. The risk of the facial nerve being destroyed during tumor removal naturally is greater when a tumor has grown to such a size that it is engulfing the facial nerve or when the nerve has

---

[1]Vestibular schwannoma is now the official name for tumors of the eighth nerve that previously were (and still are) called acoustic tumors.

become embedded in the tumor capsule. Thus, removal of tumors larger than 2.5 cm has a higher risk of impairment or permanent loss of facial function than is the case of removal of smaller tumors.

The surgical removal of a tumor might result in a total and permanent loss of facial function even in cases in which the facial nerve is located outside of the capsule of the vestibular schwannoma. The most common reason for surgical damage to the facial nerve is that the surgeon did not know exactly where the facial nerve was located. Damage to the facial nerve might occur, even during removal of relatively small vestibular schwannoma, if the surgeon does not locate the facial nerve.

Improvements in surgical techniques and the introduction of intraoperative monitoring of facial function have improved this situation considerably, and the facial nerve is now rarely severely damaged during removal of tumors 2.5 cm in size or smaller when using monitoring techniques.

Electrical stimulation of the facial nerve intracranially using a handheld stimulating electrode, in conjunction with recording facial muscle contractions, has proven to be an important tool in identifying the nerve during removal of vestibular schwannoma. Recording of electromyographic (EMG) potentials from facial muscles is the most common way to measure the degree of activation of the facial nerve *(53,54,101–108)*. Earlier, mechanical sensors were used to detect the contraction of facial muscles *(108,109)*. Regardless of how facial muscle contractions are recorded, all of these methods involve probing the surgical field for the presence of the facial nerve so that the tumor mass can be removed without injuring the facial nerve.

Although intraoperative monitoring of the facial nerve was described as early as 1898 (see ref. 110) and electrical stimulation in connection with visual detection of contractions of the facial muscles was described almost half a century ago (111,112), it was not until the mid-1980s that intraoperative

monitoring of facial function came into general use during removal of vestibular schwannoma, as some investigators recognized that there was a need for better ways to detect contractions of facial muscles. To address this need, Delgado et al. (101) developed a method to record electrophysiologic responses from facial muscles (EMG); these investigators displayed and photographed EMG potentials on an oscilloscope observed by an assistant. They did not, however, use this method to help locate the facial nerve in the operative field, but, rather, to compare the waveform of the EMGs recorded during the operation for the purpose of detecting injuries to the facial nerve. Several years later, Sugita and Kobayashi (108) recognized the need for better communication between the surgeon and the person monitoring the EMG potentials regarding the significance of the contractions of facial muscles. These investigators found a way to make the contractions of facial muscles audible by using small accelerometers placed on the face to record the movements of the facial muscles. The electrical potentials generated by the accelerometers could then be amplified and presented through a loudspeaker. Later, other investigators described different methods to record facial movements in order to detect activation of the facial nerve (109,113).

Recording facial EMGs is now the prevailing method for recording facial muscle activity in operations to remove vestibular schwannoma, and presenting facial EMG recordings through a loudspeaker is now commonly done when operating near the facial nerve.

Recording Facial EMG. Because the purpose of monitoring facial nerve function (by recording facial EMGs) during operations to remove vestibular schwannoma is to identify all parts of the facial nerve, EMG potentials can be recorded differentially on a single channel, with one electrode placed in the mentalis/orbicularis oris muscles of the lower face and the other electrode placed in the orbicularis oculi/superior frontalis muscles to represent the upper face

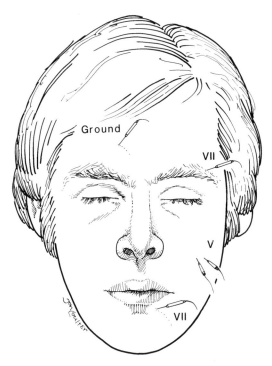

Figure 11.1: Schematic showing the placement of electrodes for recording responses from the facial muscles. The electrodes marked VII are to be connected to the differential input of the EMG amplifier. Also shown is the placement of electrodes for selective recording from the masseter muscle for monitoring the motor portion of the trigeminal nerve (CN V).

(**Fig. 11.1**). Such electrode placement makes it possible to record, on one single channel, EMG activity that is elicited by electrical stimulation of the facial nerve intracranially from muscles that represent most of the branches of the facial nerve. Such electrode placement also makes it possible to monitor muscle activity that results from mechanical stimulation of the facial nerve and activity that results from injury to the facial nerve (spontaneous activity). Needle electrodes such as platinum needle electrodes (Type E2; Grass Instrument Co., Braintree, MA) or similar disposable needle electrodes are suitable for such recordings and they should be secured by a good quality adhesive tape that has micropores (e.g., Blenderm surgical tape™, 3M Center, St. Paul, MN).

Making the recorded EMG activity audible is important because it provides valuable feedback to the surgeon, thereby helping to avoid injury to the facial nerve during removal of tumor tissue located close to the facial nerve. The audio-amplifier should be equipped with a circuitry that suppress the stimulus artifact *(54)*. There are complex computer-controlled systems on the market that allow an EMG signal to trigger a tone signal. Such systems are complex to use and offer little, if any, advantage over a simple system consisting of an amplifier and a (computer) display.

Some investigators have advocated independently recording facial muscle activity from two or more of the muscle groups that are innervated by different branches of the facial nerve on separate recording channels *(86)*. However, such dual recording has little advantage over a single-channel recording, obtained differentially between electrodes placed as described earlier, which provides information relevant to the function and preservation of all branches of the facial nerve.

When the facial muscle responses are recorded differentially between electrodes placed in the upper and lower face (**Fig. 11.1**), the responses from mastication muscles will also be included in the recording. The mastication muscles are innervated by the motor portion of the trigeminal nerve, and when operating on a large vestibular schwannoma, it might not be totally obvious from visual inspection of the surgical field which of the two nerves—the motor portion of the trigeminal nerve or the facial nerve—is being stimulated electrically. A tumor can push the facial nerve rostrally so that it becomes located close to the trigeminal nerve. However, the EMG responses from the muscles that are innervated by the trigeminal nerve can easily be differentiated from EMG responses generated by muscles that are innervated by the facial nerve because the latencies are different. Electrical stimulation of the motor portion of CN V intracranially elicits a muscle response in the masseter muscle with a latency of less than 2 ms, whereas the earliest response from the

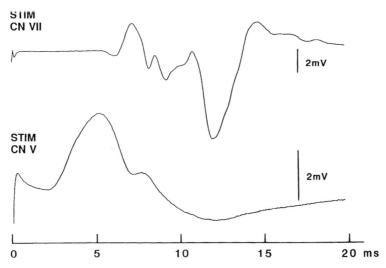

Figure 11.2: Upper curve: EMG potentials recorded differentially from electrodes placed in the superior orbicularis oculi/frontalis muscles and in the mentalis/orbicularis oris muscles (**Fig. 7.1**) in response to electrical stimulation of the facial nerve intracranially using a monopolar electrode. The stimuli were rectangular impulses of 150-μs duration presented at 5 pps and the stimulus strength was 1.0 V. **Lower curve:** EMG responses recorded from the same electrodes as shown in the upper curve, but when the motor portion of the fifth nerve was stimulated intracranially. The stimuli were rectangular impulses of 150-μs duration presented at 5 pps and the stimulus strength was 1.2 V. The results in both curves were obtained in a patient undergoing a microvascular decompression operation.

facial muscles to stimulation of the facial nerve intracranially is approx 6 ms (7 ms to its first peak) (*see* **Fig. 11.2**). Thus, EMG responses that appear with latencies longer than 5 ms are inevitably caused by contraction of facial muscles, whereas EMG responses with latencies shorter than 3 ms are caused by contraction of the masseter muscles or the temporalis muscles and, thus a result of stimulation of the trigeminal motor nerve.

It is also possible to differentiate between the responses of the muscles that are innervated by the facial nerve and those that are innervated by the trigeminal nerve by using an additional recording channel to record from the masseter muscle. Two needle electrodes placed close to each other in the masseter muscle and connected to a differential amplifier can serve that purpose (**Fig. 11.1**). With this electrode placement, the additional channel will only record from the masseter muscles, and the facial muscles will not contribute noticeably to the response.

Another advantage of having the facial EMGs displayed on a computer screen (in addition to making it possible to obtain latency measurements) is the possibility to observe the waveform of the response and determine its amplitude. When using supramaximal stimulation of the facial nerve, the amplitude of the EMG response is an approximate measure of how many nerve fibers have been activated (*see* Chap. 3). Observing the change (reduction) in the amplitude of the EMG response during an operation therefore provides information about the degree of injury to the facial nerve.

Monitoring the Facial Nerve During Removal of Large Tumors. In the beginning of an operation to remove a large vestibular schwannoma, electrical stimulation can be used to find regions of the tumor that do not contain any portion of the facial nerve. This enables the surgeon to remove large portions of the tumor without risk of injuring the facial nerve and it

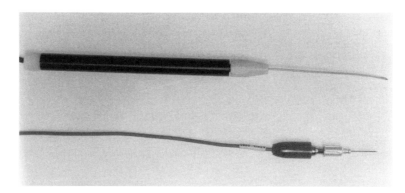

Figure 11.3: Monopolar handheld stimulating electrode.

reduces the operating time considerably. As removal of the tumor progresses, the goal is to continually identify the facial nerve so that surgical injury to the nerve can be avoided.

For finding a region of a tumor where there is no nerve present, a monopolar stimulating electrode (**Fig. 11.3**) connected to a stimulator that produces a relatively constant voltage of electrical stimulation is suitable *(54)*. When this technique is used in the first part of an operation to remove a medium-to-large tumor, considerable time is saved because large portions of the tumor can be removed without the risk of injuring the facial nerve *(54)*. In fact, a tumor mass located in the cerebellopontiue angle (CPA) should never be removed without first probing the portion of the tumor in question with the facial nerve stimulator; the tumor removal should only proceed if it is found to be unresponsive to electrical stimulation.

When the facial nerve is involved in a tumor, nerve tissue often cannot be distinguished visually from the surrounding tumor tissue; the only way to identify all parts of a nerve is by electrical stimulation. Such electrical probing of the surgical field must be done frequently so that the location of the nerve is always known during all phases of the tumor removal.

The facial nerve is often spread out in large tumors and it might have many separate fascicles and appear diffuse. Therefore, it is necessary to probe all parts of the tumor with the electrical stimulator to ensure that the entire facial nerve has been correctly identified; any nerve tissue that gives a facial response must be identified before tumor tissue is removed.

Some investigators have promoted the use of a bipolar stimulating electrode in connection with operations to remove vestibular schwannoma *(114)*. A bipolar stimulating electrode has greater spatial selectivity and is useful for finding the exact location of the facial nerve. A bipolar electrode is also ideal for determining which of two nerves located close to each other is the facial nerve. A bipolar stimulating electrode, however, is not suited for identifying regions of a tumor where no portion of the facial nerve is present. It would be ideal to have both monopolar and bipolar stimulating electrodes available during operations to remove vestibular schwannoma, but if simplicity is important, a monopolar electrode is the best choice.

Careful monitoring of facial muscle function should also be done during removal of the portions of a tumor located inside the internal auditory meatus and the facial nerve should be identified by electrically stimulation.

Mechanically Induced Facial Nerve Activity. When the facial nerve is directly involved in a tumor, it is often very fragile and does not have the visual appearance of a nerve. Therefore, removal of a tumor in which such a nerve is embedded is an extremely delicate process. Safe removal of such an adherent tumor can be greatly facilitated by continuously monitoring EMG-recorded responses while operating, because a slightly injured facial nerve will generate EMG activity in response to even slight mechanical manipulation. Removal of a tumor that is adherent to the facial nerve will cause clear and often strong EMG activity. A slightly injured nerve is sensitive to mechanical manipulation and gives off neural activity that elicits muscle contractions when the nerve is being manipulated *(115)*. By listening to the EMG responses made audible, the surgeon can tell when a manipulation might have caused damage to the nerve, and he/she can then stop or alter the manipulation *(54,104)*.

Mechanical stimulation of an injured motor nerve often causes sustained activity in the respective muscle that might last a few seconds, and sometimes longer, after it has been manipulated *(46,53,104)*. Similar mechanical stimulation of a normal (not injured) nerve might not result in any EMG activity or it might result in an EMG response that lasts only as long as the stimulation lasts.

The mechanically evoked muscle activity from surgical manipulation will cease within a short time after manipulation of a slightly injured facial nerve is discontinued, but if the nerve is severely injured, the induced muscle activity will continue for many seconds, or even minutes, after cessation of manipulation of the nerve. Such prolonged activity should be a warning to the surgeon that the manipulation has caused injury to the facial nerve that could impair facial function temporarily or even permanently. Patients who have had several episodes of sustained EMG activity during tumor removal will have more or less pronounced facial weakness postoperatively.

Monitoring facial EMG without electrically stimulating the facial nerve intracranially cannot identify the anatomical location of an uninjured facial nerve because manipulation of an uninjured nerve causes little, if any, EMG activity. This means that normal nerves can be severed or severely injured by mechanical manipulation without producing any noticeable EMG activity. The fact that it is possible to injure the facial nerve severely without generating noticeable EMG activity means that there is no substitute for electrical stimulation to identify a nerve when the nerve is located in the operative field.

The same recording electrodes and equipment as used to record evoked EMG potentials can naturally be used for continuous monitoring of the EMG activity from mechanical stimulation of the facial nerve, but it necessitates the display of "free-running EMG" during periods when electrical stimulation is not used. This possibility is included in most commercial intraoperative recording equipment.

Facial muscle contractions that are the result of injury to the facial nerve or are caused by mechanical stimulation of the nerve might not be evident by observing the patient's face, but they can easily be detected by recording EMG potentials and presented through a loudspeaker. The technique of gently scraping the tumor mass off the facial nerve while continuously listening to the EMG activity from facial muscles acts as feedback to the surgeon and can help to avoid serious and permanent injury to the facial nerve.

Heat as a Cause of Injury to the Facial Nerve. Sustained muscle activity can also result from electrocoagulation when heat spreads to the facial nerve. To reduce the risk of facial nerve injury electrocoagulation should be done with the lowest level of coagulation current and the coagulation should be applied for short periods, with intervals to allow for cooling of the tissues adjacent to the site of electrocoagulation.

Drilling the bone of the internal auditory meatus can also cause heat than can spread to the facial nerve and become a risk of injury to the facial nerve, as indicated by evoking EMG activity in facial muscles. Efficient cooling by irrigation with fluid of a suitable (low) temperature while drilling the bone of the internal auditory meatus can reduce the risk of injury to the facial nerve. Precooling the bone that is to be drilled can also be beneficial in such situations. Continuously monitoring facial EMG is a valuable tool for detecting when the facial nerve has been heated to a degree that poses a risk of permanent injury to the nerve.

Irrigation of a slightly injured facial nerve with saline, the temperature of which is below normal body temperature, often gives rise to facial muscle activity that lasts for many seconds. There is no evidence, however, that such EMG activity is a sign of risk to the function of the facial nerve. Irrigation with a fluid whose temperature is above normal body temperature imposes a serious risk to all neural tissue with which the fluid comes into contact and thus should be avoided at all times.

Identification of the Location of Injury

An injury to the facial nerve in patients with vestibular schwannoma is usually focal in nature and can be identified by comparing the latencies of the EMG responses to electrical stimulation at different locations along the nerve's intracranial course. The latency of the response typically increases in a stepwise fashion when the stimulating electrode is moved from a location that is distal to the injured section of the nerve to a location that is proximal to the injured section. When stimulation is performed proximal to an injured section of a nerve, the waveform of the recorded EMG potentials is often different (broader with multiple peaks, as seen on a computer screen) from those recorded when the nerve is stimulated at a location that is distal to the injured section. When made audible, the sounds of EMG responses are often distinctly different in response to stimulation at two such locations. These differences make it possible to identify the location of injured portions of the facial nerve.

When electrical stimulation is used to find the anatomical location of a conduction block in the facial nerve, it is important to understand that a nerve is an electrical conductor. Parts of a nerve that do not conduct nerve impulses actively conduct electrical impulses passively. When a monopolar, stimulating electrode is used and too high a stimulus intensity is utilized, it is possible that electrical stimulation of an injured part of the facial nerve might elicit an EMG response, because the stimulus current is conducted passively to the part of the nerve that is intact and conducts nerve impulses. When no response is obtained upon stimulating the facial nerve at a certain location, the stimulus intensity should not be increased too much, because this might result in misleading results because of such passive conduction of the stimulus current.

The EMG activity that is evoked by stimulation of the trigeminal nerve can be distinguished from that evoked by stimulation of the facial nerve on the basis of the latency of the responses even when the EMG activity from face muscles is recorded on a single channel, as shown in **Fig. 11.1.** EMG activity that is caused by injury or evoked by mechanical stimulation of the facial nerve cannot be distinguished from that caused by injury or evoked by mechanical stimulation of the trigeminal motor nerve by merely observing the response. Recording from the masseter muscle on a separate channel (*see* CN V in **Fig. 11.1**) offers the possibility of discriminating between muscle activity from the trigeminal nerves and that from the facial nerves evoked by mechanical stimulation of one of these two nerves as well as spontaneous activity that might be a sign of injury.

Indications for Grafting of the Facial Nerve

In situations where the response to facial nerve stimulation is lost during tumor removal and it is judged that the cause is conduction block in the facial nerve, the surgeon must make a decision regarding grafting the facial nerve in the same operation or wait and see if the function of the facial muscles recovers postoperatively. There are advantages in doing the grafting in the actual tumor operation, but it must be remembered that the absence of response to electrical stimulation of the facial nerve actually does not provide information regarding recovery of facial function. Neurapraxia and axonotmesis cannot be distinguished from more severe kinds of nerve injuries (neurotmesis) on the basis of a electrophysiological test. This means that electrophysiological tests cannot provide guidance regarding the prognosis for recovery of the facial nerve. Visual inspection must be the guide for decisions about whether to do a grafting in the tumor operation.

In summary, continuous monitoring of facial EMG in conjunction with frequent electrical stimulation of the intracranial portion of the facial nerve is critical in reducing the risk of injury to the facial nerve during operations to remove vestibular schwannoma. Using the techniques just described, total tumor removal is often possible with preservation of facial function, even in large vestibular schwannoma.

Other Tumors of the Skull Base

In operations to resect large tumors of the skull base, it is beneficial to be able to monitor the function of the facial nerve intraoperatively (together with several other cranial nerves). The same technique for identifying the facial nerve as described for use during removal of vestibular schwannoma is useful in other skull base tumors, which are often large by the time they are diagnosed and operated on and, therefore, the anatomy is often greatly distorted, resulting in uncertainty about the identity of cranial nerves. During such operations, other cranial nerves are being monitored, and the number of recording electrodes placed on the face could be large.

Other Tumors of the Cerebellopontine Angle. Although vestibular schwannoma are, by far, the most common type of tumor in the CPA, other tumors can occur in this area and removal of such tumors could place the facial nerve at risk. However, meningiomas in the CPA seldom involve the facial nerve to the same extent as do vestibular schwannoma, but intraoperative monitoring of the facial nerve during operations on meningiomas using a technique similar to that used during removal of vestibular schwannoma might be beneficial in reducing the risk of injury to the facial nerve from mechanical manipulation or from heat from electrocoagulation.

Epidermoid cysts (or cholesteatomas) and other rare masses might also be located in the CPA, and although they seldom involve the facial nerve directly, the availability of facial nerve stimulation and recording of facial EMG potentials might be useful in their removal and it might facilitate preservation of the facial nerve in such operations.

Tumors of the facial nerve itself (facial nerve neuroma) occur rarely, and it is usually not possible in these cases to save the facial nerve. For such cases, it is important that the surgeon has expertise in nerve grafting. A facial nerve stimulator is helpful in identifying the facial nerve and in finding the location of a possible conduction block in order to appropriately place a nerve graft.

Other Operations Involving the Intracranial Portion of the Facial Nerve

There are several other operations in which it is valuable to be able to identify the intracranial portion of the facial nerve. Patients with hemifacial spasm (HFS) have a blood vessel in close contact with the intracranial portion of their facial nerve near the brainstem (root exit zone [REZ]). When this blood vessel is moved away from the facial nerve and a soft implant is placed between the vessel and the nerve (microvascular decompression [MVD]), such patients are cured (*see* Chap. 15). Because monitoring the abnormal muscle response that is used to guide the surgeon in the operation involves recording facial EMG potentials, the same setup can be used for monitoring intraoperative injuries to the facial nerve in such patients. Continuous monitoring of facial muscle EMG makes it possible to detect spontaneous facial muscle activity that might be caused by surgical manipulation of the facial nerve, as was described earlier. Surgical manipulation and, particularly, heating from electrocoagulation can result in continuous EMG activity, as can compression of the facial nerve from, for instance, too large of an implant being placed between the facial nerve and the offending blood vessel.

When the facial nerve is not visible in the operative field or when there is doubt about which of several cranial nerves is the facial nerve, intraoperative neurophysiological monitoring as described earlier is beneficial. For example, it is important to be able to identify the facial nerve in operations to section the vestibular nerve to treat intractable vertigo.

Another example of an operation where the facial nerve might be at risk is MVD of the eighth or fifth nerve to treat vertigo or trigeminal neuralgia (*see* Chap. 14). Identification of the facial nerve is difficult in some of these operations solely on anatomical grounds and visual inspection. Electrical stimulation in connection with recordings of facial EMG potentials offers an easy way to positively identify the facial nerve. This is particularly important when the operation is complicated, for example, when patients have been operated on previously and scar tissue has developed or when there are other reasons for anatomical abnormalities. In such cases, extensive dissection would often be necessary to determine the identity of the different nerves anatomically by visual inspection only, whereas it is easy to identify the facial nerve by using electrical stimulation.

Monitoring the Extracranial Portion of the Facial Nerve

The facial nerve is also at risk of being injured when it is dissected and manipulated along its peripheral course in the face, as well as where it travels in its bony canal (the Fallopian canal) before reaching the stylomastoid foramen. The same technique for identifying the facial nerve as described earlier in this chapter can be used to reduce the risk of injury to the peripheral branches of the facial nerve. For example, removal of tumors of the parotid gland could result in injury to the facial nerve, but with proper identification of the various branches of the facial nerve that might be involved in the tumor, it is often possible to avoid injury to any branch of the facial nerve (116). When the area around a parotid tumor is dissected, a facial nerve stimulator should be used to identify the different branches of the facial nerve.

It is important to note that the latency of the EMG responses to stimulation of the peripheral portion of the facial nerve is much shorter than it is in response to stimulation of the facial nerve intracranially. Thus, a facial nerve stimulator that makes use of an artifact suppression circuit to inactivate the audio-amplifier during the period when the artifact occurs might also suppress some of the actual EMG response if the setting of the duration of the suppression is the same as used for intracranial stimulation of the facial nerve. Displaying of EMG potentials on a computer screen is usually not affected by

artifact suppression and the entire response will show on the screen, even if the duration of artifact suppression is set too long to make it audible.

It is important to identify the facial nerve in other kinds of operations that involve the face. Operations such as those to correct temporomandibular joint disorders might result in injury to a branch of the facial nerve from the incision because the facial nerve sometimes has an abnormal course. In repairing trauma to the face, it is important to be able to identify the facial nerve to minimize the risks of injuring it.

After an accident, or after certain operations, neuroma might form on the facial nerve; an operation might be required just to remove such neuroma. The location of neuroma that lie in the path of nerve conduction ("neuroma in continuity") can be determined intraoperatively by recording EMG potentials while stimulating the nerve electrically at different locations along its path. This is discussed in more detail in Chap. 13 in connection with intraoperative measurements of neural conduction in peripheral nerves.

MONITORING THE MOTOR PORTION OF CN V

To monitor the motor portion of CN V, similar techniques can be used, as those described for intraoperative monitoring of the facial nerve. It was mentioned earlier in this chapter that the responses from the muscles of mastication that are innervated by the motor portion of the trigeminal nerve (CN V) can be observed by recording the muscle response from a pair of recording needle electrodes placed in the masseter muscle (**Fig. 11.1**). The response from intracranial stimulation of the trigeminal nerve has a much shorter latency than that of the facial nerve (**Fig. 11.2**).

MONITORING OF CRANIAL NERVES III, IV, AND VI

Skull base tumors can invade the cavernous sinus and thereby directly involve several cranial

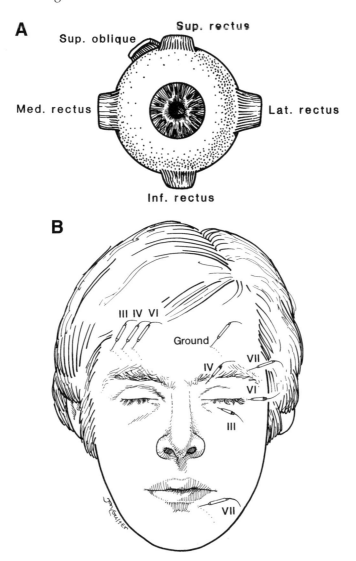

Figure 11.4: (A) Anatomy of the orbit showing the extraocular muscles; **(B)** schematic showing the electrode placement for recording EMG responses from the extraocular muscles and facial muscles (CN VII).

motor nerves, particularly those innervating the extraocular muscles (CN III, CN IV, and CN VI). Loss of function of the trochlear nerve (CN IV), which innervates the superior oblique muscle, is inconvenient to the patient but does not interfere significantly with the use of the eye in question. Loss of function of the abducens nerve (CN VI), which innervates the lateral (or external) rectus muscle, impairs the use of the affected eye noticeably. Loss of function of the oculomotor nerve (CN III), which innervates all the other extraocular muscles (**Fig. 11.4A**), is a serious complication because it essentially results in functional blindness of the affected eye. CN III has autonomic fibers that control the size of the pupil and the ciliary muscle that controls accommodation. Loss of these parts of CN III contributes to the impairment of vision of the affected eye.

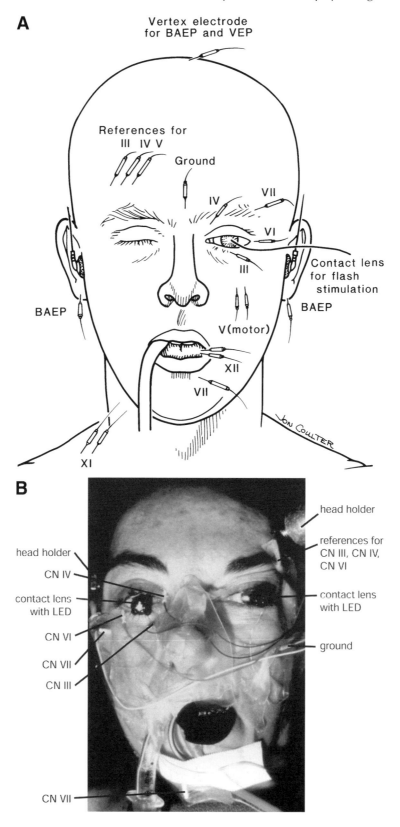

Tumors of the skull base tend to be large and they, therefore, often distort the anatomy. For this reason, one of the main purposes of intraoperative neurophysiological monitoring in operations to remove skull base tumors is to aid the surgeon in identifying the anatomical location of the cranial nerves that are involved.

To record EMG potentials from extraocular muscles, needle electrodes can be placed in the lateral rectus muscle (CN VI), the inferior rectus muscle (CN III), and the superior oblique muscle (CN IV) *(117)*. Fine, platinum needle electrodes (Type E2; Grass Instrument Co., Braintree, MA) or similar disposable needle electrodes are placed in, or near, these muscles percutaneously as shown in **Figs. 11.4B** and **11.5**. It is not necessary for the electrodes to penetrate the respective muscles because the electrodes only need to be close to the muscles to produce EMG responses with amplitudes sufficient to be visible on a computer screen without any averaging. Care must be taken not to injure the eye globe. These risks can be minimized by placing the electrodes so that they point away from the globe and securing them in that position using a good quality plastic adhesive tape (e.g., Blenderm^R; 3M, Center, St. Paul, MN). Reference electrodes are placed on the forehead on the opposite side so that they do not record activity of the facial muscles on the affected side (**Fig. 11.4B**).

Identifying the anatomical location of the cranial nerves that innervate the extraocular muscles can be done by probing the surgical field by a handheld monopolar stimulating electrode (**Fig. 11.3**) while recording EMG potentials from the extraocular muscles *(117,118)* (**Figs. 11.4B** and **11.5**). Similar stimulation parameters such as those described for stimulation of the facial nerve are suitable, although a slightly higher stimulus strength

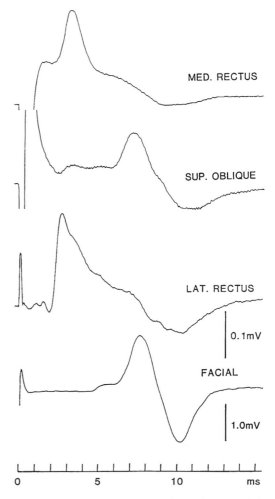

Figure 11.6: Examples of EMG potentials recorded from the extraocular muscles and from the facial muscles with electrodes placed similar to those in **Fig. 11.4**. The stimulation was applied to the intracranial portions of the respective nerves using a monopolar electrodes (as shown in **Fig. 11.3**).

might be required (1–1.5 V when using impulses of 100-μs duration and a semi-constant-voltage generator). Using a bipolar stimulating electrode

---

Figure 11.5: (*Opposite page*) (**A**) Schematic of placement of electrodes for monitoring cranial nerves. Electrode placements for ABR and visual evoked potentials were also recorded. Note the earphone and the contact lenses with light emitting diodes for monitoring visual evoked potentials. (Reprinted from: Møller AR. Intraoperative monitoring of evoked potentials: an update. In: Wilkins RH, Rengachary SS, eds. *Neurosurgery Update I: Diagnosis, Operative Technique, and Neurooncology.* New York, NY: McGraw-Hill; 1990:169–176, with permission from McGraw-Hill.) (**B**) Electrode placement in a patient in whom intraoperative recordings were made from the extraocular muscles and the facial muscles.

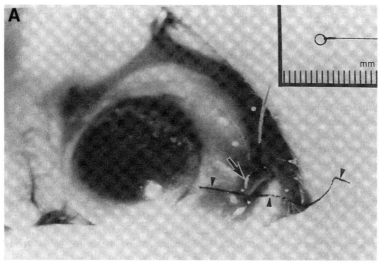

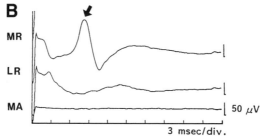

Figure 11.7: (**A**) Ring electrode for recording EMG potentials from extraocular muscles. (Reprinted from: Sekiya T, Hatayama T, Iwabuchi T, Maeda S. A ring electrode to record extraocular muscle activities during skull base surgery. *Acta Neurochir. (Wien)* 1992;117:66–69, with permission from Springer-Verlag.) (**B**) Recordings from two extraocular muscles using the electrode shown in (**A**) and recordings from the masseter muscle. MR: Medial rectus muscles; LR: Lateral rectus muscle; MA: masseter muscles. (Reprinted from: Sekiya T, Hatayama T, Iwabushi T, Maeda S. Intraoperative recordings of evoked extraocular muscle activities to monitor ocular motor function. *Neurosurgery* 1993;32:227–235, with permission from Williams and Wilkins.)

has the same advantages and disadvantages as described for monitoring the facial nerve.

The recorded potentials from the extraocular muscles have amplitudes from 0.2 to 1 mV (**Fig. 11.6**). In addition to displaying the recorded EMG responses of the respective muscles on a computer screen (**Fig. 11.6**) it is advantageous to make the responses audible— one at a time—in the same way as described for potentials recorded from the facial muscles.

Recently, Sekiya and co-workers *(120)* have described methods to record EMG potentials from extraocular muscles using noninvasive

electrodes. These electrodes (**Fig. 11.7A**) are in the form of small wire loops that are placed under the eyelids. This method provides an important alternative to using invasive methods to record EMG potentials from the extraocular muscles. The amplitudes of the EMG potentials recorded with these electrodes (**Fig. 11.7B**) are somewhat smaller than those that can be recorded from needle electrodes (**Fig. 11.6**), but the potentials are large enough to be visualized directly on a computer screen without any averaging and the EMG potentials can be made audible.

MONITORING LOWER CRANIAL MOTOR NERVES

Monitoring of lower cranial nerves (CN IX, CN X, CN XI, and CN XII) *(122–124)* is valuable in connection with removal of many kinds of skull base tumors *(118)*. The motor portion of the glossopharyngeal nerve (CN IX) can be monitored intraoperatively *(122–124)*, although CN IX only innervates one muscle, the stylopharyngeal muscle. Recording from this muscle, or its vicinity, can be done by placing a pair of recording electrodes in the soft palate on the side to be operated. The electrodes should be placed only after the patient is intubated and all other tubes that are inserted through the mouth are in place. The electrodes can be secured in place by anchoring the electrode leads to the face by adhesive tape. The EMG potentials recorded in response to simulation of the glossopharyngeal nerve intracranially typically have latencies of approx 7 ms *(122)*. Because the glossopharyngeal nerve is involved in the control of the vascular system, caution should be exercised when stimulating this nerve electrically, and cardiovascular signs should be watched closely.

A branch of CN X, the recurrence nerve, is a motor nerve that innervates the laryngeal muscles. Monitoring of this motor portion of the vagus nerve can be done by recording EMG potentials from larynx musculature, such as the vocalis musculature *(122,123)*. Some investigators have placed EMG electrodes in the laryngeal musculature, but that requires the use of a laryngoscope and some technical skill. The electrodes can be placed in the vocal cords or, even better, in the supraglottic larynx (false vocal cords) *(122,123)*.

The EMG potentials can also be recorded from larynx muscles by electrodes that are placed percutaneous in the cricothyroid muscle *(124)*. The cricothyroid muscle responds to stimulation of both the recurrence laryngeal nerve and the superior laryngeal nerve (which is a branch of CN X). Verification of correct electrode placement can be done in the awake patient, by having the patient vocalize a high-pitched sound and recording EMG activity, which shows maximal amplitude when the recording electrodes are correctly placed. Some experience makes it possible to place such electrodes correctly in anesthetized patients. Monitoring EMG from laryngeal muscles can also be done by using metallic recording tape wrapped around the tracheal tube acting as EMG electrodes *(122)*.

Because the vagus nerve innervates many systems in the abdomen and is involved with respiratory, cardiac, and intestinal functions, electrical stimulation of CN X should be done with caution.

The spinal accessory nerve (CN XI) can be monitored intraoperatively by recording from the sternocleidomastoid muscle or the trapezius muscle, which are both innervated by CN XI (**Fig. 11.5A**). The EMG responses from these muscles can easily be recorded by placing a pair of electrodes into the respective muscles. When stimulating CN XI electrically, however, there is need for caution because such stimulation could cause so strong a contraction that a rupture of tendons or a dislocation of joints might occur or the patient might move on the operating table in a way that poses a risk during the time that intracranial procedures are in progress.

The hypoglossal nerve (CN XII) innervates the tongue, and if its function is lost bilaterally, a serious handicap will develop as a result of atrophy of the tongue, such as difficulty with, or inability to, speak and swallow. Monitoring of CN XII can be done by recording EMG potentials from the tongue (**Fig. 11.8**). Monitoring the hypoglossal nerve should be done when operating in the area of the clivus and foramen magnum; such monitoring can often help save this small nerve from being injured. Recording EMG potentials from the tongue while probing the surgical field with a hand-held electrical stimulating electrode makes it possible to locate CN XII. Monitoring of the response to such stimulation can also verify the integrity of this nerve *(117,123)*.

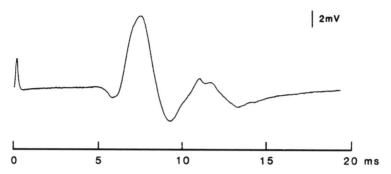

Figure 11.8: Example of EMG recordings from two needle electrodes that were placed on the side of the tongue in response to electrical stimulation of CN XII intracranially. These recordings were obtained during an operation to remove a large chordoma in which the hypoglossal nerve was embedded. The stimuli were rectangular impulses of 150-μs duration presented at 5 pps and the stimulus strength was 1.2 V.

TRANSCRANIAL MAGNETIC OR ELECTRIC STIMULATION

Transcranial magnetic stimulation was introduced for stimulating peripheral nerves as well as the motor cortex transcranially, as described in Chap. 10. Transcranial electrical stimulation *(34,43)* is in use for the same purpose (Chap. 10). Transcranial magnetic stimulation has not been used routinely for stimulation of the trigeminal and facial nerves. Some basic properties of magnetic stimulation have, however, been studied in connection with the use of magnetic stimulation in the operating room *(64,90,125–128)*. These studies have provided some insight in the mechanisms of stimulating cranial nerves by magnetic stimulation. Magnetic stimulation of these nerves could be of importance in diagnostics.

References to Section III

1. Kuypers HGJM. Anatomy of the descending pathways. In: Brookhart JM, Mountcastle VB, eds. *Handbook of Physiology: The Nervous System.* Bethesda, MD: American Physiological Society; 1981:597–666.
2. Brodal P. *The Central Nervous System.* New York: Oxford University Press; 1998.
3. Møller AR. *Neural Plasticity and Disorders of the Nervous System.* Cambridge: Cambridge University Press; 2005, in press.
4. Yoshida M, Rabin A, Anderson A. Monosynaptic inhibition of pallidal neurons by axon collaterals of caudatonigral fibers. *Exp. Brain Res.* 1972;15:33–47.
5. Albin RL, Young AB, Penney JB. The functional anatomy of basal ganglia origin. *Trends Neurosci.* 1989;12:366–375.
6. Jankovic J. Tics in other neurological disorders. In: Kurlan R, ed. *Handbook of Tourette's Syndrome and Related Tic and Behavioral Disorders.* New York, NY: Marcel Dekker; 1993: 167–182.
7. Alexander GE, Crutcher MD, DeLong MR. Basal ganglia–thalamocortical circuits: parallel substrates for motor, oculomotor, "prefrontal" and "limbic" functions. *Prog. Brain Res.* 1990; 85:119–146.
8. Alexander GE, Crutcher MD. Functional architecture of basal ganglia circuits: neural substrate of parallel processing. *Trends Neurosci.* 1990;13:266–271.
9. Blandini F, Tassorelli C, Greenamyre JT. Movement disorders. In: Dani SU, Hori A, Walter GF, eds. *Principle of Neural Aging.* Amsterdam: Elsevier; 1997.
10. Bennett DA, Beckett LA, Murray AM, et al. Prevalence of parkinsonian signs and associated mortality in a community population of older people. *N. Engl. J. Med.* 1996;334:71–76.
11. DeLong MR. Primate models of movement disorders of basal ganglia origin. *Trends Neurosci.* 1990;13:281–285.
12. Temel Y, Visser-Vandewalle V. Surgery in Tourette syndrome. *Mov. Disord.* 2004;19:3–14.
13. Daube JR, Reagan TJ, Sandok BA, Westmoreland BF. *Medical Neurosciences*, 2nd ed. Rochester, MN: Mayo Foundation; 1986.
14. Porter R, Lemon R. Cortical function and voluntary movement. Oxford: Clarendon; 1993.
15. White SR, Neuman RS. Facilitation of spinal motoneuron by 5-hydroxytryptamine and noradrenaline. *Brain Res.* 1980;185:1–9.
16. Davis M. The role of the amygdala in fear and anxiety. *Ann. Rev. Neurosci.* 1992;15: 353–375.
17. Humphrey DR, Corrie WS. Properties of pyramidal tract neuron system within functionally defined subregion of primate motor cortex. *J. Neurophysiol.* 1978;41:216–243.
18. Burke D. Spasticity as an adaptation to pyramidal tract injury. In: Waxman SG, ed. *Functional Recovery in Neurological Disease.* New York, NY: Raven; 1988.
19. Pierrot-Deseilligny E. Propriospinal transmission of part of the corticospinal excitation in humans. *Muscle Nerve* 2002;26:155–172.
20. Nicolas G, Marchand-Pauvert V, Burke D, Pierrot-Deseilligny E. Corticospinal excitation of presumed cervical propriospinal neurons and its reversal to inhibition in humans. *J. Physiol.* 2001;533:903–919.
21. Andersen P, Hagan PJ, Phillips CG, Powell TPS. Mapping by microstimulation of overlapping projections from area 4 to motor units of the baboon's hand. *Proc. R. Soc. London Ser. B* 1975;188:31–60.
22. Wiesendanger M. The pyramidal tract. its structure and function. In: Towe AL, Luschei ES, eds. *Handbook of Behavioral Neurobiology.* New York, NY: Plenum; 1981:401–490.
23. Penfield W, Boldrey E. Somatic motor and sensory representation in the cerebral cortex of man as studied by electrical stimulation. *Brain* 1937;60:389–443.
24. Penfield W, Rasmussen T. The cerebral cortex of man: a clinical study of localization of function. New York, NY: Macmillan; 1950.
25. Edgeley SA, Eyre JA, Lemon R, Miller S. Excitation of the corticospinal tract by electromagnetic

and electrical stimulation of the scalp in the macaque monkey. *J. Physiol. (Lond.)* 1990;425: 301–320.

26. Amassian VE, Quirk GJ, Stewart M. A comparison of corticospinal activation by magnetic coil and electrical stimulation of monkey motor cortex. *Electroenceph. Clin. Neurophysiol.* 1990;77:390–401.

27. Kitagawa H, Møller AR. Conduction pathways and generators of magnetic evoked spinal cord potentials: a study in monkeys. *Electroenceph. Clin. Neurophysiol.* 1994;93: 57–67.

28. Deletis V. Intraoperative neurophysiology and methodologies used to monitor the functional integrity of the motor system. In: Deletis V, Shils JL, eds. *Neurophysiology in Neurosurgery.* Amsterdam: Academic; 2002:25–51.

29. Kaneko K, Kawai S, Funchigami Y, Morieta H, Ofuji A. The effect of current direction induced by transcranial magnetic stimulation on corticospinal excitability in human brain. *Electroenceph. Clin. Neurophysiol.* 1966;101:478–482.

30. Maccabee PJ, Amassian VE, Zimann P, Wassermann EM, Deletis V. Emerging application in neuromagnetic stimualtion. In: Levin K, Luders H, eds. *Comprehensive Clinical Neurophysiology.* Philadelphia, PA: W.B. Saunders; 1999:325–347.

31. Hicks R, Burke D, Stephen J, Woodforth I, Crawford M. Corticospinal volleys evoked by electrical stimulation of human motor cortex after withdrawal of volatile anaesthetics. *J. Physiol.* 1992;456:293–404.

32. Deletis V. Intraoperative monitoring of the functional integrety of the motor pathways. In: Devinsky O, Beric A, Dogali M, eds. *Advances in Neurology: Electrical and Magnetic Stimulation of the Brain.* New York, NY: Raven; 1993;201–214.

33. Lazzaro Di V, Oliviero A, Pilato F, et al. Corticospinal volleys evoked by transcranial stimulation of the brain in concious humans. *Neurol. Res.* 2003;25:143–150.

34. Barker AT, Jalinous R, Freeston IL. Non-invasive magnetic stimulation of the human motor cortex. *Lancet* 1985;1:1106–1107.

35. Amassian VE. Animal and human motor system neurophysiology related to intraoperative monitoring. In: Deletis V, Shils JL, eds. *Neurophysiology in Neurosurgery.* Amsterdam: Academic; 2002:3–23.

36. Møller AR. *Sensory Systems: Anatomy and Physiology.* Amsterdam: Academic; 2003.

37. Sloan T, Angell D. Differential effect of isoflurane on motor evoked potentials elicited by transcortical electric or magnetic stimulation. In: Jones SS, Boyd S, Hetreed M, Smith NJ, eds. *Handbook of Spinal Cord Monitoring.* Hingham, MA: Kluwer Academic; 1993: 362–367.

38. Sloan T. Anesthesia and motor evoked potential monitoring. In: Deletis V, Shils JL, eds. *Neurophysiology in Neurosurgery.* Amsterdam: Elsevier Science; 2002.

39. Rösler KM. Transcranial magnetic brain stimulation: a tool to investigate central motor pathways. *News Physiol. Sci.* 2001;16:297–302.

40. Jankowska E, Lundberg A. Interneurons in the spinal cord. *Trends Neurosci.* 1981;4:230–233.

41. Wolpaw JR, O'Keefe JA. Adaptive plasticity in the primate spinal stretch reflex: evidence of a two-phase process. *J. Neurosci.* 1984;4: 2718–2724.

42. Brown RH, Nash CL. Current status of spinal cord monitoring. *Spine* 1979;4:466–478.

43. Merton PA, Morton HB. Electrical stimulation of human motor and visual cortex through the scalp. *J. Physiol.* 1980;305:9P–10P.

44. Marsden CD, Merton PA, Morton HB. Direct electrical stimulation of corticospinal pathways through the intact scalp in human subjects. *Adv. Neurol.* 1983;39:387–391.

45. Sloan TB, Heyer EJ. Anesthesia for intraoperative neurophsysiologic monitoring of the spinal cord. *J. Clin. Neurophysiol.* 2002;19:430–443.

46. Daube J, Harper C. Surgical monitoring of cranial and peripheral nerves. In: Desmedt J, ed. *Neuromonitoring in Surgery.* Amesterdam: Elsevier Science; 1989:115–138.

47. Tabaraud F, Boulesteix JM, Moulies D, et al. Monitoring of the motor pathway during spinal surgery. *Spine* 1993;18:546–550.

48. Burke D, Hicks R, Stephen J, Woodforth I, Crawford M. Assessment of corticospinal and somatosensory conduction simultaneously during scoliosis surgery. *Electroenceph. Clin. Neurophysiol.* 1992;85:388–396.

49. Deletis V. Intraoperative monitoring: motor evoked potentials methodology. In: Deletis V, Shils JL, eds. *Proceedings, Intraoperative Neurophysiological Monitoring in Neurosurgery.* New York, NY: Hyman-Newman Institute for Neurology and Neurosurgery; 2004:24–30.

50. Edmonds HL, Paloheimo MPJ, Backmann MH, et al. Transcranial magnetic motor evoked potentials (tc MMEP) for functional monitoring of motor pathways during scoliosis surgery. *Spine* 1989;14:683–686.

51. Stecker MM. Transcranial electric stimulation of motor pathways: a theoretical analysis. *Comput. Biol. Med.* 2005;35:133–155.

52. Deletis V, Rodi Z, Amassian VE. Neurophysiological mechanisms underlying motor evoked potentials (MEPs) elicited by a train of electrical stimuli: Part 2. Relationship between epidurally and muscle recorded MEPs in man. *Clin. Neurophysiol.* 2001;112:445–452.

53. Yingling C, Gardi J. Intraoperative monitoring of facial and cochlear nerves during acoustic neuroma surgery. *Otolaryngol. Clin. North Am.* 1992;25:413–448.

54. Møller AR, Jannetta PJ. Preservation of facial function during removal of acoustic neuromas: use of monopolar constant voltage stimulation and EMG. *J. Neurosurg.* 1984;61:757–760.

55. Prass R, Lueders H. Constant-current versus constant-voltage stimulation. *J. Neurosurg.* 1985;62:622–623.

56. Rattay F. Ways to approximate current-distance relations for electrical stimulated fibres. *J. Theor. Biol.* 1987;125:339–349.

57. Journée HL. The biological interface and hardware of electrical stimulation. In: Deletis V, Shils JL, eds. *Proceedings, Intraoperative Neurophysiological Monitoring in Neurosurgery.* New York, NY: Hyman-Newman Institute for Neurology and Neurosurgery; 2004:128–131.

58. Novak K, De Camargo AB, Neuwirth M, Kothbauer K, Amassian VE, Deletis V. The refractory period of fast conducting corticospinal tract axons in man and its implications for intra-operative monitoring of motor evoked potentials. *Clin. Neurophysiol.* 2004;115:1931–1941.

59. Hausmann ON, Min K, Boos N, Ruetsch YA, Erni T, Curt A. Transcranial electrical stimulation: significance of fast versus slow charge delivery for intra-operative monitoring. *Clin. Neurophysiol.* 2002;113:1532–1535.

60. Nowak LG, Bullier J. Axons, but not cell bodies, are activated by electrical stimulation in cortical gray matter. I. Evidence from chronaxie measurements. *Exp. Brain Res.* 1998;118:477–488.

61. Ojemann GA. Effect of cortical and subcortical stimulation on human language and verbal memory. *Res. Pub. Assoc. Res. Nerv. Ment. Dis.* 1988;66:101–115.

62. Amassian VE, Eberle L, Maccabee PJ, Cracco RQ. Modelling magnetic coil excitation of human cerebral cortex with a peripheral nerve immersed in a brain-shaped volume conductor: the significance of fiber bending in excitation. *Electroenceph. Clin. Neurophysiol.* 1992;85:291–301.

63. Werhahn KJ, Fong JKY, Meyer BU, et al. The effect of magnetic coil orientation on the latency of surface EMG and single motor unit responses in the first dorsal interosseous muscle. *Electroenceph. Clin. Neurophysiol.* 1994;93: 138–146.

64. Schmid UD, Møller AR, Schmid J. Transcranial magnetic stimulation of the facial nerve: intraoperative study on the effect of stimulus parameters on the excitation site in man. *Muscle Nerve* 1992;15:829–836.

65. Sloan TB, Rogers JN. Inhalational anesthesia alters the optimal interstimulus interval for multipulse transcranial motor evoked potentials in the baboon. *J. Neurosurg. Anesth.* 1996;8:346.

66. Day BL, Thompson PD, Dick JPR, Nakashima K, Marsden CD. Different sites of action of electrical and magnetic stimulation of the human brain. *Neurosci. Lett.* 1987;75:101–106.

67. Tsubokawa T. Clinical value of multi-modality spinal cord evoked potentials for prognosis of spinal cord injury. In: Vigouroux RP, Harris P, eds. *Thoracic and Lumbar Spine and Spinal Cord Injuries.* New York: Springer-Verlag; 1987:65–92.

68. Kernel D, Wu CP. Responses of the pyramidal tract to stimulation of the baboon's motor cortex. *J. Physiol. (Lond.)* 1967;191:653–672.

69. Katayama Y, Tsubokawa T, Maejima S, Hirayama T, Yamamoto T. Corticospinal direct response in humans: identification of the motor cortex during intracranial surgery under general anesthesia. *J. Neurol. Neurosurg. Psychiatry* 1988;51:50–59.

70. Patton HC, Amassian VE. The pyramidal tract: its excitation and functions. In: *Handbook of Physiology and Neurophysiology, Vol 11.* Washington, DC: American Physiology Society; 1960:837–861.

71. Tamaki T, Takano H, Takakuwa K. Spinal cord monitoring: basic principles and experimental aspects. *Central Nervous Syst. Trauma* 1985; 2:137–149.

72. Kothbauer KF. Motor evoked potential monitoring for intramedullary spinal cord tumor surgery. In: Deletis V, Shils JL, eds. *Neurophysiology in*

Neurosurgery. Amsterdam: Academic; 2002: 73–92.

73. Calancie B, Harris W, Broton JG, Alexeeva N, Green BA. "Threshold-level" multipulse transcranial electrical stimulation of motor cortex for intraoperative monitoring of spinal motor tracts: description of method and comparison to somatosensory evoked potential monitoring. *J. Neurosurg.* 1998;90:457–470.

74. Koyanagi I, Iwasaki Y, Isy T, Abe H, Akino M, Kuroda S. Spinal cord evoked potential monitoring after spinal cord stimualtion durong surgery of spinal cord tumors. *Neurosurgery* 1993;33:451–460.

75. Kai Y, Owen JH, Lenke LG, Bridwell KH, Oakley DM, Sugioka Y. Use of sciatic neurogenic motor evoked potentials versus spinal potentials to predict early-onset neurologic deficits when intervention is still possible during overdistraction. *Spine* 1993;18:1134–1139.

76. Leppanen R, Madigan R, Sears C, Maguire J, Wallace S, Captain J. Intraoperative collision studies demonstrate descending spinal cord stimulation evoked potentials and ascending somatosensory evoked potentials are medicated through common pathways. *J. Clin. Neurophysiol.* 1999;16:170.

77. Toleikis JR, Skelly JP, Carlvin AO, Burkus JK. Spinally elicited peripheral nerve responses are sensory rather than motor. *Clin. Neurophysiol.* 2000;111:736–742.

78. Minahan RE, Sepkuly JP, Lesser RP, et al. Anterior spinal cord injury with preserved neurogenic "motor"-evoked potentials. *Clin. Neurophysiol.* 2001;112:1442–1450.

79. Machida M, Weinstein MC, Yamada T, Kimura J. Spinal cord monitoring: electrophsysiological measures of sensory and motor function during spinal surgery. *Spine* 1985;10:407–413.

80. Owen JH, Bridwell KH, Grubb R, et al. The clinical application of neurogenic motor evoked potentials to monitor spinal cord function during surgery. *Spine* 1991;16:S385–S390.

81. Thomsen K, Christensen FB, Eiskjaer SP, et al. The effect of pedicle screw instrumentation on functional outcome and fusion rates in posterolateral lumbar spinal fusions: a prospective randomized clinical study. *Spine* 1997;22:2813–2822.

82. Bose B, Wierzbowski LR, Sestokas AK. Neurophysiological monitoring of spinal nerve root function during instrumented posterior lumbar spine surgery. *Spine* 2002;27:1444–1450.

83. Toleikis JR, Skelly JP, Carlvin AO, et al. The usefulness of electrical stimulation for assessing pedicle screw placements. *J. Spinal Disord.* 2000;13:283–289.

84. Toleikis JR. Neurophysiological monitoring during pedicle screw placement. In: Deletis V, Shils JL, eds. *Neurophysiology in Neurosurgery.* Amsterdam: Elsevier; 2002:231–264.

85. Maguire J, Wallace S, Madiga R, Leppanen R, Draper V. Evaluation of intrapedicular screw position using intraoperative evoked electromyography. *Spine* 1995;20:1068–1074.

86. Yingling C. Intraoperative monitoring in skull base surgery. In: Jackler RK, Brackmann DE, eds. *Neurotology.* St. Louis, MO: Mosby; 1994:967–1002.

87. Mills KR, McLeod C, Sheffy J, Loh L. The optimal current direction for excitation of human cervical motor roots with a double coil magnetic stimulator. *Electroenceph. Clin. Neurophysiol.* 1993;89:138–144.

88. Kimura J, Mitsudome A, Yamada T, Dickens QS. Stationary peaks from moving source in far-field recordings. *Electroenceph. Clin. Neurophysiol.* 1984;58:351–361.

89. Lueders H, Lesser RP, Hahn JR, Little JT, Klein AW. Subcortical somatosensory evoked potentials to median nerve stimulation. *Brain* 1983;106:341–372.

90. Schmid UD, Møller AR, Schmid J. The excitation site of the trigeminal nerve to transcranial magnetic stimulation varies and lies proximal or distal to the foramen ovale: an intraoperative electrophysiological study in man. *Neurosci. Lett.* 1992;141:265–268.

91. Yamada H, Transfeldt EE, Tamaki T, et al. The effects of volatile anesthetics on the relative amplitudes and latencies of spinal and muscle potentials evoked by transcranial magnetic stimulation. *Spine* 1994;19:1512–1517.

92. Sloan T. Evoked potentials. In: Albin MS, ed. *A Textbook of Neuroanesthesia with Neurosurgical and Neuroscience Perspectives.* New York, NY: McGraw-Hill; 1996:221–276.

93. Glassman SD, Shields CB, Linden RD, et al. Anesthetic effects on motor evoked potentials in dogs. *Spine* 1993;18:1083–1089.

94. Loughnan B, Anderson S, Hetreed M, Weston PF, Boyd SG, Hall GM. Effects of halothane on motor evoked potential recorded in the extradural space. *Br. J. Anaesth.* 1989;63:561–564.

95. Mavroudakis N, Vandesteene A, Brunko E. Spinal and brain-stem SEPs and H reflex during

enflurane anesthesia. *Electroenceph. Clin. Neurophysiol.* 1994;92:82–85.

96. Amassian VE, Stewart M, Quirk GJ, Rosenthal JL. Physiological basis of motor effects on a transient stimulation to cerebral cortex. *Neurosurgery* 1987;20:74–93.

97. Hicks R, Woodforth I, Crawford M, et al. Some effects of isoflurane on I waves of the motor evoked potential. *Br. J. Anaesth.* 1992;69:130–136.

98. Taylor BA, Fennelly ME, Taylor A, Farrell J. Temporal summation—the key to motor evoked potential spinal cord monitoring in humans. *J. Neurol.* 1993;56:104–106.

99. Neuloh G, Schramm J. Intraoperative neurophysiological mapping and monioring for supratentorial procedures. In: Delecrin J, Shils JL, eds. *Neurophysiology in Neurosurgery.* Amsterdam: Elsevier; 2002:339–401.

100. Taniguchi M, Schram J, Cedzich C. Recording of myogenic motor evoked potential (mMEP) under general anesthesia. In: Schramm J, Moller AR, eds. *Intraoperative Neurophysiological Monitoring.* Berlin: Springer-Verlag; 1991:72–87.

101. Delgado T, Buchheit W, Rosenholtz H, Chrissian S. Intraoperative monitoring of facial muscle evoked responses obtained by intracranial stimulation of the facial nerve: a more accurate technique for facial nerve dissection. *Neurosurgery* 1979;4:418–421.

102. Kartush J, Bouchard K. Intraoperative facial monitoring. Otology, neurotology, and skull base surgery. In: Kartush J, Bouchard K, eds. *Neromonitoring in Otology and Head and Neck Surgery.* New York, NY: Raven; 1992:99–120.

103. Leonetti J, Brackmann D, Prass R. Improved preservation of facial nerve function in the infratemporal approach to the skull base. *Otolaryngol. Head Neck Surg.* 1989;101:74–78.

104. Prass RL, Lueders H. Acoustic (loudspeaker) facial electromyographic monitoring. Part I. *Neurosurgery* 1986;19:392–400.

105. Harner S, Daube J, Beatty C, Ebersold M. Intraoperative monitoring of the facial nerve. *Laryngoscope* 1988;98:209–212.

106. Linden R, Tator C, Benedict C, Mraz C, Bell I. Electro-physiological monitoring during acoutic neuroma and other posterior fossa surgery. *J. Sci. Neurol.* 1988;15:73–81.

107. Benecke J, Calder H, Chadwick G. Facial nerve monitoring during acoustic neuroma removal. *Laryngoscope* 1987;97:697–700.

108. Sugita K, Kobayashi S. Technical and instrumental improvements in the surgical treatment of acoustic neurinomas. *J. Neurosurg.* 1982;57: 747–752.

109. Silverstein H, Smouha E, Jones R. Routine identification of the facial nerve using electrical stimualtion during otological and neurotological surgery. *Laryngoscope* 1988;98: 726–730.

110. Krauze F. *Surgery of the Brain and Spinal Cord*, 1st English edition: Rebman, Cy; 1912.

111. Olivecrone H. Die Trigeminusneuralgie und iher Behandlung. *Nervenartz* 1941;14:49–57.

112. Rand RW, Kurze TL. Facial nerve preservation by posterior fossa transmeatal microdissection in total removal of acoustic tumours. *J. Neurol. Neurosurg. Psychiatry* 1965;28:311–316.

113. Shibuya M, Matsuga N, Suzuki Y, Sugita K. A newly designed nerve monitor for microneurosurgery: bipolar constant current nerve stimualtor and movement detector with pressure sensor. *Acta Neurochir.* 1993;125: 173–176.

114. Babin RM, Jai HR, McCabe BF. Bipolar localization of the facial nerve in the internal auditory canal. In: Graham MD, House WF, eds. *Disorders of the Facial Nerve: Anatomy, Diagnosis, and Management.* New York: Raven; 1982:3–5.

115. Howe JE, Loeser JD, Calvin JH. Mechanosensitivity of dorsal root ganglia and chronically injured axons: a physiologic basis for radically pain of nerve root compression. *Pain* 1977;3:25–41.

116. Schwartz D, Rosenberg S. Facial nerve monitoring during parotidectomy. In: Kartush J, Bouchard K, eds. *Intraoperative Monitoring in Otology and Head and Neck Surgery.* New York, NY: Raven; 1992:121–130.

117. Møller AR. Electrophysiological monitoring of cranial nerves in operations in the skull base. In: Sekhar LN, Schramm VL Jr, eds. *Tumors of the Cranial Base: Diagnosis and Treatment.* Mt. Kisco, NY: Futura; 1987:123–132.

118. Sekhar LN, Møller AR. Operative management of tumors involving the cavernous sinus. *J. Neurosurg.* 1986;64:879–889.

119. Møller AR. Intraoperative monitoring of evoked potentials: an update. In: Wilkins RH, Rengachary SS, eds. *Neurosurgery Update I: Diagnosis, Operative Technique, and Neurooncology.* New York, NY: McGraw-Hill; 1990:169–176.

120. Sekiya T, Hatayama T, Iwabuchi T, Maeda S. A ring electrode to record extraocular muscle activities during skull base surgery. *Acta Neurochir.* (Wien) 1992;117:66–69.

121. Sekiya T, Hatayama T, Iwabushi T, Maeda S. Intraoperative recordings of evoked extraocular muscle activities to monitor ocular motor function. *Neurosurgery* 1993;32: 227–235.

122. Lanser M, Jackler R, Yingling C. Regional monitoring of the lower (ninth through twelfth) cranial nerves. In: Kartush J, Bouchard K, eds. *Intraoperative Monitoring in Otology and Head and Neck Surgery.* New York, NY: Raven; 1992:131–150.

123. Yingling CD, Ashram YA. Intraoperative monitoring of cranial nerves in skull base surgery. In: Jackler RK, Brackmann D, eds. *Neurotology*, 2nd ed. Philadelphia: Elsevier–Mosby; 2005:958–993.

124. Stechison M. Vagus nerve monitoring: a comparison of percutaneous versus vocal fold electrode recording. *Am. J. Otol.* 1995;16: 703–706.

125. Schmid UD, Møller AR, Schmid J. Transcranial magnetic stimulation excites the labyrinthine segment of the facial nerve: an intraoperative electrophysiological study in man. *Neurosci. Lett.* 1991;124:273–276.

126. Murray NMF, Hess CW, Mills KR, Schriefer TN, Smith SJM. Proximal facial nerve conduction using magnetic stimulation. *Electroenceph. Clin. Neurophysiol.* 1987;66:71.

127. Maccabee PJ, Amassian VE, Cracco RQ, Cracco JB, Anziska BJ. Intracranial stimulation of the facial nerve in human with the magnetic coil. *Electroenceph. Clin. Neurophysiol.* 1988;70:350–354.

128. Rösler KM, Hess CW, Schmid UD. Investigation of facial motor pathways by electrical and magnetic stimualtion: Sites and mechanisms of excitation. *J. Neurol. Neurosurg. Psychiatry* 1989;52:1149–1156.

Chapter 12
Anatomy and Physiology of Peripheral Nerves
Chapter 13
Practical Aspects of Monitoring Peripheral Nerves

The subject of monitoring cranial motor nerves to reduce or prevent the risk of injury was discussed in Chaps. 10 and 11. This section will discuss intraoperative monitoring of the function of peripheral nerves. Perhaps of greater importance will be the discussion regarding diagnostic aids, in operations to repair injured peripheral nerves, employed intraoperatively through the use of electrophysiological methods. This assignment of importance stems from the fact that the severity of lesions of peripheral nerves cannot be assessed by visual inspection and the physiological diagnosis intraoperatively is essential for deciding the strategy of an operation. Although such tasks can be performed with basic neurophysiological equipment, the interpretation of the results of recordings from peripheral nerves requires detailed knowledge about the anatomy and the normal function of peripheral nerves. Understanding of the effect of various forms of insults on the function of peripheral nerves is also important for providing intraoperative electrophysiological support during surgical repair of injured nerves.

Anatomy and Physiology of Peripheral Nerves

Introduction
Anatomy
Pathologies of Nerves
Signs of Injuries to Nerves

INTRODUCTION

This chapter describes the normal anatomy and function of somatic peripheral nerves and different forms of injuries that can occur from trauma and other forms of insults. Because intraoperative monitoring of nerves of the autonomic system has not found practical use, this topic is not covered in detail. Chapter 13 provides a description of the practical aspects of intraoperative monitoring and diagnosis of pathologies of peripheral nerves.

ANATOMY

Peripheral nerves of the body are spinal nerves that originate or terminate in the spinal cord; some cranial nerves that originate or terminate in the brainstem also give rise to peripheral nerves (*see* Appendix). Most peripheral nerves contain somatic motor fibers, sensory nerve fibers, proprioceptive fibers, and pain fibers, and some spinal nerves contain visceral and autonomic nerve fibers. In general, sensory fibers of peripheral nerves enter the spinal cord as dorsal roots, and motor fibers exit the spinal cord as ventral roots.

Classification of Peripheral Nerves

Sensory and motor nerves are mostly composed of myelinated nerve fibers. Most mixed

From: *Intraoperative Neurophysiological Monitoring: Second Edition*
By A. R. Møller
© Humana Press Inc., Totowa, NJ.

nerves also contain nerve fibers that carry pain signals and fibers that belong to the autonomic nervous system. Whereas sensory and motor nerves and some pain fibers are myelinated fibers, some pain fibers and autonomic fibers are unmyelinated.

Myelinated fibers can be divided into three main groups according to the diameter of their axons, usually labeled Aα Aβ, and Aδ fibers; unmyelinated fibers are C fibers. The conduction velocity of nerve fibers is proportional to the diameter of their axons (**Table 12.1**). Motor nerve fibers belong to the Aα groups and most sensory nerves belong to the Aβ fiber types, whereas pain fibers belong to the Aδ and C groups.

When peripheral nerves enter or exit the spinal cord or the brainstem the myelin changes from peripheral myelin to central myelin. Central myelin is generated by oligodendrocytes, whereas the myelin of the peripheral portion of nerves is generated by Schwann cells. The transition zone between the peripheral and the central part of nerves occurs near their entry to the central nervous system (CNS) and is known as the Obersteiner–Redlich zone.

Axons of the peripheral portion of nerves are covered by endoneurium to form nerve fibers, and nerve fibers are organized in bundles (fascicles) that are covered by a sheath of perineurium (**Fig 12.1**). The peripheral portion of nerves can consist of a single funiculus or it can be composed of several funiculi (bundles) that are covered by perineurium. Epineurium covers nerve trunks (*1*).

Table 12-1
Conduction Velocity in Nerve Fibers of Different Types

Fiber type	Function	Average axon diameter (mm)	Average conduction velocity (m/s)
Aα	Motor nerves, primary Muscle-spindle afferents	15	100 (70–120)
Aβ	Mechanoreceptor afferents	8	50 (30–70)
Aδ	Temperature and pain afferents	<3	15 (12–30)
C	Pain afferents Sympathetic postganglionic fibers (unmyelinated)	~1	1 (0.5–2)

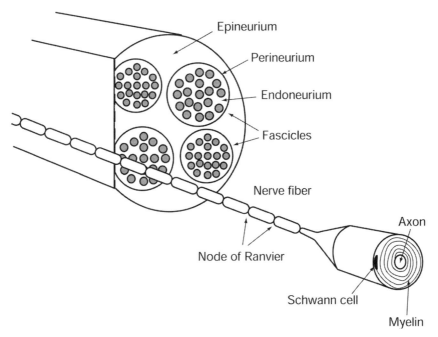

Figure 12.1: Anatomy of a typical peripheral portion of a nerve. (Reprinted from: Møller AR. *Neural Plasticity and Disorders of the Nervous System*. Cambridge: Cambridge University Press; 2005, with permission from Cambridge University Press, after ref. *1*.)

Funiculi in the peripheral portion of nerves have an undulated course (**Fig. 12.2**). That allows the nerves to be stretched without inducing stress on the individual axons, but traction that exceeds the stretched length of a nerve will cause some of the typical injuries, which often occur as a result of trauma *(1)*.

In the central portion of a nerve, the endoneurium, which consists of collagen fibrils, has finer fibrils than in the peripheral portion, and the perineurium and epineurium are absent.

Therefore, the central part of nerves lacks some of the protection that peripheral portions have. Because the central portion of nerves lacks a funicular support structure and undulations are absent (**Fig. 12.2**), the central portion of nerves is more fragile and sensitive to traction than their peripheral counterparts.

The transition zone between the peripheral and central portion of nerves (the Obersteiner–Redlich zone) has been studied especially in cranial nerves, where it has been shown to be

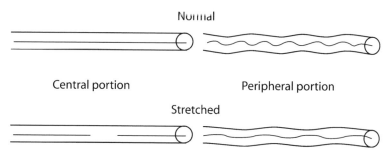

Figure 12.2: Effect of traction and injury on the central and the peripheral portion of a nerve. (Reprinted from: Møller AR. *Neural Plasticity and Disorders of the Nervous System.* Cambridge: Cambridge University Press; 2005, with permission from Cambridge University Press, after ref. *1.*)

sensitive to irritation from (e.g., blood vessels) (*see* Chap. 15). This region of nerves is the common anatomical location of schwannoma, such as vestibular schwannoma of the auditory vestibular nerve. Spinal nerves can also have schwannoma, especially in connection with a genetic defect, neurofibromatosis type 2 (NF2).

Sensory Nerves

The fibers of sensory spinal nerves are bipolar nerve fibers that have their cell bodies in the dorsal root ganglia (DRG). Sensory nerves enter the dorsal horn of the spinal cord (**Fig 12.3**) as dorsal root fibers. Low-threshold cutaneous receptors are innervated by Aβ fibers (6–12 μm in diameter) with conduction velocities between 30 and 70 m/s (**Table 12.1**). Proprioceptive fibers from muscle spindles and tendon organs and receptors monitoring joint movements are large (Aα) fibers, and pain fibers are the smallest myelinated fibers (Aδ). Unmyelinated fibers (C fibers) also mediate pain *(2)*.

Motor Nerves

The motor nerve fibers that leave the spinal cord as ventral spinal roots mostly belong to the Aα group of nerve fibers. The cell bodies (alpha motoneurons) of axons that innervate skeletal muscles are located in lamina IX of the ventral horn of the spinal cord (**Fig. 12.3**) *(4)*. The nerve fibers that innervate the intrafusal muscle (Aα fibers) travel together with other motor fibers, and their cell bodies are

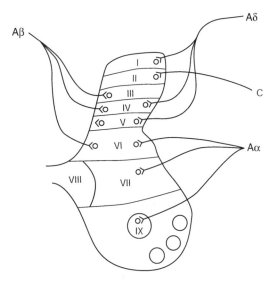

Figure 12.3: Different types of sensory nerve fiber terminating on cells in the different lamina of the horn of the spinal cord (Rexed's classification *[3]*). (Reprinted from: Møller AR. *Neural Plasticity and Disorders of the Nervous System.* Cambridge: Cambridge University Press; 2005, with permission from Cambridge University Press.)

located in lamina IX of the ventral horn of the spinal cord *(4)*.

Autonomic Nerves

So far, the autonomic nervous system has had little importance in intraoperative monitoring, but development of new methods for testing the autonomic nervous system might make it possible to monitor the autonomic nerves intraoperatively.

The fibers of nerves of the autonomic nervous system are unmyelinated (C fibers) or myelinated fibers of small diameter (Aδ fibers). They enter the spinal cord through dorsal roots; from there, they make contact with cells in the dorsalmost parts of the dorsal horn with their cell bodies being in the DRG. Parasympathetic efferents that innervate the bladder and some genital organs originate in the dorsal roots of the S₃ and S₄ segments of the spinal cord (2,4). The afferent sympathetic innervation of viscera (visceral afferents) in the abdomen forms the greater and lesser splanchnic nerves. Afferent sympathetic nerve fibers that innervate the lower body pass uninterrupted through the sympathetic trunk enter the spinal cord at T₁₁–L₄ levels through dorsal roots and terminate in the dorsalmost part of the spinal cord, whereas the vagus nerve (CN X) provides most of the parasympathetic innervation of visceral organs (2,4). Parasympathetic afferents from S₃ and S₄ segments innervate the bladder and the genital organs. Generally, afferents from visceral nociceptors follow sympathetic nerves, whereas autonomic afferents from other receptors follow parasympathetic nerves (4). This would mean that the vagus nerve does not carry nociceptor afferents, which has been disputed because it has been shown that vagal stimulation can affect nociception (5,6).

PATHOLOGIES OF NERVES

Trauma can cause specific injuries to nerves, and nerves can be injured because of disorders, some of which can destroy the myelin (demyelination). Inflammation and age also cause changes in the morphology and the function of peripheral nerves.

Traumatic injuries could affect a limited portion of a (single) nerve (focal injuries), whereas disorders (and age) more likely affect one or more entire nerves (mononeuropathy or polyneuropathy) (2).

Focal Injuries

Some investigators have classified the focal morphological changes that typically occur in nerves from traumatic injuries into three main types: neurapraxia, axonotmesis, and neurotmesis. Others have divided such injuries in five groups (7) (**Fig. 12.4**).

Neurapraxia is the mildest form of focal lesions of a nerve (Sunderland grade 1 [7]) (**Fig. 12.4**). It involves partial or complete conduction failure without any detectable structural changes. A nerve can recover totally from neurapraxia without any intervention.

Stretching or compression of a nerve containing axons of different diameter affects large-diameter axons more than smaller ones, whereas the effect of local anesthetics on nerves is the opposite. Thus, there is greater effect on neural transmission in small (pain) fibers than larger fibers, and thereby, local anesthetics can provide absence of pain while tactile sensation is maintained. Traction or heating can injure nerves to various degrees, and the injury can be either temporary or permanent. If the injury is slight (neurapraxia; Sunderland grade 1), full function of the nerve will return within a certain time, ranging from several hours to a few days.

Interruption of axons of a nerve without damage to its supporting structures is known as axonotmesis (Sunderland grade 2). Axonotmesis could be caused by insults such as crushing or pinching of a nerve, or it could occur after stretching a nerve. If such lesion occurs distally to the location of the cell body, the parts of the axons that are distal to the lesion will begin to degenerate immediately after the lesion has occurred (Wallerian degeneration[1]) (8). However, it is important to keep in mind that the distal portion of the nerve can conduct nerve

[1]Degenerative changes in a segment of a nerve fiber (axon and myelin) that occurs when continuity with its cell body is interrupted.

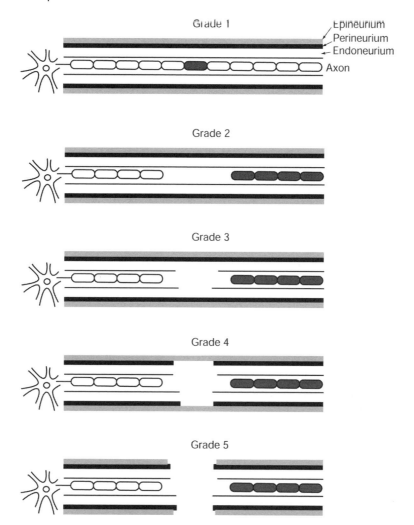

Figure 12.4: Illustration of a nerve with a conduction block without morphological changes (neurapraxia, Sunderland grade 1, and different types of nerve injuries (Sunderland grades 2, 3, 4, and 5) *(7)*. (Reprinted from: Møller AR. *Neural Plasticity and Disorders of the Nervous System.* Cambridge: Cambridge University Press; 2005, with permission from Cambridge University Press.)

impulses for 24–72 h after an injury. The degeneration of the distal portion is usually complete within 48–72 h after the injury, at which time the nerve will no longer conduct nerve impulses. Interruption of axons proximal to the cell body causes similar degeneration of the part of the axons that are proximal to the injury.

If trauma to a nerve also involves the support structure of the injury, it is known as neurotmesis (Sunderland grade 3, 4, and 5 *[7]*) **(Fig. 12.4)**. The lightest form of neurotmesis (Grade 3)

involves a mixture of axon damage and some damage to the support structure (loss of Schwann cell basal lamina endoneural integrity). This form of injury might resolve by partial regeneration of axons that can occur without intervention and some function might be regained. Grade 4 describes more serious injuries, where scar formation occurs over the entire cross-section of a nerve. In this kind of injury, the continuity of the nerve is maintained but spontaneous regeneration is blocked by scar tissue. When a total transection of a nerve occurs, it is labeled a Grade 5 injury. This form of injury requires surgical intervention (grafting) to regain function.

The central portions of nerves are more vulnerable to injuries than the peripheral portions because of the lack of support structures, but trauma to a central portion of a nerve produces injury similar that of the peripheral portion. The absence of the undulation of the central portion of nerves adds to the vulnerability of the central portion of nerves to stretching **(Fig. 12.2)**.

Regeneration of Injured Nerves

When peripheral nerves are injured to the degree that the axons have been interrupted, yet the support structure remains intact (axonotmesis), the axons will regenerate. This involves sprouting of axons, which begin to grow (sprout) away from its cell body and toward their normal target using the preserved support structure as a conduit. The regeneration proceeds at a speed of approx 1 mm per day. Not all of the new motor axons will eventually reach their targets and form new motor endplates. If the interruption of a bipolar (sensory) axon occurs at a location that is proximal to the cell body, the axon will grow centrally and make contact with the cells in the spinal cord (or brainstem) to which they were originally connected. Lesions that are located distal to the cell body of axons of sensory nerves will cause the axons to grow toward their sensory receptors. New sensory receptors must be created when sensory nerve fibers, such as those innervating cutaneous receptors, reach their normal targets. Axons of motor nerves that are interrupted will grow toward the muscles that the nerves normally innervated.

Recovery of function after interruption of axons of a motor nerve requires formation of new motor endplates. Sprouting of motor nerves consists of multiple fine fibers, many of which would fail to create functional motor endplates. To obtain muscle function, some of these fine filaments must therefore be eliminated *(9)*. This

normally occurs when the outgrowing axon reaches the muscle that it innervated before it was interrupted.

Axons will also regenerate (sprout) after more severe injuries to a nerve (neurotmesis), but the success of the sprouts' venture to reach their target depends on the condition of the support structure of the injured nerve. Sufficient regrowth might occur if some of the support structure is intact and enough recovery of function may occur. Grades 4 and 5 lesions, however, require grafting, either end to end or with another nerve, that serves to provide the support structures that can act as conduits for the regenerating axons. Such regenerated nerves have fewer functional nerve fibers than they had before the injury, and many of the new axons will activate their targets incorrectly. Misdirected and incomplete regeneration of sensory nerves could cause abnormal sensory input, or partial to complete deprivation of input to the CNS *(10)*.

Scar tissue that forms after injuries could act as an obstacle to regeneration. Sprouting of axons could also cause formation of neurinoma, which can cause various symptoms such as pain.

SIGNS OF INJURIES TO NERVES

Intraoperative signs of injuries to peripheral nerves are changes in the response to electrical stimulation, spontaneous or mechanically evoked activity from the motor portion of peripheral nerves, and of course, if the injury is severe, conduction block.

Slight injury to a peripheral nerve causes decreased conduction velocity that manifests electrophysiologically as increased latency of compound action potentials (CAPs) recorded from one location of a nerve while the nerve is stimulated electrically at another location. Slight injury might also cause a broadening of the CAPs if the conduction velocity is decreased unevenly among the nerve fibers that make up the nerve in question. A severer injury causes greater change in the waveform of the CAP, and a total conduction block results in a single positive deflection when recorded by a monopolar recording electrode (*see* Chap. 3).

Mechanosensitivity of Injured Nerves

Normal peripheral nerves are rather insensitive to moderate mechanical stimulation, but slightly injured nerves can be very sensitive to mechanical stimulation and surgical manipulations, and touching injured nerves with surgical instruments can result in contraction of muscles that are innervated with the nerve in question (*see* Chap. 11). Similar mechanical stimulation of an uninjured nerve elicits little or no muscle contractions, clearly indicating that the sensitivity to mechanical stimulation of a nerve is related to injury.

Clinically, mechanical sensitivity of peripheral nerves is often present in carpel tunnel syndrome. Tapping on the skin over the median nerve produces a tingling sensation (paresthesia) in the parts of the hand where the skin is innervated by the injured nerve Tinel's sign[2]. Mechanosensitivity of dorsal root ganglia is also common and involved in some forms of pain *(11)*.

---

[2]A tingling sensation from percussion of the skin over a peripheral nerve.

13

Practical Aspects of Monitoring Peripheral Nerves

Introduction

Intraoperative Measurement of Nerve Conduction

INTRODUCTION

Monitoring of neural conduction is important for detecting surgically induced injuries to nerves and it is a prerequisite for reducing the risks of postoperative deficits. Several different techniques can be used for such monitoring. One method utilizes stimulation of a nerve and recording of the compound action potential (CAP) from another location on the nerve. Other methods use recording of somatosensory evoked potential or the F response[1] and H response.[2] These methods can be used for detecting partial or complete failure of neural conduction and for measurements of changes in neural conduction velocity. Such measures are important for detecting injuries caused by surgical manipulations. Similar electrophysiological methods can be used for finding the anatomical location of injuries to nerves (*see* Chap. 14). Intraoperative measurement of conduction of peripheral nerves plays an important role in guiding the surgeon in repair of injured nerves (discussed in Chap. 15).

INTRAOPERATIVE MEASUREMENT OF NERVE CONDUCTION

The principles are to stimulate a nerve electrically and record the response from the same nerve at a distance from where it is being stimulated. In the clinic, nerve conduction studies often use recordings of the responses from muscles (electromyography [EMG]) in response to electrical stimulation of a mixed nerve *(12)*, but that method only tests motor nerves and in the operating room it requires the patient to be anesthetized without the use of muscle relaxants. Quantitative information about abnormalities in the function of nerves, including abnormal neural conduction velocity, can better be obtained by recording of nerve action potentials (CAPs). This method can be used to determine the neural conduction velocity in all large fibers in a mixed nerve and it can provide quantitative assessment of the function of peripheral nerves. Such assessments include both motor and sensory fibers, but only large fibers (Aα and Aβ fibers) can be studied in that way. (The conduction velocity of slower conducting fibers [Aδ and C fibers] in mixed nerves can be determined by collision techniques that are used in clinical diagnostics, but such methods are rarely used intraoperatively because of their complexity.) Recording of the CAP does not require that muscle relaxants be avoided.

---

[1]The F-response is caused by backfiring of motoneurons. The F-response is recorded in a similar way as the H response (p. 187), by stimulating mixed nerves electrically and recording from muscles that are innervated by the nerve that is stimulated *(12)*.

[2]The H reflex is the responses of the stretch reflex *(2)*.

From: *Intraoperative Neurophysiological Monitoring: Second Edition*
By A. R. Møller

Recordings of CAP From Peripheral Nerves

The most characteristic effect on the response from a nerve from insults such as those that might occur during surgical operation is increased latency, indicating that the conduction velocity is reduced. A decrease in the amplitude of the negative peak (and increased amplitude of the initial positive component) of the recorded CAP in response to supramaximal stimulation is an indication that fewer nerve fibers are currently being activated. Broadening of the negative peak of the CAP and decrease of its amplitude are signs of temporal dispersion of the unit action potentials in the individual nerve fibers that contribute to the CAP. This occurs when the conduction velocity of the different axons of a nerve is affected (decreased) to different degrees.

Because various diseases (such as diabetes mellitus) and age-related changes often cause decreased nerve conduction velocity, the conduction velocity of a nerve suspected to be injured should be compared with that obtained before the operation or it should be compared with that of another nerve in the region or on the other side of the body of the individual before it can be judged that surgical injury is the cause of an observed reduced conduction velocity. Obtaining a baseline determination of the conduction velocity of the nerve that is to be monitored is naturally superior to these mentioned methods, but it is not always possible.

Other Methods for Assessing Injuries to Peripheral Nerves

Methods such as recording of the F response or the H response can be used for detecting injuries to peripheral nerves. The F response can be used to monitor the conduction velocity selectively in the motor axons of the proximal part of mixed nerves, whereas the H response measures the conduction velocity of both sensory (proprioceptive) and motor fibers. Both of these measures are affected by anesthesia and muscle relaxants and, therefore, have limited use for intraoperative monitoring. Monitoring of the SSEP can be used for detecting changes in conduction velocity of sensory nerve.

Identification of the Anatomical Location of Nerve Injuries

Measurements of neural conduction velocity in peripheral nerves (sensory, motor, or mixed nerves) can be used to identify the location of pathology and to determine its nature. Such intraoperative diagnosis can guide the surgeon in operations to repair peripheral nerves and it is possible to identify the anatomical location of an injured segment of a nerve because of its decreased conduction velocity (*see* Chap. 15).

Assessing Nerve Injuries

When using electrophysiological methods for assessing the location of injury to peripheral nerves, it is important to recognize that the distal portion of a transected peripheral nerve will continue to conduct nerve impulses for a period of time up to 72 h after the injury. This means that it is possible to elicit contractions of muscles from electrical stimulation of a motor nerve at locations that are distal to the lesion.

Localizing the Place of Injury. Neurophysiological methods make it possible to localize the exact place where a nerve is injured. This is done by stimulating the nerve in question electrically and recording from different locations along the nerve. Similar basic electrophysiological techniques make it possible to determine if an injured nerve is beginning to regenerate. These methods are superior to other often-used methods involving recordings of EMG potentials. Decisions about how a particular nerve would best respond to resection and repair compared to more conservative treatment such as neurolysis can be made right at the operating table using such basic electrophysiological methods (described in Chap. 15).

Determination of Neural Conduction Velocity. The CAP recorded from a long nerve with a monopolar electrode is a triphasic potential (*see* Chap. 3), and the latency of the response is usually determined as the time between the onset of the stimulus and the earliest negative peak of the response. The neural conduction velocity of the nerve between these two locations is obtained by dividing the distance between the stimulating and recording electrodes by the value of the latency of the response. The conduction velocity of peripheral nerves is usually given in meters per second, which corresponds to dividing the distance in millimeters by the latency in milliseconds.

Because neural conduction occurs with almost the same velocity in both directions along a peripheral nerve (the difference being less than 10%), it does not affect the results markedly whether the nerve is stimulated proximal or distal to the location where the recording is being performed.

Measurements of conduction velocity in a peripheral nerve, such as that described earlier, can be performed without exposing the nerve by properly placing needle electrodes percutaneously for recording and stimulation. This requires a high degree of certainty in identifying the nerve that is to be tested. However, in many cases, such as, in connection with injuries in the brachial plexus, it is not possible to ensure that the proper nerve is being tested. In such cases, it is necessary to expose the nerve surgically so that the injured nerve can be properly identified and there is no doubt which nerve is being tested (Chap. 15).

References to Section IV

1. Sunderland S. Cranial nerve injury. Structural and pathophysiological considerations and a classification of nerve injury. In: Samii M, Jannetta PJ, eds. *The Cranial Nerves.* Heidelberg: Springer-Verlag; 1981:16–26.
2. Møller AR. *Neural Plasticity and Disorders of the Nervous System.* Cambridge: Cambridge University Press; 2005 in press.
3. Rexed BA. Cytoarchitectonic atlas of the spinal cord. *J. Comp. Neurol.* 1954;100:297–379.
4. Brodal P. *The Central Nervous System.* New York, NY: Oxford University Press; 1998.
5. Berthoud HR, Neuhuber WL. Functional and chemical anatomy of the afferent vagal system. *Auton. Neurosci.* 2000;85:1–17.
6. Fu QG, Chandler MJ, McNeill DL, Foreman RD. Vagal afferent fibers excite upper cervical neurons and inhibit activity of lumbar spinal cord neurons in the rat. *Pain* 1992;51: 91–100.
7. Sunderland S. A classification of peripheral nerve injuries producing loss of function. *Brain* 1951;74:491–516.
8. Chaudhry V, Cornblath DR. Wallerian degeneration in human nerves; Serial electrophysiological studies. *Muscle Nerve* 1992;15:687–693.
9. Happel L, Kline D. Intraoperative neurophysiology of the peripheral nervous system. In: Deletis V, Shils JL, eds. *Neurophysiology in Neurosurgery.* Amsterdam: Academic; 2002:169–195.
10. Lundborg G. Brain plasticity and hand surgery: an overview. *J. Hand Surg (Brit)* 2000;25: 242–252.
11. Howe JE, Loeser JD, Calvin JH. Mechanosensitivity of dorsal root ganglia and chronically injured axons: a physiologic basis for radically pain of nerve root compression. *Pain* 1977;3: 25–41.
12. Aminoff MJ. *Electromyography in Clinical Practice.* New York: Churchill Livingstone; 1998.

INTRAOPERATIVE RECORDINGS THAT CAN GUIDE
THE SURGEON IN THE OPERATION

Chapter 14
   Identification of Specific Neural Tissue
Chapter 15
   Intraoperative Diagnosis and Guide in Operations

The previous sections have concerned the use of electrophysiological methods in reducing the risk of permanent postoperative neurological deficits as a result of surgical manipulation of neural tissue. In this section, we will discuss a different use of electrophysiology in the operating room, namely for identification of specific neural structures, beginning with localization of nerves and extending to electrophysiological mapping of the spinal cord and the floor of the fourth ventricle. The use of electrophysiological techniques for that purpose is in steady increase and it can be expected to find use in the future in many other kinds of operation that involve the nervous system. The use of electrophysiology for the purpose of guiding the surgeon in an operation requires other kinds of knowledge and skill than intraoperative monitoring that is done for reducing the risk of postoperative neurological deficits. The following chapters provide the physiological and practical basis for that.

14

Identification of Specific Neural Tissue

Introduction
Localization of Motor Nerves
Mapping of Sensory Nerves
Mapping of the Spinal Cord
Mapping of the Floor of the Fourth Ventricle
Localization of the Somatosensory and Motor Cortex (Central Sulcus)
Type of Stimulation
Anesthesia Requirements

INTRODUCTION

The most direct way that intraoperative neurophysiological recordings can guide the surgeon in an operation is in identifying a specific nerve. This is of great importance when trying to identify cranial nerves in cases where the anatomy is distorted by a pathological process. Previous operations might have changed the anatomy, making it difficult to identify specific nerves solely on the basis of visual observation in a surgical field. Tumors and malformations of various kinds can have distorted the anatomy so that it becomes difficult to identify specific neural tissue. These problems could occur in connection with cranial nerves and peripheral nerves. Neurophysiologic methods can identify nerves in such situations, and in other situations, neurophysiological methods can confirm the anatomy.

Intraoperative neurophysiological recording can help to identify structures of the central nervous system (CNS) such as the central fissure that separates the sensory and motor cortical areas. This is of particular importance when a tumor is to be removed or when brain tissue is to be removed to treat intractable epileptic

From: *Intraoperative Neurophysiological Monitoring: Second Edition*
By A. R. Møller
© Humana Press Inc., Totowa, NJ.

seizures. Neurophysiological methods are also used for mapping of the floor of the fourth ventricle and to guide the surgeon in specific operations (*see* Chap. 15).

LOCALIZATION OF MOTOR NERVES

In this part of the chapter, localization of cranial motor nerves and peripheral motor nerves will be discussed. Earlier in this volume, we have shown an example of how intraoperative monitoring can reduce the risk of injury to nerves that innervate the extraocular muscles (CN III, CN IV, and CN VI) and the facial nerve (CN VII) (*see* Chap. 11).

Localization of Cranial Motor Nerves

Cranial motor nerves may become displaced by tumors, such as skull base tumors that often distort the anatomy to such an extent that it is difficult to identify the nerves visually on the basis of anatomical knowledge alone. Cranial nerves are often directly involved in tumors, thereby adding to the difficulty of identification (1–6). Identifying the facial nerve is particularly important in removal of vestibular schwannoma for preservation of facial function. It is sometimes equally important to be able to identify regions of a tumor where no nerve is apparent, so that these regions of the tumor can be removed without injuring the particular nerve (Chap. 11).

Motor nerves are commonly identified by probing specific region of the surgical field with a stimulating electrode and recording of electromyographic (EMG) potentials from the muscle (or one of the muscles) that the nerve in question innervates. Ideally, the EMG potentials from a muscle should be recorded differentially between two electrodes placed in the same muscle to avoid potentials that are generated by other muscles being included in the recording. When only one electrode can be placed in a muscle because of limited access, the reference electrode should be placed as far as possible from the muscles from which the recordings are made and from other muscles that might be activated. For example, when recordings are made from the extraocular muscles, it is important that the reference electrodes be placed on the opposite side of the face to the extraocular muscles from which recording is made. If the reference electrodes were to be placed on the same side of the face, they would record EMG potentials from facial and mastication muscles that might be elicited by electrical stimulation in the operative field that could activate nerves that innervate facial and mastication muscles. If the reference electrodes were placed near these muscles, EMG potentials from stimulating the facial or trigeminal motor nerves would be indistinguishable from the EMG response from the extraocular muscles that were elicited by stimulating CN III, CN IV, and CN VI.

Because there is usually more than one nerve that needs to be identified, it is beneficial to have the EMG potentials of different muscles displayed in several separate recording channels. Modern equipment allows for displaying many records simultaneously. This allows for many nerves at different anatomical sites to be tested within a short time, and the test can be repeated as often as necessary without causing significant delay of the operation.

Practical Aspects on Identification of Motor Nerves. It is important to make sure that the stimulator and the EMG amplifiers, as well as the recording electrodes, are functioning adequately. The appearance of a stimulus artifact in the recording of EMG potentials that can be observed when the handheld stimulating electrode is first brought into contact with the tissue to be tested is an important indicator that the entire system is working correctly, but it is not sufficient proof. A small stimulus artifact might be seen even when there is no contact between the stimulator and the patient. The stimulus artifact should increase in amplitude when the stimulating electrode is brought into contact with the tissue in the surgical field if the electrode is delivering an electrical current to the tissue that is being probed. As soon as it is possible during the operation, it is advisable to test the entire system by stimulating a motor nerve that innervates the muscle from which the EMG potentials are being recorded.

The return electrode for the stimulator could easily become dislodged if it is a hypodermic needle placed directly in the wound. In such a case, there will be no, or only a small, stimulus artifact in the recording. Therefore, it is also important during the operation to always check the stimulus artifact whenever electrical stimulation is being done. To do this, the entire response should be displayed together with the EMG potentials. When an audio-monitor is used to make the EMG potentials audible, the initial few milliseconds of the responses are "cut out" to avoid audible interference from the stimulus artifact (*see* Chap. 18), but this should only be done in the signal that is directed to the audio-amplifier and not to the signal that is displayed on the computer display.

Although it is true that in many cases touching a motor nerve with a surgical instrument results in a stimulation of the nerve and an EMG potential can be recorded, this does not always happen. Therefore, one should never rely on such mechanical stimulation for the purpose of locating a cranial motor nerve. Only electrical stimulation should be used for this purpose, and it is important to use the electrical stimulating electrode often when trying to locate a nerve in a surgical field.

Surgical dissecting instruments that can be connected to a nerve stimulator are available *(7)*. Such instruments are helpful for properly identifying a motor nerve by touching it with a surgical instrument without having to take a different instrument (stimulating electrode) for probing the surgical field for the presence of a motor nerve.

Choice of Stimulation. For probing a surgical field for the presence of motor nerves, a relatively low-impedance stimulator[1] *(3,8)* is the most suitable kind of stimulator. The stimulus impulses that are applied to a nerve should have a negative polarity. Rectangular impulses with a duration of 100 μs and a strength of 0.1–0.4 V will normally elicit EMG responses from muscles that are innervated by a motor nerve when a monopolar stimulating electrode is placed directly in contact with the nerve in question, or in its immediate vicinity such as the facial nerve. The cranial nerves that innervate the extraocular muscles are slightly less sensitive to electrical stimulation than is the facial nerve (*see* Chap. 11). Should the nerve in question be covered by tissue of any kind, such as the arachnoid membrane, a stimulus strength of 0.8–1.5 V might need to be applied to elicit a response.

Whenever electrical stimulation is used to identify a motor nerve, it must be kept in mind that all surrounding tissue and fluid are good electrical conductors that might conduct the stimulating current to a motor nerve. However, the attenuation of the stimulus current by the tissue makes such remote locations less sensitive to electrical stimulation than a nerve that is located closer to the stimulating electrode. Therefore, it is important to use the lowest possible stimulus strength for localizing a motor nerve. Also, nerves are good electrical conductors. A nerve will (passively) conduct stimulus current even when it does not conduct nerve impulses (because of injury).

Technique That Can Facilitate Finding a Nerve That Is Embedded in Tissue. If moving the stimulating electrode causes an increase in the amplitude of the recorded EMG response, then the nerve is located in the direction the electrode was moved. If moving the electrode results in a smaller response, the electrode was moved away from the nerve. The use of this method requires frequent adjustments of the stimulus strength to keep the response below its maximal amplitude, and close collaboration between the person who does the monitoring and the surgeon is necessary, but it can shorten the time it takes to locate a nerve in the surgical field considerably.

Bipolar Versus Monopolar Stimulating Electrodes. The use of a bipolar stimulating electrode will result in greater spatial selectivity *(5,7)*, but a bipolar stimulating electrode is more difficult to use and its ability to stimulate a nerve depends on its orientation. In short, a bipolar stimulating electrode is preferable if the purpose is to determine the identity of each one of two closely located nerves that are clearly visible, but a bipolar stimulating electrode is not suitable for searching for the location of a nerve in the surgical field.

Injured Nerves. Often, it is tempting to increase the stimulus strength when no response is obtained from stimulating a nerve because it is believed that the sensitivity of the nerve has decreased. However, the high stimulus strength might cause stimulation of the normal functioning portion of the nerve by (galvanic) conduction of the stimulus current and thus give a false impression that the part of the nerve that is stimulated is conducting nerve impulses. This problem is caused by the fact that an injured nerve conducts electrical current even though it does not conduct nerve impulses. The problem is most pronounced when a nerve is free from surrounding tissue or

---

[1]Even if the stimulator can deliver a (true) constant voltage, the resistance of the stimulus electrode will make the stimulus that is delivered to the tissue have a certain source resistance. A true constant-voltage stimulator means a source without any internal resistance (*see* Chap. 18).

fluid that would otherwise shunt the electrical stimulus current. It is, therefore, important to select a proper stimulus strength — just above normal threshold — when testing a nerve for its ability to conduct nerve impulses.

Mapping the Course of Peripheral Motor Nerves

There are several instances when it is valuable to map the course of peripheral nerves so that a decision can be made as to exactly where to make an incision. Skin incisions of the face are typical examples of situations where injury could occur to a branch of the facial nerve. The course of the facial nerve varies from individual to individual and mapping of the different branches of the facial nerve is, therefore, important for determining the exact anatomical location of specific branches of the facial nerve. This can be done by applying fine needle electrodes (such as Type E2 [Grass Instrument Co., Braintree, MA]) percutaneously to determine the location of the facial nerve. The return electrode for the stimulator should be placed on the other side of the face. Such mapping can be done by visual observation of contraction of muscles, but more accurate mapping can be made by recording the evoked EMG activity from respective muscles. The stimulus strength should be small enough to accurately locate a branch of the nerve, but the stimulus strength should be sufficient to avoid missing the nerve. Usually, 1.5–2 V is sufficient when using subdermal needle electrodes and when using a semi-constant-voltage stimulator. If a constant-current stimulator is used, a stimulus strength of 0.2–0.5 mA is suitable. Such mapping is best done in an anesthetized patient, but it is important that the patient is not paralyzed.

Electrical stimulation in connection with recording EMG potentials is valuable for identifying other motor nerves intraoperatively. In operations where a peripheral nerve might be exposed, the surgical field can be probed by a handheld stimulating electrode, similar to what was described for identifying cranial nerves (*see* Chap. 11). This method for identifying motor nerves is specifically useful in connection with operations that involve the brachial plexus, where the courses of the various nerves are complex and likely to be altered by trauma or by previous operations.

Recordings From Motor Nerves

Motor nerves can be identified intracranially by stimulating their peripheral portions electrically and recording the compound action potential (CAP) from their intracranial portions (nerves conduct approximately equally well in both directions). Thus, the motor branch of CN V (portio minor) can be identified using electrical stimulation of its peripheral portion and recording CAP from the intracranial portion. The intracranial portion of the facial nerve can be identified by electrically stimulating one or more of its peripheral branches in the face and recording the resulting antidromic activity in the facial nerve intracranially. Recording of the CAP from motor nerves is more complicated than recording EMG activity from the respective muscles, but it has the advantage that it does not require that the patient is not paralyzed. It has, however, not gained much practical usage.

Safety Concerns

When electrical stimulation is used to identify motor nerves (or for monitoring the integrity of motor nerves), caution should be exercised when the particular nerve innervates large skeletal muscles. Because electrical stimulation might activate all, or nearly all, motor nerve fibers maximally and simultaneously, the contraction might be strong enough to injure the muscle or cause joint dislocations. To avoid this, it is necessary to begin to stimulate motor nerves (for instance, CN XI) with a weaker stimulus and then to increase the stimulus strength slowly while keeping the stimulating electrode in the same position. This procedure must then be repeated for each new anatomical location that is to be tested.

MAPPING OF SENSORY NERVES

Sensory nerves can be localized by applying a sensory stimulus that is specific for the nerve to be identified (e.g., click sounds for the auditory nerve or light flashes for the optic nerve) or an nonspecific stimulus, such as electrical stimulation, for the trigeminal nerve and then record the CAP from the respective nerve. Recordings can be done using either a monopolar or a bipolar recording electrode. The use of a bipolar recording electrode makes it possible to determine the location of a nerve more accurately than using a monopolar electrode because it has a larger degree of spatial selectivity and it selectively records potentials that are the result of propagated neural activity; however, it is often difficult to use a bipolar electrode when a nerve is located within a small space.

When averaging is used to enhance the recorded evoked potentials, it is important to keep in mind that if many responses are averaged, what might be seen might be a far-field response rather than the response from a specific nerve. When recordings of CAP to identify a nerve, the amplitudes and the latencies of the potentials should be noticed. When a recording electrode is placed close to a nerve, the amplitude of the CAP can be expected to be in the range of 10–200 µV. Moving the electrode a few millimeters away from the nerve should reduce the amplitude of the potentials considerably. If the recorded potentials are caused by propagated neural activity in a nerve, the latency of the potentials is expected to change when the recording electrode is moved along the nerve. If the potentials are far-field potentials that are generated by a distant source, then the latency will not change by moving the recording electrode; only the amplitude of the recorded potentials will change.

A monopolar recording electrode will record electrical activity that is conducted passively to the recording site because any tissue is an electric conductor that can conduct evoked potentials to the recording electrode. The recording electrode placed on a nerve might pick up electrical potentials that are generated by other structures and (passively) conducted to the recording site by the nerve from which the recordings are being made. A bipolar recording electrode will mainly record propagated neural activity when placed on a nerve, which is another reason to use bipolar recording electrodes rather than monopolar electrodes (see Chap. 3).

The reference electrode for monopolar recording should be placed as close to the active electrode as possible in order to reduce the stimulus artifact, but such electrode placement will increase the risk that the reference electrode might pick up evoked potentials from structures that generate evoked potentials in response to the stimulus that is being used. It is not possible to determine from observing the recorded potentials whether they are picked up by the (presumed) active electrode or by the (presumed) reference electrode. Therefore, the reference electrode must be placed at a location where the stimulus cannot be expected to generate evoked potentials of any significant amplitude, as compared with those that are recorded by the active electrode (see Chap. 3).

Identifying the Different Branches of the Trigeminal Nerve

Methods for identifying the three different branches of the sensory portion (portio major) of CN V in the posterior fossa using electrophysiological techniques have been described (9). When a branch of CN V is stimulated electrically by two needle electrodes placed close to the point where the branches emerge from their respective foramina, a CAP can be recorded from the intracranial portion of CN V. For practical reasons, it is better to record from the distal branches of the trigeminal nerve while the intracranial portion is stimulated electrically using a bipolar stimulating electrode (9) (**Fig. 14.1**). This method can be used to determine where the different branches of the nerve are located in the intracranial portion of the trigeminal nerve.

Identifying the Auditory and the Vestibular Portions of CN VIII

When the central portion of the vestibular nerve is to be severed to treat disorders of the vestibular system, such as certain forms of

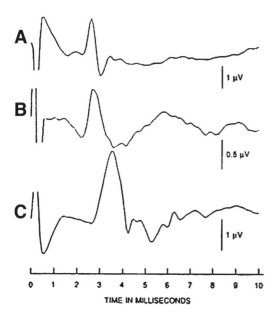

TIME IN MILLISECONDS

Figure 14.1: Recording of CAP from the trigeminal foramina (supraorbital, infraorbital, and metal) while stimulating the rostral–medial, medial–lateral, and caudal–lateral portions of the trigeminal nerve intracranially with a monopolar stimulating electrode . The stimulus strength was supramaximal (0.5–1.0 V). The recordings were made from needle electrodes placed in each of the foramina and connected to each one of three amplifiers. The reference electrodes were placed close to each of the foramina. (Reprinted from: Stechison MT, Møller AR, Lovely TJ. Intraoperative mapping of the trigeminal nerve root: technique and application in the surgical management of facial pain. *Neurosurgery* 1996;38:76–82, with permission from Lippincott Williams and Wilkins.)

Ménière's disease, it is important to determine the anatomical location of the border between the auditory and the vestibular portions of CN VIII. These two portions of CN VIII are located close together near the brainstem. Although the auditory and the vestibular portions of CN VIII have slightly different degrees of grayness, it is not always possible to determine the exact location of the demarcation between these two portions of CN VIII on the basis of visual observations alone. Recording the CAP from the auditory nerve

in response to click stimulation provides a way to determine the border between these two portions of CN VIII. A monopolar recording electrode does not have sufficient spatial selectivity for such differentiation and it is necessary to use a bipolar recording technique *(10,11)*. Placement of a bipolar recording electrode is more demanding than that of a monopolar recording electrode because of the small dimensions of CN VIII *(12)* **(Fig. 14.2)**. The necessity to have electrodes with narrow tips is also a problem, because such narrow tips can easily cause injury to the auditory–vestibular nerve.

It has been shown that the use of clicks of a relatively low stimulus strength (25 dB sensation level; SL) facilitates discrimination between the vestibular and auditory nerves *(10)* **(Fig. 14.3)**. (These authors defined stimulus level as 25 dB above the auditory brainstem response [ABR] threshold, thus probably slightly more than 25 dB above the patient's hearing threshold.) This stimulus level is 30–40 dB lower than that normally used for obtaining ABR in the operating room (usually approx 65 dB HL [hearing level] at a click repetition rate of 20 pulses per second (pps), corresponding to about 105 dB peak equivalent sound pressure level [PeSPL]; *see* Chap. 6).

Identifying Spinal Dorsal Rootlets That Carry Specific Sensory Input

When performing selective dorsal root neurectomy to treat spasticity, it is important to spare parts of the dorsal roots that mediate important functions. Each dorsal root consists of several rootlets, and the treatment requires that one or more of these are severed to reduce spasticity and it is important to spare the parts of the dorsal roots that have important functions. Usually, it is the roots from L_1 to S_2 that are candidates for such selective rhizotomy *(13,14)*. Electrical stimulation of a nerve at a peripheral location in connection with recording CAP from exposed spinal dorsal roots can be used to test whether a particular rootlet carries important sensory input and thus should not be sectioned *(14,15)*. For identification of

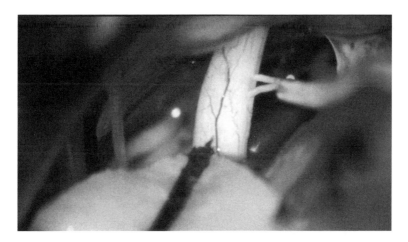

Figure 14.2: Bipolar electrode placed on the exposed eighth cranial nerve.

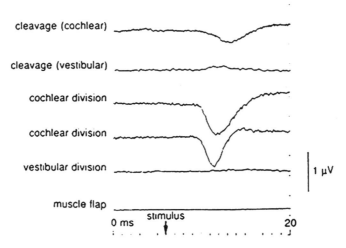

Figure 14.3: Bipolar recordings from the intracranial portion of CN VIII. The stimuli were clicks with an intensity that was 25 dB above the threshold for ABR. (Reprinted from: Rosenberg SI, Martin WH, Pratt H, Schwegler JW, Silverstein H. Bipolar cochlear nerve recording technique: a preliminary report. *Am. J. Otol.* 1993;14:362–368, with permission from Elsevier.)

rootlets that are involved in micturition and sexual function, the dorsal penile or clitoral nerves are stimulated electrically and recording of the elicited CAP is made from each rootlet before it is sectioned **(Fig. 14.4)** *(16)*.

The recordings of the CAPs are best done by a handheld bipolar electrode consisting of two wire hooks having a distance between them of about 5 mm. Each rootlet is then lifted up on this hook, so that it is free from fluid and is out of contact with other rootlets, and the respective nerve is stimulated electrically at a peripheral location *(16)* **(Fig. 14.4)**.

Because it is a matter of a negative identification of the rootlets (rootlets that do not have a response are supposed to be candidates for being severed), it is important to be sure that the stimulation is adequate to elicit a response and that the recording equipment has adequate sensitivity for the recording. Before any rootlets are severed some rootlets with a response must be identified in order to ensure

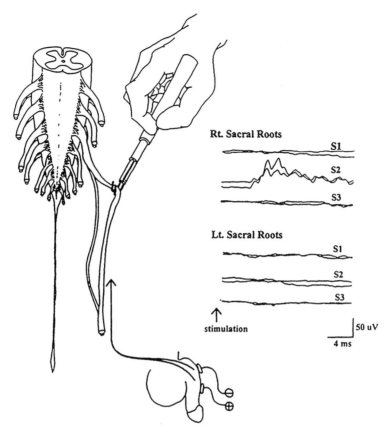

Figure 14.4: Illustration of how dorsal sacral rootlets of the cauda equine can be identified so that specific pudendal afferents can be saved during dorsal root rhizotomies. (Reprinted from: Deletis V, Vodusek DD, Abbott R, Epsetein FJ, Turndorf H. Intraoperative monitoring of the dorsal sacral roots: minimizing the risk of iatrogenic micturition disorders. *Neurosurgery* 1992;30:72–75, with permission from Lippincott Williams and Wilkins.)

that the stimulation is adequate and that the recording equipment works satisfactorily.

MAPPING OF THE SPINAL CORD

Newly developed collision techniques have made it possible to intraoperatively map the anatomical position of the corticospinal tract (CT) within a surgically exposed spinal cord and provide a semiquantitative estimate of the number of intact fibers and the number of desynchronized or blocked fibers of the CT *(17,18)*. The technique thereby expands the benefits of monitoring D waves and it provides

information about how D waves are generated (Chaps. 9 and 10). Collision techniques have been used for many years in animal studies, but it is only recently that this technique has been introduced in intraoperative neurophysiological monitoring *(17)*. The use of this technique is especially important for proper treatment of patients with intramedullary spinal cord tumors where the anatomy of the spinal cord might be distorted and the anatomical location of the CT is difficult to determine using visual inspection alone.

This D-wave collision technique involves simultaneous transcranial electrical stimulation of the motor cortex with concurrent stimulation

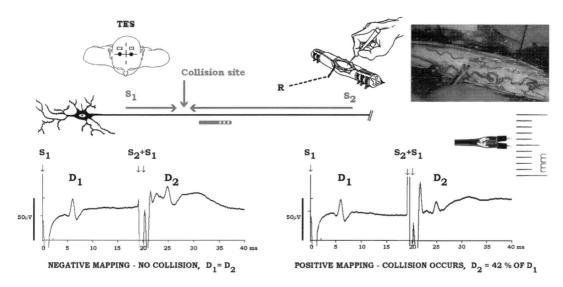

Figure 14.5: Mapping of the corticospinal tract (CT) by the D-wave collision technique. S1 = Transcranial electrical stimulation (TES); S2 = spinal cord electrical stimulation (SpES); D1 = control D wave (TES only); D2 = D wave after combined stimulation of the brain and spinal cord; R= D wave recording electrode in the spinal epidural space. **Left**: Negative mapping results (D1 = D2); **right**: positive mapping results (D wave amplitude significantly diminished after collision); **right upper corner**: position of handheld stimulating electrode over exposed spinal cord. (Reprinted from: Deletis V, Camargo AB. Interventional neurophysiological mapping and monitoring during spinal cord procedures. *Stereotact. Funct. Neurosurg.* 2001;77:25–28, with permission from Karger AG.)

of the CT in the surgically exposed spinal cord **(Fig. 14.5)**. Stimulating the exposed spinal cord is done with a small handheld probe delivering a 2-mA-intensity stimulus, then simultaneously, transcranial electrical stimulation (TES) is used to elicit a descending D wave from the motor cortex (*see* Chap. 10). This descending D wave collides with the ascending neural activity elicited by stimulation of the spinal cord and then propagates antidromically along the CT **(Fig. 14.5)** The amplitude of the D wave recorded caudal to the collision site decreases because some of the descending activity in the CT that was elicited by transcranial cortical stimulation becomes extinguished by colliding with the ascending activity elicited by stimulation of the CT of the spinal cord. This will only occur when the spinal cord stimulating probe is in close proximity to the CT and the location of the stimulating electrode that produces such decrease in the D wave is therefore the location of the CT. This technique

guides surgeons and allows them to stay clear of the CT.

MAPPING OF THE FLOOR OF THE FOURTH VENTRICLE

Operations inside the brainstem are delicate because of the many important structures that are located within a very small volume of brain tissue. Neurophysiological methods for recording and electrical stimulation are used for mapping the floor of the fourth ventricle to find safe entries to internal structures of the brainstem. Several superficial structures have been identified for that purpose *(19–23)* **(Fig. 14.6)**. Motor structures can be identified by electrically stimulating the surface of the floor of the fourth ventricle and recording the EMG responses from muscles that are innervated by the respective motor systems. Using this method, the seventh cranial nerve (CN VII) can be identified

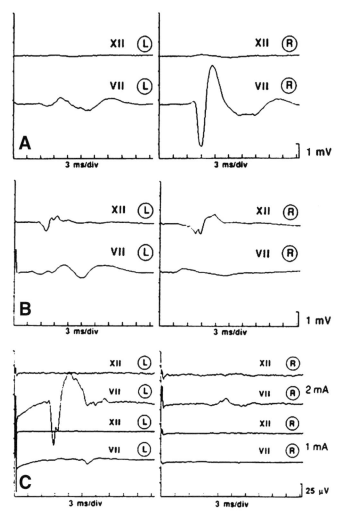

Figure 14.6: Recordings of EMG potentials from muscles innervated by CN VII and CN XII when bipolar electrical stimulation was done at different locations on the floor of the fourth ventricle. **(A)** Bipolar stimulation of the right facial colliculus and recordings from the genioglossal (CN XII) and orbicularis muscles (CN VII) on both sides. The stimulus current was 0.5 mA. **(B)** Bipolar stimulation at the left trigone of the hypoglossal (CN XII) nerve. **(C)** Bipolar stimulation of the left facial colliculus in the same patient who had a left peripheral facial paresis. The stimulus strength required to evoke a response was 2 mA because of the facial paresis. (Reprinted from: Strauss C, Romstock J, Nimsky C, Fahlbush R. Intraoperative identification of motor areas or the rhomboid fossa using direct stimulation. *J. Neurosurg.* 1993;79:393–399, with permission from Journal of Neurosurgery.)

where it comes close to the surface of the floor of the fourth ventricle. The hypoglossal nerve (CN XII) can also be identified **(Fig. 14.6)**. Both bipolar and monopolar stimulating electrodes have been used for that purpose. EMG recordings

are made from the orbicularis oculi and orbicularis oris muscles for the facial nerve, and recordings are made from the genioglossal muscle for the hypoglossal nerve **(Fig. 14.6)**. (Recording from the lateral side of the tongue

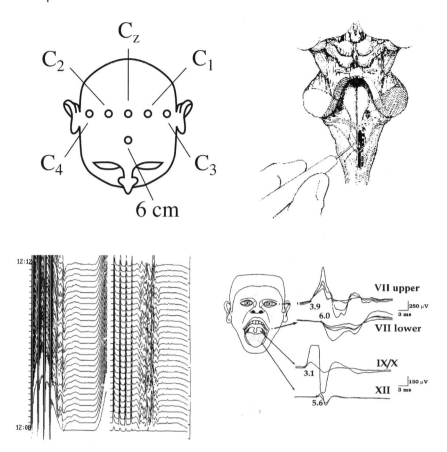

Figure 14.7: Mapping of the floor of the fourth ventricle to localize motor nuclei. **Upper row**: Placement of stimulating electrodes on the scalp and mapping of the floor of the fourth ventricle using a handheld stimulating electrode. **Lower row**: Consecutive recordings of corticobulbar transcranial motor evoked potentials and recordings from muscles innervating cranial nerves VII, IX/X, and XII. (Reprinted from: Morota N, Deletis V, Epstein FS, et al. Brain-stem mapping: Neurophysiological localization of motor nuclei on the floor of the fourth ventricle. *Neurosurgery* 1995;37:922–930, with permission from Lippincott Williams and Wilkins.)

would be a better location for recording EMG potentials.) Such recordings can distinguish between the two sides' hypoglossal nerves and indicate which side is being stimulated. Also CN IX and CN X can be identified using similar methods **(Fig. 14.7)** *(22)*.

Electrical stimulation of the floor of the fourth ventricle should be done with great caution, and the lowest possible stimulus strength should be used. The stimulus repetition rate should not exceed 10 pps, although 5 pps is generally a better choice, and short duration impulses should be used (50–100 µs duration).

LOCALIZATION OF THE SOMATOSENSORY AND MOTOR CORTEX (CENTRAL SULCUS)

Localization of the motor and sensory areas of the cerebral cortex can be done by electrically stimulating the surface of the cortex in a way similar to that done by Penfield and Rasmussen *(24)* in their pioneering work on the representation of different muscles of the body on the motor cortex, but a more practical method uses recording of cortical evoked potentials elicited by electrical stimulation of the median nerve. That can be used to find the anatomical localization of the location of the central sulcus (Rolandic fissure) *(25,26)*, which separate the primary motor and sensory areas of the cerebral cortex.

Localization of the central sulcus is based on the observation that the polarity of the recorded potentials from the sensory and the motor gyri are reversed **(Fig. 14.8)**. While stimulating the median nerve in the same way as done to record somatosensory evoked potential (SSEP) from scalp electrodes (*see* Chap. 7), the exposed surface of the cerebral cortex is mapped by placing strips of plastic material on which four or more electrodes are mounted, each of which is connected to the input of an amplifier. Usually, such recording electrodes are placed in a straight line with a distance of 1 cm between each and the electrodes are connected to separate amplifiers. Some investigators have used mats with an array of as many as 16 electrodes (4×4 or 8×8). These electrodes are then connected to an electrode box, from which individual electrodes can be selected for recording.

Because the finer details in such recordings are not of any interest, filter settings of 30–250 Hz or 30–500 Hz are suitable. The median nerve can be stimulated at a rate of 10 pps, as was described in Chap. 7. The potentials recorded directly from the surface of the somatosensory cortex are of large amplitude, usually well over 5 μV **(Fig. 14.8)**, and an interpretable response can be obtained by direct observation of the potentials or after averaging only a few responses, thus requiring less than 10 s. The recording from the electrode that is placed on the sensory cortex has a prominent negative peak with a latency of approx 20 ms **(Fig. 14.8)**. This peak is often preceded by a small positive deflection and followed by a broad positive deflection that might last more than 10 ms. Stimulation of the median nerve should be done on the side contralateral to the side on which the recordings are being made. Scalp recordings to stimulation of the ipsilateral median nerve are dominated by the N_{18} peak, which has subcortical sources (*see* Chap. 7). The negative peak **(Fig. 14.8)** is

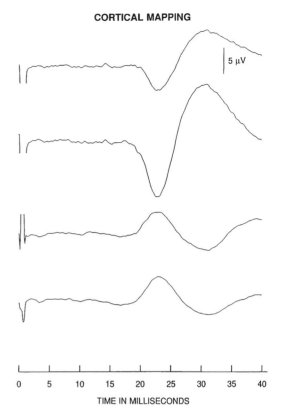

CORTICAL MAPPING

5 μV

0   5   10   15   20   25   30   35   40
TIME IN MILLISECONDS

Figure 14.8: Recordings from the exposed surface of the cerebral cortex using four electrodes placed in a straight line with a distance of 1 cm between each of the electrodes, in response to electrical stimulation of the contralateral median nerve at the wrist at a rate of 10 pps . The reference electrode was placed in the wound. The electrode strip was placed in an anterior–posterior direction, with the upper tracing originating from the most anterior electrode. The phase reversal of the recordings occurs between the two middle electrodes thus indicating that the central sulcus is located between these two electrodes. Thus, the upper two recordings were from the motor area (precentral gyrus) and the lower recording was from the sensory area. Each recording was the average of 150–250 responses. Negativity is shown as an upward deflection.

assumed to correspond to the N_{20} peak in the SSEP, as is seen in scalp recordings contralateral to the side that is stimulated.

The determination of the location of the central sulcus, as described earlier, is usually done before beginning tumor removal or other relevant operations. If the electrodes are left in place after the central sulcus has been identified, the recordings of the responses from one or more of these electrodes can then be used to monitor the integrity of the somatosensory cortex during tumor removal.

TYPE OF STIMULATION

Selecting the proper kind of electrical stimulation is important for localization of specific structures and it is important to use the appropriate stimulus strength for localizing neural tissue such as a motor nerve. If the stimulus is too weak, there might be no response, even when the stimulating electrode is close to the nerve or even when it is in contact with the nerve in question. This would result in failure to identify a nerve, which could be disastrous, as the surgeon would then be led to believe that there is no nerve present in the region that had been probed and, subsequently, manipulate the tissue that contains a nerve or potentially resect a nerve unknowingly. On the other hand, a stimulus that is too strong might spread stimulus current to nerves that are located at a distance from the site of stimulation; this could lead the surgeon to believe that

there is nerve tissue located in areas where there is, in fact, none.

Electrical stimulators are of two types. One type delivers a (nearly) constant current independent of the electrical resistance of the electrode and the tissue. The other type of stimulator delivers a constant voltage independent of the electrical resistance in the tissue stimulated *(3,8)*. The difference between these two types of stimulation is discussed in more detail in Chap. 11.

ANESTHESIA REQUIREMENTS

Mapping of the floor of the fourth ventricle depends on recording EMG potentials; this naturally cannot be done if paralyzing agents are used as a part of the anesthesia regimen (*see* Chap. 16), but mapping of the spinal cord is little affected by anesthesia and paralyzing agents. The directly recorded potentials from the exposed cortex are affected by anesthesia in a way similar to that of the SSEPs, recorded from electrodes placed on the scalp (Chap. 16). The amplitude, latency, and waveform of the potentials that are recorded from the exposed cerebral cortex are affected by the level and type of anesthesia, and the way the recorded potentials appears depends on the levels and the kind of anesthesia used.

15

Intraoperative Diagnosis and Guide in Operations

INTRODUCTION

Intraoperative neurophysiological recordings are not only beneficial for reducing the risk of postoperative deficits, but similar techniques can be used for diagnosis of peripheral nerve disorders and for guiding the surgeon in certain operations. Intraoperative measurements of neural conduction and neural conduction velocity can help to determine the nature of a specific pathology and to identify the anatomical location of the pathology of nerves. Such recordings can guide the surgeon to the proper anatomical location for surgical intervention and, indeed, might also help the surgeon choose the appropriate surgical intervention.

DIAGNOSIS OF INJURED PERIPHERAL NERVES

Before introduction of electrophysiological methods for assessing neural conduction

From: *Intraoperative Neurophysiological Monitoring: Second Edition*
By A. R. Møller
© Humana Press Inc., Totowa, NJ.

in injured peripheral nerves, surgeons were confronted with making difficult decisions regarding the repair of severe nerve injuries on the basis of visual observations and intuition. The introduction of electrophysiological methods have now made it possible to do functional testing of peripheral nerves in the operating room, and decisions about how to repair such nerves can be based on hard physiological information. Neuroma in continuity possesses a particular problem regarding choice of optimal treatment.

Neuroma in Continuity

Neuroma in continuity can occur because of injury to peripheral nerves. It is caused because of incorrect regrowth (sprouting) of regenerating nerve fibers. Accumulation of tangled regenerating nerve fibers (sprouts) builds neuroma that might compress nerve fibers that are unaffected by the lesion or that are regenerating normally. Even in small neurinoma, the nerve fibers that pass through it might be interrupted. Conversely, many nerve fibers that pass through a large neurinoma might be conducting effectively and, thus, do not need any surgical intervention.

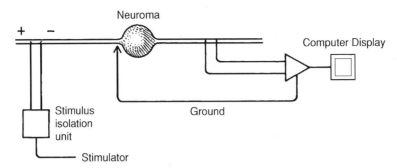

Figure 15.1: Stimulation of a peripheral nerve with a neuroma and recording from the opposite side of the neuroma.

Surgical treatment of neuroma in continuity is especially demanding and neurophysiological diagnosis performed intraoperatively is of great importance for the success of the repair of such lesions. The severity of lesions of peripheral nerves cannot be assessed by visual inspection and the aid of physiological diagnosis intraoperatively is essential. If injury to a peripheral nerve has resulted in a neuroma in continuity, it is not possible to determine preoperatively whether the nerve that is distal to the neuroma has begun to regenerate.

Such information is important for making decisions about whether to perform a nerve graft or to do nothing at all and wait for the nerve to regrow by itself and reach its target (muscles for motor nerves). Such diagnosis can only be obtained by exposing the nerve surgically at the location of the neuroma and doing neurophysiological recordings of neural conduction (27–30).

After a peripheral nerve has been dissected, a neuroma appears as a thickening of the nerve, but it is not possible to determine by inspection alone whether there is any neural conduction across the neuroma. However, this can easily be determined by electrically stimulating the nerve on one side of the neuroma and recording the compound action potential (CAP) from a location on the nerve on the other side of the neuroma (**Fig. 15.1**). If a CAP can be recorded, it is a sign that the nerve conducts nerve impulses through the neuroma, and that indicates that the nerve is in the process of regenerating and is

growing toward its target. In this case, nothing needs to be done. If no CAP can be recorded, there is no neural conduction across the neuroma and a nerve graft must then be performed in order to re-establish function.

It could be argued that surgical exploration is unnecessary in such cases, because it would eventually become obvious if the nerve were properly regenerating if a sufficient length of time was allowed to pass. However, if the nerve does not regenerate, it might be too late to perform a nerve graft by the time this fact was to become obvious because, at that time, the nerve might no longer have the ability to regenerate and, in the case of motor nerves, create new muscle endplates. Even if a nerve graft would be effective following such a time lapse, the patient would have gone without nerve function for a long time unnecessarily.

Localizing the Place of Injury

Neurophysiological methods make it possible to localize the exact place where a nerve is injured. This is done by stimulating the nerve in question electrically and recording from a location a short distance from where the nerve is stimulated. Similar basic electrophysiological techniques make it possible to determine if an injured nerve is beginning to regenerate. These methods are superior to other often-used methods involving recordings of electromyographic (EMG) potentials. Decisions about how a particular nerve would best respond to resection and repair compared to more conservative treatment

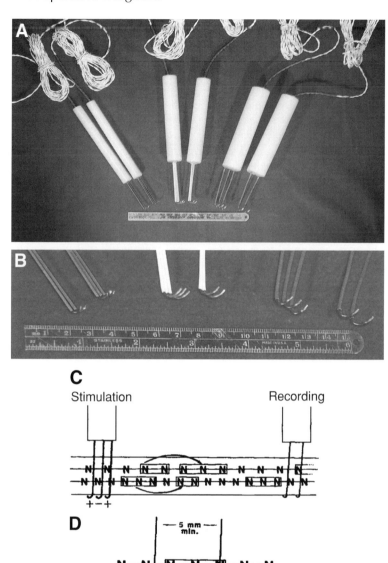

Figure 15.2: **(A)** Electrodes for stimulating and recording compound nerve action potentials (CNAPs) can be made in many sizes according to one's needs. Illustrated here, from left to right, are miniature, mid-size, and large electrodes. The stimulating electrode contains three contacts and the recording electrode contains two. **(B)** Enlargement of the electrode tips illustrating the curved hooks on which the exposed nerve can be suspended. The tip separation of the recording electrodes can be adjusted according to the nerve from which recordings are made. (From ref. *29.*) **(C)** Use of a tripolar stimulating electrode in testing a peripheral nerve. **(D)** The distance between the stimulating electrodes must include several nodes of Ranvier of the nerve that is being tested. (Adapted from: Happel L, Kline D. Nerve lesions in continuity. In: Gelberman RH, ed. *Operative Nerve Repair and Reconstruction,* Vol. 1, 1st ed. Philadelphia, PA: J.B. Lippincott.)

such as neurolysis can be made right at the operating table using such basic electrophysiological methods.

For such an intraoperative diagnosis, both the stimulating and the recording electrodes (**Fig. 15.2A**) should be placed on the same nerve a short distance from each other. Both stimulating and recording electrodes should be metal hooks (**Fig. 15.2A**). The distance between the stimulating electrodes must be long enough to include a sufficient number of nodes of Ranvier *(30)* (**Fig. 15.2D**).

When a satisfactory response is obtained from a normal nerve, the stimulating-recording electrode assembly can be moved to a section of the nerve whose function is to be diagnosed while keeping the settings for stimulation and recording the same as used for the normal nerve. If a response is observed, it proves the presence of viable axons. The decision about the treatment of the nerve is made on the basis of these observations. A flowchart for such procedures is shown in **Fig. 15.3**.

For the purpose of finding regions of a peripheral nerve that have abnormal conduction properties, the electrodes should be moved along the length of the nerve from distal to proximal. When no response is seen from a section of an injured nerve, it is a sign of a conduction block and this kind of recording procedure makes it possible to discern the part of a nerve where viable axons are present. This is a totally nondestructive type of testing that can be repeated until the results are satisfying and it does not involve risks of damage to regenerating axons. Upon visual inspection, nerves might appear to be injured but electrophysiological testing could prove otherwise, showing clear signs of axonal continuity. Similarly, lesions, that appear to be mild from visual inspection can be functionally severe. This means that the physical appearance of a nerve with regard to lesions might be misleading.

Neuromuscular blocking agents can be used during such recordings and they might even produce an advantage because they prevent muscle activation from the electrical stimulation of motor nerves.

Slightly injured nerves have a lower conduction velocity than normal nerves. Also, regenerating nerves have lower conduction velocities because the regenerated nerve fibers have smaller diameters than normal nerve fibers. The threshold for electrical stimulation of nerve fibers decreases when the duration of the electrical impulses is increased. The curve of threshold vs duration of the impulses used to stimulate a nerve is shifted toward the right for regenerated fibers (**Fig. 15.4**) because of their smaller diameters. It is seen that the current (intensity) required to achieve maximal response from a nerve is larger for short-duration impulses and that nerves with regenerated fibers require more current at a certain duration to reach the maximal response than normal nerve fibers. The difference is exaggerated for regenerated fibers. Therefore, studies of the strength–duration relationship of nerves provide information about the quality of regenerated axons.

Stimulus and Recording Parameters

It is practical first to apply the stimulation to a nerve that is known to be normal and record its response. That will make sure that the equipment is working appropriately and that the patient has normal nerve functions of nerves that are not injured. A stimulus rate of one to three per second suitable and stimulus strengths between 3 and 5 V corresponding to 0.5–2 mA can usually activate all large fibers in a mixed nerve. Filters for such recording should be set at approx 10 Hz high pass and 3 kHz low pass and a suitable gain of the amplifier should be selected.

The effect of stimulus artifacts on the recorded responses can be diminished by keeping the amplification low so that the stimulus artifact does not overload the amplifier, which will cause it to spread out in time (*see* Chap. 19). The use of good quality stimulus isolation units is important for minimizing the stimulus artifacts. Naturally, the stimulus artifacts can be reduced by increasing the distance between stimulating and recording electrodes (at least 2 cm) and separating the stimulating and recording leads. Placing a ground electrode

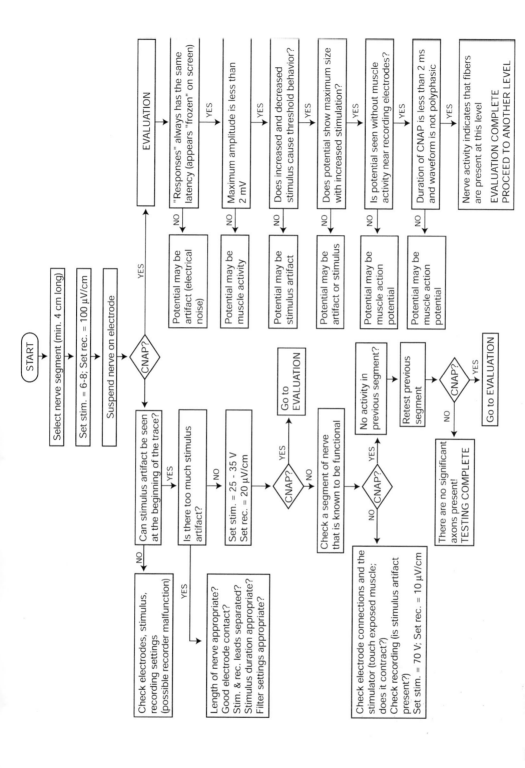

Figure 15.3: Flowchart showing options in peripheral nerve repairs. (Reprinted from: Happel L, Kline D. Intraoperative neurophysiology of the peripheral nervous system. In: Deletis V, Shils JL, eds. *Neurophysiology in Neurosurgery*. Amsterdam: Academic; 2002:169–195, with permission from Elsevier.)

255

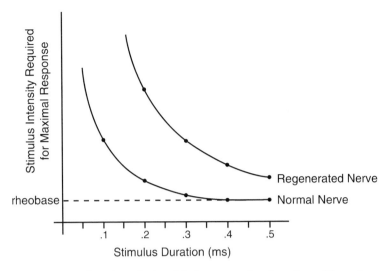

Figure 15.4: Curves showing the relationship between the duration of impulses used to electrically stimulate a nerve and the stimulus intensity required to achieve maximal response (strength–duration curves) for normal and regenerated nerve fibers. (Data from ref. *30.*)

between the recording and stimulating electrodes (**Fig. 15.1**) can help to reduce the stimulus artifact. The use of a tripolar recording electrode (**Fig. 15.2C**) instead of a bipolar stimulating electrode is even more effective in reducing the stimulus artifacts because it eliminates a current path that would include the site of the recording electrode *(29).*

IDENTIFICATION OF THE COMPRESSING VESSEL IN OPERATIONS FOR HEMIFACIAL SPASM

The microvascular decompression (MVD) operation to relieve hemifacial spasm (HFS) is one of few operations in which intraoperative neurophysiological recordings can guide the surgeon in identifying the anatomical location of the pathology. Intraoperative neurophysiological recordings can also provide evidence of a successful accomplishment of the goal of the operation.

Hemifacial spasm can be cured by moving a blood vessel off the facial nerve (MVD opera-

tion). The offending vessel (artery or vein) is most often located near the root exit zone (REZ) of the facial nerve. To cure the disorder, the vessel(s) must be moved off the nerve and an implant of a soft material (such as shredded Teflon) is placed between the nerve and the vessel(s). MVD operations normally have a high cure rate (approx 85%) (31,32). If the offending vessel is not moved off the facial nerve root, the spasm persists postoperatively and the patient must be reoperated. The reason for this has almost always been that there was more than one vessel in contact with the facial nerve root, which was not obvious from visual inspection during the first operation and, therefore, some patients had incomplete relief of their spasm.

Introduction of intraoperative recording of the abnormal muscle response in MVD operations for HFS has reduced the necessity of reoperations and improved the cure rate to more than 95% *(33).* During such operations, intraoperative neurophysiological recordings of the abnormal muscle response can help identify the blood vessel that is involved in causing the spasm and help to ensure that the therapeutic goal of the operation has been achieved before the operation has been terminated. (The abnormal muscle response *[33–35]* is also known as the "lateral spread response" *[36]* or the "delayed muscle response".) The abnormal muscle response of facial muscles appears as an EMG response from a muscle that is innervated by one branch of the facial nerve when a different branch is stimulated electrically.

Abnormal Muscle Response

When a branch of the facial nerve in a patient with HFS is stimulated electrically, not only do the muscles that are innervated by this branch of the facial nerve contract but also the muscles that are innervated by other branches of the facial nerve contract. This abnormal muscle response can thus be elicited by electrical stimulation of one branch of the facial nerve while recordings of the EMG response from muscles that are innervated by a different branch of the facial nerve are being made *(37)*. For example, the abnormal muscle response can be elicited by stimulating the temporal or zygomatic branch of the facial nerve electrically while recording EMG potentials from the mentalis muscle (**Figs. 15.5** and **15.6**) or by stimulating the marginal mandibular branch while recording from the orbicularis oculi muscles. The abnormal muscle response seems to be specific to patients with HFS and it can only be elicited from the side of the face where the spasm occurs.

The abnormal muscle response elicited by electrical stimulation of a branch of the facial nerve consists of an initial EMG potential that occurs with a latency of about 10 ms, followed by a variable series of potentials (afterdischarges) (**Fig. 15.7**). Such stimulation also evokes a (direct) response from the muscles that are innervated by the nerve that is stimulated.

When a blood vessel that is in close contact with the facial nerve and related to the patient's spasm is lifted off the nerve, the abnormal muscle response usually disappears instantaneously *(39)* (**Fig. 15.8**), but if the vessel is allowed to fall back on the nerve, the response reappears *(39)* (**Fig. 15.8**). The abnormal muscle response

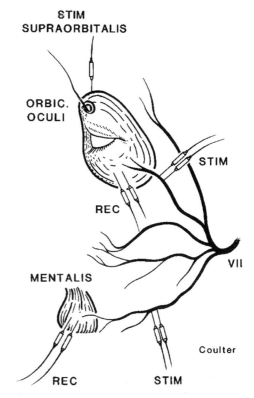

Figure 15.5: Schematic of the arrangement used for stimulating one branch of the facial nerve (the marginal mandibular or zygomatic branch) and for recording EMG potentials from muscles that are innervated by a different branch for monitoring the abnormal muscle response.

remains absent after an implant (for instance, a small piece of Teflon felt) is placed between the facial nerve and the offending blood vessel.

The abnormal muscle response is obviously a result of abnormal spread of activity from one branch of the facial nerve on the affected side to other branches of the facial nerve on the same side (crosstalk).

Evidence has been presented that the abnormal muscle response is backfiring (exaggerated F response) of motoneurons in the facial nucleus (34,40–43). These motoneurons have become hyperactive and hypersensitive by unknown processes involved in the disorders.

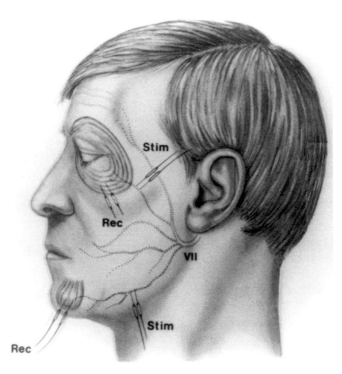

Figure 15.6: Electrode placement for monitoring the abnormal muscle response in a patient undergoing MVD to relieve HFS. (Reprinted from: Møller AR, Jannetta PJ. Synkinesis in hemifacial spasm: results of recording intracranially from the facial nerve. *Experientia* 1985;41:415–417, with permission from Birkhauser Verlag AG.)

The location of a blood vessel on the facial nerve root is obviously necessary to maintain that hyperactivity, explaining why the abnormal muscle response disappears when the blood vessel is moved off the facial nerve.

The abnormal muscle response can be recorded while the patient is awake as well as when the patient is under surgical anesthesia, provided that muscle relaxants are not used. The amplitude of the abnormal muscle response is only 5–10% of that of the direct muscle response (M response) to stimulation of the branch of the nerve that innervates the particular muscle, indicating that the abnormal muscle response only activates a small fraction of the total number of motor units. (The M response is assumed to involve most of the motor units of the muscle when the facial nerve is stimulated at a supramaximal strength.)

Use of the Abnormal Muscle Response for Monitoring MVD Operations for HFS. Because the abnormal muscle response disappears instantly when the offending vessel is moved off the facial nerve *(39)*, monitoring the abnormal muscle response can guide the surgeon in this kind of MVD operation, achieving a better success rate *(33)*. The after-discharges that follow the initial component of the abnormal muscle response (**Fig. 15.7**) often disappear or become infrequent after the dura is opened and when the facial nerve is exposed, and, usually, only the initial component with a latency of 10 ms remains. If the abnormal muscle response only decreases in amplitude when a vessel is moved off the facial nerve, it is an indication that another vessel is also affecting the facial nerve. When this other vessel is identified and moved off the facial nerve, the abnormal muscle response disappears totally.

Sti Zyg. NVII

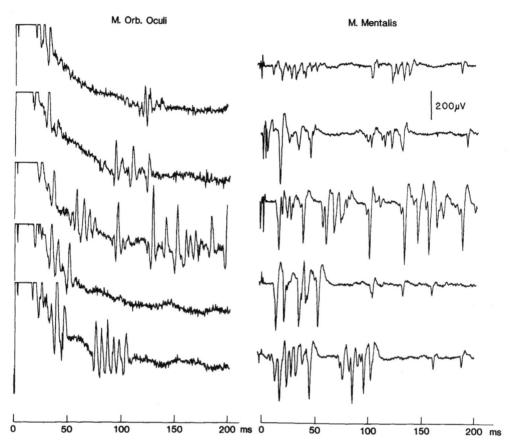

Figure 15.7: Recordings of the EMG response from the orbicularis oculi (**left**) and mentalis (**right**) muscles when the zygomatic branch of the facial nerve was stimulated electrically in a patient undergoing MVD to relieve HFS. The recordings were obtained after the patient was anesthetized but before the operation was begun. (Reprinted from: Møller AR, Jannetta PJ. Physiological abnormalities in hemifacial spasm studied during microvascular decompression operations. *Exp. Neurol.* 1986;93:584–600, with permission from Elsevier.)

In some patients, the abnormal muscle response might be absent when the stimulation is first switched on, but it can be activated by increasing the stimulus rate to 50 pps for a few seconds, after which the repetition rate might again be set at the customary rate of 2–5 pps (**Fig. 15.9**). The initial absence of the abnormal muscle response often occurs in patients who have had HFS for only a short time prior to the operation. If the amplitude of the abnormal muscle response is low in the beginning of an opera-

tion, the amplitude of the response will increase after such rapid stimulation (*41*). After-discharges also often reappear after the initial response, and spontaneous muscle contractions might also occur for a short time after rapid stimulation.

The amplitude of the abnormal muscle response often decreases when the arachnoidal membrane over the lower cranial nerves is opened and the after-discharges usually disappear at this stage of the operation (**Fig. 15.10**). If the abnormal muscle response disappears

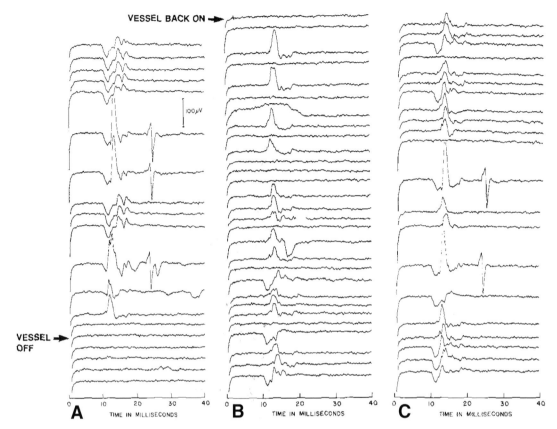

Figure 15.8: EMG recordings from a patient undergoing MVD to relieve HFS. Each graph shows consecutive recordings (beginning at the top) from the mentalis muscle in response to electrical stimulation of the zygomatic branch of the facial nerve. As indicated, the recordings in the middle of the right column were made when the vessel was lifted off the nerve. (Reprinted from: Møller AR, Jannetta PJ. Microvascular decompression in hemifacial spasm: intraoperative electrophysiological observations. *Neurosurgery* 1985;16:612–618, with permission from Lippincott Williams and Wilkins.)

totally when the dura or the arachnoidal membrane is opened and if response cannot be brought back by applying stimulation at 50 pps for a short period (**Fig. 15.9**), the offending vessel is often found to be a loose loop of an artery (either the anterior inferior cerebellar artery [AICA], or the posterior inferior cerebellar artery [PICA], or a branch of either one). The disappearance of the abnormal muscle response occurs because the loop of the vessel loses contact with the nerve when the intracisternal fluid pressure is decreased because of opening the dura or arachnoidal membrane.

In patients who have had HFS for a long time (7–15 yr), after-discharges sometimes occur after the initial component of the abnormal muscle response, even after the facial nerve has been exposed. In such patients, the offending vessel is often in firm contact (held in place by arachnoidal bands), with the proximal portion of the facial nerve near the brainstem. Such vessels must be dissected off the nerve in order to place an implant between the vessel and the nerve, involving risk of injury to the facial nerve. Monitoring of the function of the facial nerve to detect possible injuries to the nerve is indicated

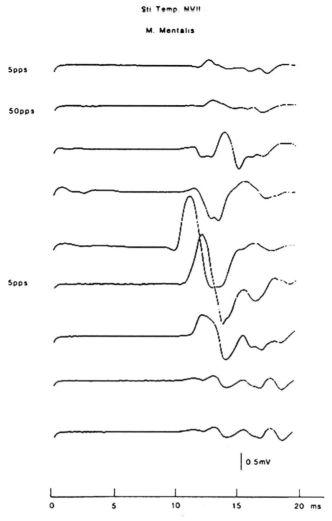

Figure 15.9: Recordings of the abnormal muscle response in a patient undergoing MVD operation to relieve HFS, obtained before the offending vessels were moved off the facial nerve. The effect of increasing the stimulus rate from 5 to 50 pps for a short period of stimulation on the abnormal muscle response is shown. (Reprinted from: Møller AR, Jannetta PJ. Physiological abnormalities in hemifacial spasm studied during microvascular decompression operations. *Exp. Neurol.* 1986;93:584–600, with permission from Elsevier.)

in such situations. The techniques described in Chap. 11 can be used for that purpose.

The abnormal muscle response might not disappear before a small artery or veins that are in close contact with the facial nerve, often where its root blends into the brainstem *(33,34)*. (Before the introduction of intraoperative monitoring of the abnormal muscle response, it was reported that such small vessels could cause the symptoms of HFS *[44]*.) When such small vessels were moved off the nerve root or coagulated (veins), the abnormal muscle response usually disappeared and the response could not be made to reappear by increasing the stimulus rate. In most cases, these patients obtained total relief from their spasms postoperatively.

A   **B**

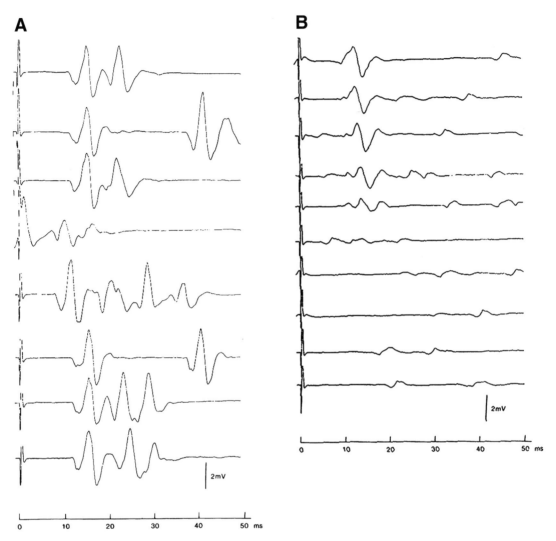

Figure 15.10: Examples of the abnormal EMG response recorded in a patient who was undergoing MVD to relieve HFS. **(A)** Shows recordings done before the dura was opened. The response appearing with a latency of approx 10 ms is the abnormal muscle response. This is followed by variable EMG activity (after-discharges). **(B)** The top recordings were obtained after the dura was opened and show only the initial component of the abnormal muscle response. The vessel was moved off the nerve when the recordings in the middle of this column were obtained. **(B)** The bottom recordings show an absence of the abnormal muscle response. The low-amplitude, spontaneous activity seen in the recordings is indicative of slight injury to the facial nerve. (Reprinted from: Shils JL, Tagliati M, Alterman RL. Neurophysiological monitoring during neurosurgery for movement disorders. In: Deletis V, Shils JL, eds. *Neurophysiology in Neurosurgery.* Amsterdam: Academic Press; 2002:405–448, with permission from Elsevier.)

If the abnormal muscle response does not disappear when a blood vessel was moved off the facial nerve, the patients' spasms often remained after the operation *(33)*.

On the basis of these findings it seems essential for curing HFS that blood vessels are moved of the facial nerve root to an extent that the abnormal muscle response can no longer be elicited *(33,45)*. If moving one vessel off the facial nerve does not eliminate the abnormal muscle response, it is important to explore the facial nerve root further, including the surface of the brainstem where the facial nerve exits to identify any vessel that might cause the spasm.

Before it can be made sure that the abnormal muscle response is absent, a sufficiently high stimulus intensity (at least 20 V, corresponding to about 5 mA) must be used, and the facial nerve must be stimulated at a high rate for a few seconds before it can be concluded that the abnormal muscle response is indeed absent *(41)* (**Fig. 15.9**).

If these maneuvers cause the abnormal muscle response to reappear, even for a short period, another vessel is most likely in contact with the facial nerve and the operation cannot be regarded to be completed before that vessel has been moved off the facial nerve. Individuals who have that kind of residual occurrence of the abnormal muscle response most likely have spasm postoperatively, but that spasm might disappear over time. If the abnormal muscle response cannot be brought back by increasing the stimulus strength and stimulus rate, there is only a very small likelihood that the patient will have residual spasm postoperatively *(33)*.

This technique has been used in many patients who were operated on for HFS *(33)* and its usefulness has been confirmed by other investigators *(45)*, who also found that monitoring the abnormal muscle response is helpful in identifying the vessel that is causing the patient's HFS. Other investigators *(42)* have found that good outcome might occur even when the abnormal muscle response is present at the end of the operations and, thus, have questioned the value of this form of intraoperative monitoring.

In addition to increasing the success rate of the MVD operation, the results of using the abnormal muscle response in operations on patients with HFS have provided evidence that there can be more than one vessel involved in generating the abnormal muscle response and thus the spasm and that vessels can be in close contact with the facial nerve without causing any noticeable problems. Recordings of the abnormal muscle response in operations to relieve HFS have also provided research opportunities that have contributed to both a better understanding of the pathophysiology of HFS and to the understanding of other disorders that are caused by similar pathologies *(43,46)*.

Technique Used to Monitor the Abnormal Muscle Response

For monitoring purposes, it is most suitable to elicit the abnormal muscle response from the temporal branch of the facial nerve, but in patients who have had HFS for many years, stimulation of the marginal mandibular branch of the facial nerve might be used as well. EMG responses recorded from the mentalis muscle and elicited by electrical stimulation of the temporal branch of the facial nerve provide the most reproducible recording of the abnormal muscle response for the purpose of intraoperative monitoring of MVD operations for HFS.

For recording the abnormal muscle response, two fine-needle electrodes should be placed approx 1 cm apart deep in the mentalis muscle. Two electrodes should be placed superficially in the orbicularis oculi muscles for recording the direct muscle response (M response) (**Fig. 15.6**). These two pairs of recording electrodes should be connected to two differential amplifiers in order to obtain differentially recorded EMG from each muscle (**Fig. 15.7**). Electrical stimulation of the temporal branch of the facial nerve is accomplished by two similar needle electrodes placed about 1 cm apart in or near the temporal branch of the facial nerve. The proper location is easily found by noting an imaginary line between the ear canal and the lateral corner of the eye and placing the stimulating electrodes about halfway between the ear and the eye on that line. The cathode (negative electrode) should be placed closest to the ear.

If the marginal mandibular nerve is to be stimulated, recordings of the abnormal muscle response should be made from muscles around the eye (orbicularis oculi muscles) (**Fig. 15.6**), and the direct muscle response (M response) should be recorded from the mentalis muscle.

Although recording of the M response is not important to intraoperative monitoring, it makes it possible to check that the stimulating electrodes are correctly placed in the appropriate branch of the facial nerve. Placing the stimulating electrodes correctly is facilitated by having the stimulator connected to the stimulating electrodes and the stimulation switched on (at a rate of 5–10 pps at about 20 V using a semi-constant-voltage stimulator) while observing the face for muscle contractions. Rectangular impulses of 100–150 µs duration should be used as the stimulus. After all of the electrodes are in place, the stimulus strength could be lowered to find the threshold for eliciting the abnormal muscle response. This is usually approx 6 V but can be as low as 1.5 V. During monitoring of the abnormal muscle response, a stimulus repetition rate of 1–2 pps and a stimulus level that is 20–30% above threshold will usually provide a stable abnormal muscle response.

The amplifiers for the EMG potentials should have filter settings at 10–3000 Hz. The recorded EMG potentials can be made audible by using a device similar to that described when discussing intraoperative monitoring during removal of acoustic tumors (*see* Chap. 11) *(8,47)*.

Intraoperative monitoring of auditory function is usually done in patients who are operated for HFS concurrently with monitoring of facial muscle contractions. The stimulation of the facial nerve should not be a submultiple of the stimulus rate for the auditory stimulation to avoid interference with the recording of auditory potentials.

PHYSIOLOGICAL GUIDANCE OF PLACEMENT OF STIMULATING ELECTRODES AND FOR MAKING LESIONS IN THE BRAIN

Identifying specific tissue in operations where lesions are to be made in central nervous system (CNS) structures has become an important part of practical use of neurophysiological methods in the operating room. It places particular demand on the physiologist who carries out such procedures regarding knowledge about anatomy and physiology of the systems

in question. Most of the procedures are done in awake patients, which places additional obligations on everybody who are present in the operating room.

The targets for lesions and implantation of stimulating electrodes (for deep brain stimulation [DBS]) are now mostly different nuclei of the basal ganglia and the thalamus. The purpose is mainly treatment of movement disorders and pain. Implantation of electrodes for chronic stimulation (DBS) has replaced many forms of making small lesions in these structures. Implantation of electrodes in the cerebral cortex for promoting expression of neural plasticity in stroke victims *(48)* and for treatment of tinnitus *(49)* and pain *(50)* are methods that are in the state of development in clinical useful methods. Implantation of electrodes for stimulation of the dorsal column of the spinal cord for pain *(51,52)* and for stimulation of the vagus nerve for epilepsy and pain *(53)* have been in use for some years.

Although the anatomical location of lesions or implantation of electrodes in the basal ganglia and the thalamus are determined grossly by imaging techniques such as magnetic resonance imaging (MRI), the exact location for lesions or for implantation of electrodes for DBS is normally made using neurophysiological recordings as guidance. Neurophysiological guidance using neurophysiological recordings is also important for placement of auditory brainstem implants (cochlear nucleus implants) *(54)*.

Implantation of Electrodes in the Basal Ganglia and Thalamus

The proper target for implantation of electrodes for DBS can be determined by recordings of electrical activity from cells of these nuclei *(55)*. Other groups *(56)* have used a similar technique for guidance of the placement of lesions in specific structures of the basal ganglia. Understanding the anatomy and physiology of the specific parts of the thalamus and the basal ganglia (Chap. 9) is essential for the success of such procedures.

For the purpose of finding the correct location for lesions or implantation of electrodes for DBS, microelectrodes are used to record responses from single nerve cells or small groups of nerve cells (multiunit recordings). The methods that are used for recordings from deep brain structures in humans for these purposes were developed by Albe-Fessard and her co-workers (57) for research purposes. The recent extensive practical use of these methods in humans have provided opportunities for research purposes, and much of our present knowledge about the normal and the pathological function of the basal ganglia and parts of the thalamus have been acquired in that way. The use of these methods in clinical settings have produced a wealth of information not only about the normal functions of these structures but also about the pathophysiology of movement disorders (56,58–65).

Localization of Specific Basal Ganglia Structures in Movement Disorders. For location of the sites for implantation of DBS electrodes, the goal is to find the anatomical location with the best therapeutical effect and the least side effect. For that purpose, microelectrodes are inserted using stereotaxic methods and the responses are observed as the electrode is advanced through the structures that are the targets for implantations or lesions. Sometimes more than one path has to be used to find the optimal location for implantation of the electrodes for permanent stimulation or for making lesions. The identification of the specific target for implantation (or lesions) is made on the basis of electrical activity recorded by microelectrodes that either record from single neural elements (mostly cell bodies) or from a small group of cells (multiunit recording). Two kinds of activity is recorded: spontaneous activity and activity elicited by specific voluntary movements that the patient is asked to do. The target is determined on the basis of empirical data and experience because our understanding of the function of these structures and their involvement in movement disorders is still incomplete.

Microelectrodes have been used for many years in animal experiments and two types

are used: glass pipets and metal electrodes. Metal microelectrodes were developed by David Hubel. The tips of such electrodes are uninsulated and have a diameter of a few micrometers (1 µm =1/1000 of a millimeter). For use in humans, metal electrodes have been used exclusively. Some of the first such uses were for research studies of cortical cells (66) and for studies of the somatosensory part of the thalamus (59,60). Lenz and co-workers (59,60) described the construction of microelectrodes that were suitable for use in humans. The diameter of the tip of electrodes that only record from a single nerve cell should be 1–5 µm. Electrodes with larger tips (20–50 µm) will normally record from more than one cell (multiunit recordings). The electrical impedance of such electrodes is inversely proportional to their tip diameter and could vary from 50 kΩ for a tip size on the order of 50 µm to 1 MΩ for the smallest tip size (1–3 µm), all depending on the material used and the length of the uninsulated tip. The properties of such electrodes were studied by other investigators and these studies are the basis for the present use of such electrodes in finding targets for implantation of electrodes for DBS and for making lesions in CNS structures.

Some investigators make their own electrodes, whereas others use commercially available electrodes. For example, Starr and his group (67) use glass-coated platinum/iridium microelectrodes that are commercially available (Microprobe, Inc., Gaithersburg, MD or FHC, Inc., Brunswick, ME). These electrodes have impedances between 0.4 and 1 MΩ.

Responses From Cells in the Basal Ganglia

The discharge pattern varies much from cell to cell and it is different from nucleus to nucleus (**Fig. 15.11** and **15.12**). The cells from which recording is done are often named according to their pattern of discharge, such as "burster" cells, which generate bursts of activity and "pauser cells," which have tonic discharges that are interrupted by brief pauses in

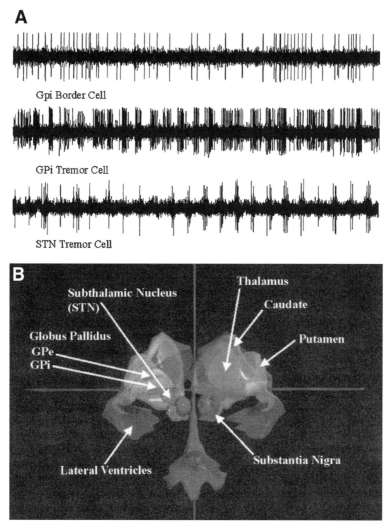

Figure 15.11: (A) Typical good quality recordings from three different cells in the basal ganglia. These recordings are single-cell recordings as seen from the fact that all spikes have the same amplitude. Notice that the level of the background noise is well below that of the spikes. The recording was 5s long. **(B)** Artist's rendition of the structures of the basal ganglia that are targets for lesions and implantation of electrodes for DBS. GPi and GPe: Globus pallidus internal and external; STN: subthalamic nucleus. (Reprinted from: Shils JL, Tagliati M, Alterman RL. Neurophysiological monitoring during neurosurgery for movement disorders. In: Deletis V, Shils JL, eds. *Neurophysiology in Neurosurgery*. Amsterdam: Academic Press; 2002:405–448, with permission from Elsevier.)

firing. Some cells will exhibit bursting activity that is superimposed on continuous activity. Different types of disorder produce specific pattern of discharges, as do different cells in the different nuclei and in different parts of the nuclei. Examples of recordings of single-cell

activity and multiunit activity are shown in **Figs. 15.12–15.14.**

Equipment for Microelectrode Recordings. The equipment used for neurophysiological guidance is more complex than that used for

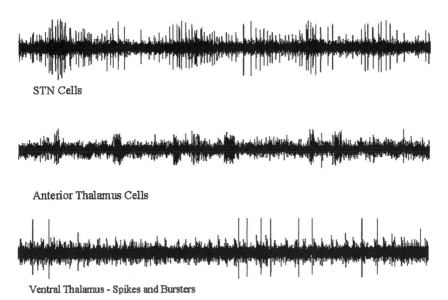

STN Cells

Anterior Thalamus Cells

Ventral Thalamus - Spikes and Bursters

Figure 15.12: Typical multiunit recording from three different locations in the thalamus. Individual units can be distinguished by the difference in the amplitude and the difference in the waveform, which is detected by modern computer software. The recording were 5s epochs. (Reprinted from: Shils JL, Tagliati M, Alterman RL. Neurophysiological monitoring during neurosurgery for movement disorders. In: Deletis V, Shils JL, eds. *Neurophysiology in Neurosurgery.* Amsterdam: Academic Press; 2002:405–448, with permission from Elsevier.)

intraoperative neurophysiological monitoring (**Fig. 15.15**). Filter settings for the amplifiers of 300 Hz to 5 kHz are suitable. The recorded activity should be made audible by a loudspeaker so everyone in the operating room can hear the activity, in addition to being displayed on a computer screen together with statistics such as mean discharge rate, and interspike interval. The software should be able to sort the different components of multiunit recordings and store data for later analysis and for use in research (**Fig. 15.15**).

Display of Results and Quality Control. During sessions to find appropriate anatomical locations for lesions or for implantation of electrodes for DBS, the discharge properties at each location should be plotted on planes that refer to relevant anatomical structures. When a location for stimulation is found, test stimulations are done to see if the anticipated effect is achieved, such as cessation of tremor or other abnormal muscle contractions.

Quality control is especially important for microelectrode recordings because of the high electrode impedance that makes such recordings prone to be contaminated with many kinds of electrical interference (**Fig. 15.16**). Making a recording in awake patients adds other sources of interference, although the movement artifact should not be a problem because the patient's head is firmly secured in a head holder. Poor recordings can also have other reasons, such as recording far from active structures or defective electrodes (**Fig. 15.16**).

MONITORING IMPLANTATION OF AUDITORY PROSTHESES

Two kinds of auditory prosthesis are in routine use: cochlear implants *(68)* are the most common and, implants to stimulate the cochlear nucleus (auditory brainstem implants [ABIs]) *(69)*. Cochlear implants were introduced by William House *(70),* and the early implants

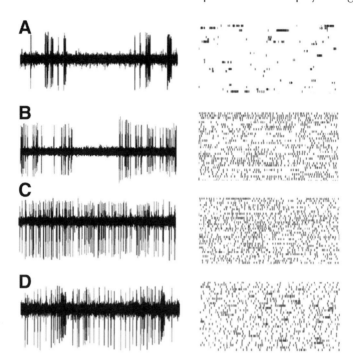

Figure 15.13: Unit recording from GPe and GPi in a patient with dystonia (1-s epochs are shown). Raster diagrams to the right: each line represents 500 ms, and a 15-s segment of the receded activity is shown. Each vertical tick mark represents a single action potential (discharge). **(A)** Recording from a GPe burster cell; **(B)** recording from a GPe pause cell; **(C)** recording from a GPi cell; **(D)** recording from "high-frequency burster" cell in the GPi. *(67)* (Reprinted with permission from *Neurosurg. Focus.*)

consisted of a single electrode placed inside the cochlea and connected to electronics that converted sounds picked up by a microphone into electrical current. Modern cochlear implants consist of an array of electrodes that are implanted in the basal portion of the cochlea *(71)*. Electrical signals are generated by a processor of sounds that reach a microphone placed near the individual's ear that activate these electrodes. Both adults who have acquired hearing loss and children who have been born deaf are now routinely given cochlear implants.

Auditory brainstem implants were introduced for use in individuals who have lost hearing on both ears from bilateral vestibular schwannoma usually from neurofibromatosis type 2 (NF2). More recently, it has been found possible to restore hearing by such cochlear nucleus implants in individuals with disorders

of the auditory nerve such as auditory nerve aplasia or severe auditory neuropathy *(72)*.

Implantation of the stimulating electrodes in the cochlea requires a minimum of electrophysiological guidance, but the correct placement of the implanted array of electrodes is usually checked using recordings of auditory brainstem response (ABR) in a way similar to that described in Chap. 6. Implantation of electrodes to stimulate the cochlear nuclei (ABIs) requires testing of the position of the implanted electrode array with regard to adequately stimulating their target neurons *(54)*, and intraoperative guidance in the placement of such implants has gained increasing use *(54,73)*.

Physiological Guidance for Placement of ABIs

Auditory brainstem implants consist of an array of 8–16 electrodes placed on a plastic

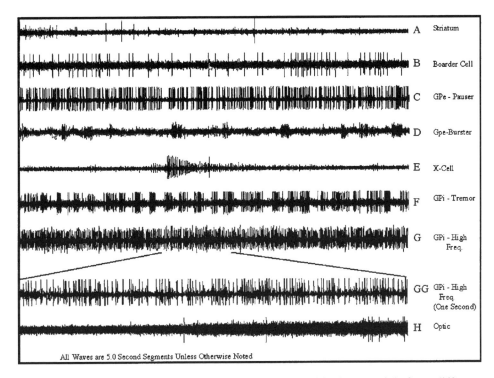

A   Striatum

B   Boarder Cell

C   GPe - Pauser

D   Gpe-Burster

E   X-Cell

F   GPi - Tremor

G   GPi - High
     Freq.

GG   GPi - High
     Freq.
     (One Second)

H   Optic

All Waves are 5.0 Second Segments Unless Otherwise Noted

Figure 15.14: Variations in the appearance of recorded multiunit potentials from different nuclei of the basal ganglia. All recordings were 5s epochs. (Reprinted from: Shils JL, Tagliati M, Alterman RL. Neurophysiological monitoring during neurosurgery for movement disorders. In: Deletis V, Shils JL, eds. *Neurophysiology in Neurosurgery,* Amsterdam: Academic Press; 2002:405–448, with permission from Elsevier.)

sheet that is placed on the surface of the cochlear nucleus *(74,75)*. The cochlear nucleus is the floor of the lateral recess of the fourth ventricle *(76)*. The proper location for the placement of the implant is not visible when implantation is done; it is reached through the foramen of Luschka, located close to the entrance/exit of cranial nerves IX and X from the brainstem *(76)*. The methods for electrophysiological guidance of placement of the stimulating array of electrodes on the surface of the cochlear nucleus consists of recording ABRs while electrical impulses are applied to one pair after another of the implanted electrodes *(54)*. The manufacturers of brainstem implants supply hardware and software that allows such testing. If some electrode pairs do not elicit a response, the implanted array of electrodes is moved and the test

repeated. This process is repeated until a satisfactory response is obtained. One of the problems in such testing is related to the stimulus artifact that is generated by the electrical stimulation, but the interference can be reduced by appropriate placement of the recording electrodes and electronic elimination of the artifacts *(54,73)*.

**GUIDE FOR PLACEMENT
OF STIMULATING ELECTRODES
IN OTHER PARTS OF THE CNS**

Electrical stimulation of the dorsal column of the spinal cord has been in used for many years *(50,51)*, but requirements for electrophysiological guidance in such implantations have not yet emerged. Electrical stimulation of various parts of the cerebral cortex is beginning

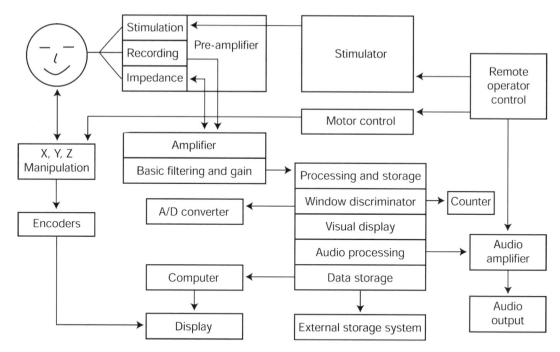

Figure 15.15: Block diagram of components of equipment involved in neurophysiological guidance for lesions and electrode implantation such as in the basal ganglia and thalamus. (Reprinted from: Shils JL, Tagliati M, Alterman RL. Neurophysiological monitoring during neurosurgery for movement disorders. In: Deletis V, Shils JL, eds. *Neurophysiology in Neurosurgery.* Amsterdam: Academic Press; 2002:405–448, with permission from Elsevier.)

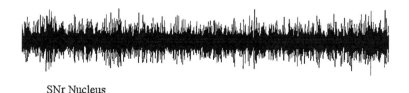

SNr Nucleus

Figure 15.16: Example of a recording of poor quality. The electrode tip was probably too large (50 μm) as also reflected by its low impedance (50 kΩ). The recording is a 5-s epoch. (Reprinted from: Shils JL, Tagliati M, Alterman RL. Neurophysiological monitoring during neurosurgery for movement disorders. In: Deletis V, Shils JL, eds. *Neurophysiology in Neurosurgery.* Amsterdam: Academic Press; 2002:405–448, with permission from Elsevier.)

to gain clinical usage. Thus, it has been shown that electrical stimulation of the motor cortex has beneficial effects in the treatment of severe pain *(50)*. Such implantations have been made on the basis of imaging data only. Stimulation of the auditory cortex for tinnitus *(77)* and stimulations of other parts of the cortex to enhance expression of neural plasticity for rehabilitation of stroke victims *(48)* are examples of such new usages of chronic electrical stimulation of the CNS using implanted electrodes. Methods for physiological guidance for such implantations have not yet become established, but the so-called functional MRI has been used *(49)*.

ANESTHESIA REQUIREMENTS

Testing of peripheral nerves is not affected by commonly used anesthetics unless muscles responses are recorded, in which case muscle relaxants must be excluded from the used anesthesia regimen.

Muscle relaxants cannot be used where monitoring the abnormal muscle response in MVD operations for HFS. Even the use of partial muscle relaxation severely hampers the monitoring of the abnormal muscle response. Therefore, when the abnormal muscle response is to be monitored the patient should be anesthetized without the use of any endplate-blocking agents. The abnormal muscle response is only slightly affected by commonly used anesthetics. The best anesthesia regimen consists of an initial administration of succinylcholine with 3 mg of tubocurarine for induction and intubation. The anesthesia throughout the operation is then maintained with inhalation agents and narcotics. No further muscle relaxants should be administered. Agents such as intravenous barbiturates or propofol are also suitable.

Electrophysiological guidance for finding the targets in the thalamus and basal ganglia for lesions and implantation of electrodes for DBS is usually done in awake patients, but when done in children, it might be necessary to use some form of anesthesia. Propofol (*see* Chap. 16) is often used for placement of the stereotaxic frame and terminated before recordings are done. For children who need anesthesia during the recordings, propofol and inhalation agents have been found less suitable than anesthesia maintained with ketamine and remifentanyl (a synthetic opioid) *(67)*.

Guidance of implantation of ABIs use recordings of ABR, which is insensitive to anesthetics and muscle relaxants.

References to Section V

1. Sekhar LN, Møller AR. Operative management of tumors involving the cavernous sinus. *J. Neurosurg.* 1986;64:879–889.
2. Møller AR. Electrophysiological monitoring of cranial nerves in operations in the skull base. In: Sekhar LN, Schramm VL Jr, eds. *Tumors of the Cranial Base: Diagnosis and Treatment.* Mt. Kisco, NY: Futura; 1987:123–132.
3. Yingling C. Intraoperative monitoring in skull base surgery. In: Jackler RK, Brackmann DE, eds. *Neurotology.* St. Louis, MO: Mosby; 1994:967–1002.
4. Yingling C, Gardi J. Intraoperative monitoring of facial and cochlear nerves during acoustic neuroma surgery. *Otolaryngol. Clin. North Am.* 1992;25:413–448.
5. Lanser M, Jackler R, Yingling C. Regional monitoring of the lower (ninth through twelfth) cranial nerves. In: Kartush J, Bouchard K, eds. *Intraoperative Monitoring in Otology and Head and Neck Surgery.* New York, NY: Raven; 1992:131–150.
6. Daube J. Intraoperative monitoring of cranial motor nerves. In: Schramm J, Moller A, eds. *Intraoperative Neurophysiologic Monitoring in Neurosurgery.* Heidelberg; Springer-Verlag; 1991:246–267.
7. Kartush J, Bouchard K. Intraoperative facial monitoring. Otology, neurotology, and skull base surgery. In: Kartush J, Bouchard K, eds. *Neuromonitoring in Otology and Head and Neck Surgery.* New York, NY: Raven; 1992:99–120.
8. Møller AR, Jannetta PJ. Preservation of facial function during removal of acoustic neuromas: Use of monopolar constant voltage stimulation and EMG. *J. Neurosurg.* 1984;61:757–760.
9. Stechison MT, Møller AR, Lovely TJ. Intraoperative mapping of the trigeminal nerve root: technique and application in the surgical management of facial pain. *Neurosurgery* 1996;38:76–82.
10. Rosenberg SI, Martin WH, Pratt H, Schwegler JW, Silverstein H. Bipolar cochlear nerve recording technique: a preliminary report. *Am. J. Otol.* 1993;14:362–368.
11. Colletti V, Fiorino FG. Electrophysiologic identification of the cochlear nerve fibers during cerebellopontine angle surgery. *Acta Otolaryngol. (Stockh.)* 1993;113:746–754.
12. Møller AR, Colletti V, Fiorino FG. Neural conduction velocity of the human auditory nerve: bipolar recordings from the exposed intracranial portion of the eighth nerve during vestibular nerve section. *Electroenceph. Clin. Neurophysiol.* 1994;92:316–320.
13. Sindou M, Mertens P. Selective spinal cord procedures for spasticity and pain. In: Deletis V, Shils JL, eds. *Neurophysiology in Neurosurgery.* Amsterdam: Academic; 2002:93–117.
14. Deletis V. Intraoperative neurophysiology and methodologies used to monitor the functional integrity of the motor system. In: Deletis V, Shils JL, eds. *Neurophysiology in Neurosurgery.* Amsterdam: Academic; 2002:25–51.
15. Fasano VA, Broggi G, Zeme S. Intraoperative electrical stimulation for functional posterior rhizotomy. *Scand. J. Rehabil. Med.* 1988;17:149–154.
16. Deletis V, Vodusek DD, Abbott R, Epsetein FJ, Turndorf H. Intraoperative monitoring of the dorsal sacral roots: Minimizing the risk of iatrogenic micturition disorders. *Neurosurgery* 1992;30:72–75.
17. Deletis V, Camargo AB. Interventional neurophysiological mapping and monitoring during spinal cord procedures. *Stereotact. Funct. Neurosurg.* 2001;77:25–28.
18. Deletis V. Intraoperative monitoring: motor evoked potentials methodology. In: Deletis V, Shils JL, eds. *Proceedings, Intraoperative Neurophysiological Monitoring in Neurosurgery.* New York, NY: Hyman-Newman Institute for Neurology and Neurosurgery; 2004:24–30.
19. Strauss C, Romstock J, Nimsky C, Fahlbush R. Intraoperative identification of motor areas or the rhomboid fossa using direct stimulation. *J. Neurosurg.* 1993;79:393–399.
20. Strauss C. The anatomical aspects of a surgical approach through the floor of the fourth ventricle. *Acta Neurochir. (Wien)* 1998;140:1099.
21. Sala F, Lanteri P. Brain surgery in motor areas: the invaluable assistance of intraoperative neurophysiological monitoring. *J. Neurol. Sci.* 2003;47:79–88.
22. Morota N, Deletis V, Epstein FS, et al. Brainstem mapping: Neurophysiological localization

of motor nuclei on the floor of the fourth ventricle. Neurosurgery 1995;37:922–930.

23. Kyoshima K, Koboyashi S, Gibo H, Kuroyanagi Y. A study of safe entry zones via the floor of the fourth ventricle for brain-stem lesions. *J. Neurosurg.* 1993;78:987–993.

24. Penfield W, Rasmussen T. *The Cerebral Cortex of Man: A Clinical Study of Localization of Function.* New York, NY: Macmillan; 1950.

25. Lueders H, Dinner DS, Lesser RP, Morris HH. Evoked potentials in cortical localization. *J. Clin. Neurophysiol.* 1986;3:75–84.

26. Goldring S, Gregorie EM. Surgical management of epilepsy using epidural recordings to localize the seizure focus. Review of 100 cases. *J. Neurosurg.* 1984;60:457–466.

27. Landi A, Copeland SA, Wynn, Parry CB, Jones SJ. The role of somatosensory evoked potentials and nerve conduction studies in the surgical management of brachial plexus injuries. *J. Bone Joint Surg. (Brit.)* 1980;62B:492–496.

28. Kline DG, Judice DJ. Operative management of selected brachial plexus lesions. *J. Neurosurg.* 1983;58:631–649.

29. Happel L, Kline D. Intraoperative neurophysiology of the peripheral nervous system. In: Deletis V, Shils JL, eds. *Neurophysiology in Neurosurgery.* Amsterdam: Academic; 2002:169–195.

30. Happel L, Kline D. Nerve lesions in continuity. In: Gelberman RH, ed. *Operative Nerve Repair and Reconstruction,* Volume 1, 1st ed. Philadelphia, PA: J.B. Lippincott; 1991:601–616.

31. Barker FG, Jannetta PJ, Bissonette DJ, Shields PT, Larkins MV. Microvascular decompression for hemifacial spasm. *J. Neurosurg.* 1995;82:201–210.

32. Møller AR. The cranial nerve vascular compression syndrome: I. A review of treatment. *Acta Neurochir. (Wien)* 1991;113:18–23.

33. Møller AR, Jannetta PJ. Monitoring facial EMG during microvascular decompression operations for hemifacial spasm. *J. Neurosurg.* 1987;66:681–685.

34. Møller AR, Jannetta PJ. On the origin of synkinesis in hemifacial spasm: results of intracranial recordings. *J. Neurosurg.* 1984;61:569–576.

35. Nielsen V. Pathophysiological aspects of hemifacial spasm. Part I. Evidence of ectopic excitation and ephaptic transmission. *Neurology* 1984;34:418–426.

36. Nielsen VK. Pathophysiology of hemifacial spasm: II. Lateral spread of the supraorbital nerve reflex. *Neurology* 1984;34:427–431.

37. Esslen E. Der Spasmus facialis—eine Parabiosserscheinung: Elektrophysiologische Untersuchnungen zum Enstehungsmechanismus des Facialisspasmus. *Dtsch Z. Nervenheil.* 1957;176: 149–172.

38. Møller AR, Jannetta PJ. Synkinesis in hemifacial spasm: results of recording intracranially from the facial nerve. *Experientia* 1985;41:415–417.

39. Møller AR, Jannetta PJ. Microvascular decompression in hemifacial spasm: Intraoperative electrophysiological observations. *Neurosurgery* 1985;16:612–618.

40. Møller AR, Jannetta PJ. Blink reflex in patients with hemifacial spasm: Observations during microvascular decompression operations. *J. Neurol. Sci.* 1986;72:171–182.

41. Møller AR, Jannetta PJ. Physiological abnormalities in hemifacial spasm studied during microvascular decompression operations. *Exp. Neurol.* 1986;93:584–600.

42. Hatem J, Sindou M, Vial C. Intraoperative monitoring of facial EMG responses during microvascular decompression for hemifacial spasm. Prognostic value for long-term outcome: a study in a 33-patient series. *Br. J. Neurosurg.* 2001:496–499.

43. Møller AR. Cranial nerve dysfunction syndromes: pathophysiology of microvascular compression. In: Barrow DL, ed. *Surgery of Cranial Nerves of the Posterior Fossa. Neurosurgical Topics Book 13.* Park Ridge. IL: American Association of Neurological Surgeons; 1993:105–129.

44. Jannetta PJ. Hemifacial spasm caused by a venule: case report. *Neurosurgery* 1984;14: 89–92.

45. Haines SJ, Torres F. Intraoperative monitoring of the facial nerve during decompressive surgery for hemifacial spasm. *J. Neurosurg.* 1991;74:254–257.

46. Møller AR. Neural plasticity and disorders of the nervous system. Cambridge: Cambridge University Press; 2005, in press.

47. Prass RL, Lueders H. Acoustic (loudspeaker) facial electromyographic monitoring. Part I. *Neurosurgery* 1986;19:392–400.

48. Brown JA, Lutsep HL, Cramer SC, Weinand M. Motor cortex stimulation for enhancement of recovery after stroke: case report. *Neurol. Res.* 2003;25:815–818.

49. De Ridder D, De Mulder G, Walsh V, et al. Transcranial magnetic stimulation for tinnitus: a clincial and pathophysiological approach. *J. Neurosurg.* 2004;100:560–564.

50. Meyerson BA, Lindblom U, Linderoth B, Lind G. Motor cortex stimulation as treatment of trigeminal neuropathic pain. *Acta Neurochir.* 1993;58(Suppl.):150–153.

51. Meyerson BA, Linderoth B. Mechanism of spinal cord stimulation in neuropathic pain. *Neurol. Res.* 2000;22:285–292.

52. Yakhnitsa V, Linderoth B, Meyerson BA. Spinal cord stimulation attenuates dorsal horn hyperexcitability in a rat model of mononeuropathy. *Pain* 1999;79:223–233.

53. Kirchner A, Birklein F, Stefan H, Handwerker HO. Left vagus nerve stimulation suppresses experimentally induced pain. *Neurology* 2000;55:1167–1171.

54. Waring MD. Intraoperative electrophysiologic monitoring to assist placement of auditory brain stem implant. *Ann. Otol. Rhinol. Laryngol.* 1995;166(Suppl.):33–36.

55. Shils JL, Tagliati M, Alterman RL. Neurophysiological monitoring during neurosurgery for movement disorders. In: Deletis V, Shils JL, eds. *Neurophysiology in Neurosurgery.* Amsterdam: Academic; 2002:405–448.

56. Vitek JL, Bakay RAE, Hashimoto T, et al. Microelectrode-guided pallidotomy: technical approach and application for treatment of medically intractable Parkinson's disease. *J. Neurosurg.* 1998;88:1027–1043.

57. Albe-Fessard D, Sarfel G, Guiot G, et al. Electrophysiological studies of some deep cerebral structures in man. *J. Neurosci.* 1966;3:37–51.

58. Vitek JL, Chockkan V, Zhang JY, et al. Neuronal activity in the basal ganglia in patients with generalized dystonia and hemiballismus. *Ann. Neurol.* 1999;46:22–35.

59. Lenz FA, Dostrovsky JO, Kwan HC, Tasker RR, Yamashiro K, Murphy JT. Methods for microstimulation and recording of single neurons and evoked potentials in the human central nervous system. *J. Neurosurg.* 1988;68: 630–634.

60. Lenz FA, Dostrovsky JO, Tasker RR, Yamashiro K, Kwan HC, Murphy JT. Single-unit analysis of the human ventral thalamic nuclear group: somatosensory responses. *J. Neurophysiol.* 1988;59:299–316.

61. Lenz FA, Tasker RR, Kwan HC, et al. Single unit analysis of the human ventral thalamic nuclear group: correlation of thalamic "tremor cells" with the 3–6 Hz component of parkinsonian tremor. *J. Neurosci.* 1988;8: 754–764.

62. Lenz FA, Kwan HC, Dostrovsky JO, Tasker RR. Characteristics of the bursting pattern of action potentials that occurs in the thalamus of patients with central pain. *Brain Res.* 1989;496: 357–360.

63. Lenz FA, Martin R, Kwan HC, Tasker RR, Dostrovsky JO. Thalamic single-unit activity occurring in patients with hemidystonia. *Stereotact. Funct. Neurosurg.* 1990;54–55:159–162.

64. Lenz FA, Kwan HC, Dostrovsky JO, Tasker RR, Murphy JT, Lenz YE. Single unit analysis of the human ventral thalamic nuclear group. Activity correlated with movement. *Brain* 1990;113:1795–1821.

65. Lenz FA, Jaeger CJ, Seike MS, et al. Thalamic single neuron activity in patients with dystonia: dystonia-related activity and somatic sensory reorganization. *J. Neurophysiol.* 1999;82: 2372–2393.

66. Ojemann GA, Creutzfeldt O, Lettich E, Haglund MM. Neuronal activity in human lateral temporal cortex related to short-term verbal memory, naming and reading. *Brain* 1988;111:1383–1403.

67. Starr PA, Turner RS, Rau G, et al. Microelectrode-guided implantation of deep brain stimulators into the globus pallidus internus for dystonia: techniques, electrode locations, and outcomes. *Neurosurg. Focus* 2004;17:20–31.

68. Copeland BJ, Pillsbury HC. Cochlear implantation for the treatment of deafness. *Annu. Rev. Med.* 2004;55:157–167.

69. Toh EH, Luxford WM. Cochlear and brainstem implantation. *Otolaryngol. Clin. North Am.* 2002;35:325–342.

70. House WH. Cochlear implants. *Ann. Otol. Rhinol. Laryngol.* 1976;85(Suppl. 27):3–91.

71. Zeng FG. Trends in cochlear implants. *Trends Amplif.* 2004;8:1–34.

72. Colletti V, Fiorino FG, Sacchetto L, Miorelli V, Camer M. Hearing habilitation with auditory brainstem implantation in two children with cochlear nerve aplasia. *Int. J. Pediatric Otorhinolaryngol.* 2001;60:99–111.

73. Waring MD. Auditory brain-stem responses evoked by electrical stimulation of the cochlear nucleus in human subjects. *Electroenceph. Clin. Neurophysiol.* 1995;96: 338–347.

74. Portillo F, Nelson RA, Brackmann DE, et al. Auditory brain stem implant: electrical stimulation of the human cochlear nucleus. *Adv. Oto-Rhino-Laryngol.* 1993;48:248–252.

75. Brackmann DE, Hitselberger WE, Nelson RA, et al. Auditory brainstem implant: 1. Issues in surgical implantation. *Otolaryngol. Head Neck Surg.* 1993;108:624–633.

76. Kuroki A, Møller AR. Microsurgical anatomy around the foramen of Luschka with reference to intraoperative recording of auditory evoked potentials from the cochlear nuclei. *J. Neurosurg.* 1995;82:933–939.

77. De Ridder D, De Mulder G, Walsh V, Muggleton N, Sunaert S, Møller A. Magnetic and electrical stimulation of the auditory cortex for intractable tinnitus. *J. Neurosurg.* 2004;100: 560–564.

PRACTICAL ASPECTS OF ELECTROPHYSIOLOGICAL RECORDING IN THE OPERATING ROOM

Many practical aspects must be considered to achieve the goals of intraoperative neurophysiological monitoring and other uses of neurophysiological methods in the operating room. Matters such as anesthesia and the choice of equipment and its use are fundamental to the success of using electrophysiological methods in the operating room. The following chapters provide basic information of common anesthesia techniques used in operations where the nervous system is involved. Another chapter provides information regarding the working of the electrophysiological equipment commonly used for electrophysiological studies in the operating room and the different methods of analysis of neuroelectrical data that is used in the operating room are discussed. The persons who do intraoperative monitoring should understand that mistakes in the use of these methods could occur, and how such mistakes can be reduced as much as possible is discussed in one of the chapters that follows. Correcting such problems as those caused by electrical interference is necessary for successful use of electrophysiology in an operating room that has many different sources of electrical interference. The people who use electrophysiological techniques in the operating room must therefore have sufficient knowledge about how electrical interference can reach the monitoring equipment and how its effect on electrophysiological recordings can be reduced so that interpretable records can be obtained promptly. Chapter 17 addresses these problems and provides suggestions of how to do troubleshooting and suggests remedies for these problems. It is also an important task of those who use these methods in the operating room to evaluate the benefits of intraoperative neurophysiological monitoring and other electrophysiological methods in improving medical care by reducing the risk of postoperative deficits and thereby improving the outcome of operations on the nervous system. This matter is also covered in Chap. 19.

16

Anesthesia and Its Constraints in Monitoring Motor and Sensory Systems

INTRODUCTION

Because anesthesia could affect the results of intraoperative monitoring, it is important that the person who is performing the intraoperative neurophysiological monitoring understand the basic principles of anesthesia. The person who is responsible for monitoring should communicate with the anesthesiologist to obtain information regarding the type of anesthesia that is to be used, if there are changes made in the anesthesia during the operation, and, if so, what other drugs might be administered during the operation.

Maintaining a stable level of anesthesia is important and administration of drugs should be by continuous infusion; bolus administration should be avoided. The effect of anesthesia on specific kinds of monitoring has been discussed in the preceding chapters. In this chapter, we will discuss the various types of anesthesia most commonly used in connection with operations where intraoperative neurophysiological monitoring of motor and sensory systems are used (for details about anesthesia in neurosurgery, *see* ref. *1*. The classical text is ref. *2*).

BASIC PRINCIPLES OF ANESTHESIA

The two primary purposes of general anesthesia are to make the patient unconscious and to

provide analgesia (freedom from pain). A third purpose is to keep the patient muscle relaxed, thus keeping the patient from moving during the operation. In the Western world, general anesthesia is predominantly accomplished by administering pharmacological agents using either an inhalation or intravenous delivery method. Two or more agents are often used together for additive or (synergistic) action to achieve one of the anesthesia goals, as well as to reduce the side effects from a particular agent.

Different Kinds of Anesthesia

Anesthesia agents used in connection with common operations can be divided into inhalation and intravenous anesthesia types. Often a combination of these two types is used. More recently, total intravenous anesthesia (TIVA) has won popularity.

Inhalation Anesthesia

Inhalation anesthesia is the oldest form of general anesthesia. In its modern forms, it usually consists of at least two different agents, such a nitrous oxide and a halogenated agent, administered together with pure oxygen. The relative potency of inhalation agents is described by their MAC[1] value.

Halogenated agents such as halothane (which is used rarely now), enflurane, isoflurane,

From: *Intraoperative Neurophysiological Monitoring: Second Edition*
By A. R. Møller
© Humana Press Inc., Totowa, NJ.

---

[1]One MAC (minimal end-alveolar concentration) is the equivalent of the sum of the effect of the anesthetics administered that prevent a response to painful stimuli in 50% of individuals.

and so forth will cause increased central conduction time (CCT) for somatosensory evoked potentials (SSEPs) and essentially make it impossible to elicit motor evoked potentials by single-impulse stimulation of the motor cortex (transcranial magnetic or electrical stimulation). This unfortunate effect is present even at low concentrations.

Intravenous Anesthesia

Some intravenous agents have almost always been used together with inhalational agents, but, recently, the TIVA regimen has become increasingly prevalent. One reason for that is that the inhalational agents, including nitrous oxide, are obstacles when electromyographic (EMG) responses are to be monitored in connection with transcranial stimulation of the motor cortex. It is an advantage that the mechanism of action of intravenous agents appears to be different from that of inhalational agents in such a way that benefits monitoring EMG and of MEPs (*see* Chap. 10).

Analgesia. Achieving analgesia (pain relief) is a primary component of anesthesia, and for many years, opioids have been used in the anesthesia regimen together with agents such as inhalation agents for achieving unconsciousness *(3)*. One of the oldest synthetic opioids is fentanyl, but now several different agents with similar action are in use for that purpose, such as alfentanil, sufentanil, and remifentanil. Muscle responses evoked by transcranial cortical stimulation (electrical and magnetic) are only slightly affected by opioids. The effects of opioids can be reversed by administering naloxone, suggesting that the effect is related to µ-receptor activity. Intravenous sedative agents are frequently used to induce or supplement general anesthesia, particularly with opioids or ketamine, when inhalational agents are not utilized.

Ketamine is a valuable component of anesthetic techniques allowing recording responses that might be depressed by other anesthetics. Ketamine could heighten synaptic function rather than depress it (probably through its interaction with the NMDA receptor) and it could provoke seizure activity in individuals with epilepsy but not in normal individuals. Ketamine has been reported to increase cortical somatosensory evoked potential (SSEP) amplitude and to increase the amplitude of muscle and spinal recorded responses following spinal stimulation and it could potentiate the H reflex. Ketamine has minimal effects on muscle responses evoked by transcranial cortical stimulation. Because of that, ketamine combined with opioids has become a valuable adjunct during some TIVA techniques for recording muscle responses. The fact that ketamine could cause severe hallucinations postoperatively and increase intracranial pressure has reduced its use in anesthesia.

Opioids provide analgesia but do not provide sufficient degrees of sedation, relief of anxiety, and loss of memory during operations (amnesia). Hence, TIVA usually includes some sedative–hypnotic agents such as barbiturates (thiopental) and benzodiazepines such as midazolam. Propofol is an agent that is in increasing use because it provides excellent anesthesia and limited effect on MEPs.

Barbiturates that are often used for induction of general anesthesia have effects similar to that of inhalation agents on evoked potentials. For example, muscle responses to transcranial stimulation are unusually sensitive to barbiturates and the effect lasts a long time, making barbiturates a poor choice in connection with monitoring MEPs.

Etomidate is another popular agent to be used in intravenous anesthesia. It enhances synaptic activity at low doses; thus, opposite to the action of barbiturates and benzodiazepines, it might produce seizures in patients with epilepsy when given in low doses (0.1 mg/kg) and it might produce myoclonic activity at induction of anesthesia. The ability to enhance neural activity or reduce the depressant effects of other drugs has been used to enhance the amplitude of both sensory and motor evoked responses. The enhancing of evoked activity occurs at doses similar to those that produce the desired degree of sedation and loss of recall of memory when used in TIVA.

Benzodiazepines, notably midazolam, are often used in connection with TIVA in many kinds of operations because they provide excellent sedation and they suppress memories (recall). Benzodiazepines can also reduce the risk of hallucinations caused by ketamine.

Muscle Relaxants

Muscle relaxants are usually not regarded as anesthetics but often combined with agents (intravenous or inhalation) that produce unconsciousness and freedom of pain. Muscle relaxants are part of a common anesthesia regimen—so-called "balanced anesthesia" (neurolept anesthesia)—that includes a strong narcotic for analgesia plus a muscle relaxant to keep the patient from moving, together with a relatively weak anesthetic such as nitrous oxide.

Muscle relaxants used in anesthesia are of two different types, each affecting muscle responses differently: one blocks transmission in the neuromuscular junction (muscle endplate) and the other type depolarizes the muscle endplate, thereby preventing it from activating the muscle. The oldest neuromuscular blocking agent is curare, but that has been replaced by a long series of steroid-type endplate blockers with different action durations. Pancuronium bromide (Pavulon®) was one of the earliest of this series and the effects of pancuronium bromide last more than 1 h when a dose that causes total paralysis is administered. Other and newer drugs of the same family have a shorter duration of action (about 0.5 h for vecuronium bromide, [Norcuron®] and atracurium [Tracurium®]).

The most often used muscle-relaxing agent that paralyzes by depolarizing the muscle endplate is succinylcholine. The muscle-relaxing effect of succinylcholine lasts only a very short time.

EFFECTS OF ANESTHESIA ON RECORDING NEUROELECTRICAL POTENTIALS

Successful neurophysiological monitoring often depends on the avoidance of certain types of anesthetic agent; for instance, it is not possible to record EMG potentials if the patient is paralyzed, as is the case for many commonly used anesthesia regimens. Recording of cortical evoked potentials is affected by most of the agents commonly used in surgical anesthesia. Monitoring motor evoked responses elicited by transcranial magnetic or electrical stimulation of the motor cortex requires special attention on anesthesia and the use of a special anesthesia regimen is necessary.

Recording of Sensory Evoked Potentials

It is advantageous to reduce the use of halogenated agents and nitrous oxide in anesthesia when cortical evoked potentials are monitored. Monitoring of short-latency sensory evoked potentials is not noticeably affected by any type of inhalation anesthesia; therefore, short-latency sensory evoked potentials should be used whenever possible for intraoperative monitoring instead of cortical evoked potentials. Auditory brainstem responses (ABRs), which are short-latency evoked potentials, are practically unaffected by inhalation anesthetics and can be recorded regardless of the anesthesia used. Short-latency components of SSEPs are not affected by inhalation anesthetics, but only upper limb SSEPs have clearly recordable short-latency components. Short-latency SSEPs evoked by stimulation of the median nerve are suitable for monitoring the brachial plexus and the cervical portion of the spinal cord, but they are not useful for monitoring the spinal cord below the C_6 vertebra or for monitoring central structures such as the somatosensory cortex. Therefore, it is usually the long-latency components, which are generated in the cortex, that are used for intraoperative monitoring of SSEP.

The general effect of anesthetics is a lowering of the amplitude and a prolongation of the latency of an individual component of the recorded potentials *(4)* (*see* Chap. 7, **Fig. 7.10**). The effect is different for different components of the evoked potentials, as the potentials are affected by inhalation anesthetics or barbiturates to varying degrees *(5)* and the effect varies from patient to patient, with children being generally more sensitive than adults (6).

Because these components are affected by inhalation anesthetics it is important to discuss with the anesthesiologists in order to select a type of anesthesia that allow such monitoring.

Recording of EMG Potentials

Response from muscles (electromyographic [EMG] potentials or mechanical response) cannot be recorded in the presence of muscle relaxants. It is usually necessary to use a muscle-relaxing agent for intubation. When EMG recordings are to be done during an operation, it is suitable to use succinylcholine together with 3 mg of d-tubocurarine (curare) or short-acting endplate blockers, such as atracurium (Tracurium) or vecuronium bromide (Norcuron) during intubation. This will allow monitoring of muscle potentials 30–45 min after the administration of the drug, providing that only the minimal amount of the drug is given and that it is given only once for intubation.

If a short-acting endplate-blocking agent is used, it is important to be aware that the paralyzing action disappears gradually and at a rate that differs from patient to patient. The rate at which muscle function is regained depends on the age, weight, and so forth of the patient, what other diseases might be present, and what other medications might have been administered.

During the time that the muscle-relaxing effect is decreasing, stimulation of a motor nerve with a train of electrical shocks (such as the commonly used "train of four" test) will give rise to a relatively normal muscle contraction in response to the initial electrical stimulus, but the response to subsequent impulses decreases and will be less than normal.

The effect of muscle relaxants of the endplate-blocking type can be shortened ("reversed") by administering agents such as neostigmine, which inhibits the breakdown of acetylcholine and thereby makes better use of the acetylcholine receptor sites that are not blocked by the muscle relaxant that is used. However, a prerequisite for the use of such "reversing" agents is that a fair amount of muscle response (10–20%) has returned before reversing is attempted. It is also important to note that such reversing does not immediately return the muscle function to normal, as the effect of the muscle relaxant will last for some time.

When muscle relaxation is not used during an operation, the patient could have noticeable spontaneous muscle activity, which increases the background noise level in recordings of different kinds of neuroelectrical potential. This is important when monitoring of evoked potentials of low amplitude, such as ABR, is to be done. The resulting background noise will prolong the time over which responses must be averaged in order to obtain an interpretable recording. The muscle activity often increases as the level of anesthesia lessens. If the muscle activity becomes strong, it might be a sign that the level of anesthesia is too low. Early information about such increases in muscle activity is naturally important to the anesthesiologist so that he/she can adjust the level of anesthesia before the patient begins to move spontaneously. In this way, electrophysiological monitoring can often provide valuable information to the anesthesiologist, because if anesthesia becomes light, spontaneous muscle activity frequently manifests in the recording of evoked potentials from scalp electrodes a long time before any movement of the patient is noticed. To do that, the output of the physiological amplifier must be watched continuously to detect any muscle activity.

Intraoperative monitoring that involves recording EMG potentials from muscles is becoming more and more common in the complex neurosurgical operations that can now be performed and demands on the selection of an appropriate anesthesia regimen have, therefore, increased. A close collaboration between the anesthesia team and the neurophysiologist in charge of intraoperative neurophysiological monitoring can often solve such problems.

17

General Considerations About Intraoperative Neurophysiological Monitoring

Introduction
How to Reduce Mistakes
Electrical and Magnetic Interference in the Operating Room
Electrical Safety in the Operating Room

INTRODUCTION

Intraoperative neurophysiological monitoring is a technique used to assist in the prevention of accidents in surgical operations, or rather reduce the risks of accidents. In order that intraoperative neurophysiological monitoring can serve that purpose adequately, it is important to reduce the risk of human mistakes, equipment failure, or electrode failure, which can jeopardize proper execution of intraoperative neurophysiological monitoring.

If the recorded responses are obscured by noise, the records cannot be interpreted, or if electrodes lose contact or equipment fails, the planned monitoring cannot be done adequately. Other obstacles to successful monitoring are mistakes such as incorrect placement of electrodes for recording and stimulation or setting up the equipment incorrectly. Of course, misinterpretation of recorded potentials is also a serious obstacle to successful monitoring that can often be related to inadequate training of the individual who performs monitoring.

Clinical setups for recording neuroelectrical potentials are usually fixed installations, but neurophysiological monitoring equipment that is used in the operating room is almost always moved into the operating room for the particu-

From: *Intraoperative Neurophysiological Monitoring: Second Edition*
By A. R. Møller
© Humana Press Inc., Totowa, NJ.

lar operation, and cables between the equipment and the patient are placed for each individual case. This is yet another difference between the clinical laboratory and the operating room and such differences contribute to mistakes and breakage of cables and equipment.

The operating room is an electrically hostile environment, which differs from the clinical neurophysiological laboratory where recording of electromyographic (EMG) responses and sensory evoked potentials such as auditory brainstem responses (ABRs), somatosensory evoked potentials (SSEPs), visual evoked potentials (VEPs), and EMG recordings are obtained in electrically and acoustically shielded rooms. In the operating room, many different kinds of electronic equipment are connected to the patient. Equipment used to monitor the patient's vital parameters, for electrocoagulation, drilling of bone, and so forth all could interfere with neurophysiological monitoring. In the clinic, usually only the equipment used for the recordings in question is connected to the patient.

Intraoperative neurophysiological monitoring cannot be done correctly if electrical interference in the operating room prevents obtaining interpretable records. We will discuss in this chapter how to identify the source of electrical interference that might influence monitoring, how to reduce such electrical interference, and how to reduce its effect on electrophysiological recordings in the operating room.

Other practical matters such as the requirements of the stimulating and recording equipment, selection of optimal recording and stimulus parameters, and methods for processing the recorded potentials are matters that are discussed in Chap. 18, which also describes techniques for stimulation of the nervous system and techniques for data acquisition and processing of the neuroelectrical potentials that are recorded in intraoperative neurophysiological monitoring.

HOW TO REDUCE MISTAKES

Mistakes and errors are a natural phenomenon that can only be avoided by making it physically impossible to make them. That means that mistakes could be regarded as a law of nature that, unlike man-made laws, cannot be broken. This is also often referred to as Murphy's Law and states, "If something can go wrong, it will do so." It could happen as frequently as 1 in 10 or as infrequently as 1 in 1000 or 1 in a million, but anything that can go wrong will do so sooner or later.

How to Make It Impossible to Make Mistakes

One example of how a specific mistake can be avoided by making it physically impossible comes from the recording of ABRs (*see* Chap. 6). Such potentials are evoked by (click) sounds that are delivered by an earphone placed in the ear. If the purpose is to monitor the function of the auditory nerve in operations in the cerebellopontine angle, the sound should be delivered to the ear on the side of the operation. If earphones for monitoring ABRs in such operations are placed in both ears, there will always be a certain risk that the ear on the unoperated side is being selected for stimulation by mistake, although it is thought that it was the operated (correct) side that was being stimulated. Such a mistake might be made when connecting the earphone to the stimulator or by mistakenly switching the stimulus to the wrong ear during the operation. The mistake is not obvious from observing the recorded ABR, because the waveforms of the

ABR recorded from both sides are similar, regardless of from which ear they were elicited. Such a mistake will make it impossible to detect any change in the function of the auditory nerve on the operated side. The recordings obtained to contralateral stimulation will not show any change if the auditory nerve is injured, not even if it was severed. It will make monitoring useless in detecting injuries to the auditory nerve for which it was intended and it provides a false security to the surgeon. It is a typical example of how false-negative responses (no change in the recorded potentials is noted, despite the fact that that an injury has occurred) are obtained and it might cause the patient to lose hearing on the operated ear permanently without being detected during the operation. The mistake could have been prevented if the operated ear was the sole ear to have been equipped with an earphone, so that it would have been physically impossible to stimulate the wrong ear. Therefore, an earphone should never be placed in the ear on the unoperated side if it is not strongly indicated to do so for monitoring reasons.

Similar reasoning applies to other areas of intraoperative neurophysiological monitoring. For example, when monitoring SSEPs in an operation on one side of the spinal cord, the stimulating electrodes should only be placed on peripheral nerves on the same side as the operation. If placed on both sides, there is a risk that the SSEPs that are being observed are being elicited from the unoperated side, because the stimulus has been mistakenly applied to the peripheral nerve on the wrong side of the body.

Stimulating nervous tissue with dangerously high currents is another mistake that can have catastrophic consequences but that can be avoided by making it physically impossible to apply dangerously high stimulus currents. This is best done by limiting the output of the stimulator so that it cannot produce stimuli that are dangerously high. Such precaution is not often taken because of the desire of versatility of stimulators. Because the limits for dangerously high stimulus current is different for different types of stimulation, such as stimulation of peripheral nerves compared to stimulation in the brain, precautions that involve limiting the output of stimulators are rarely taken.

How to Reduce the Risk of Mistakes

If it is not possible to make mistakes impossible, measures should be taken to make it as unlikely as possible that something goes wrong. In many situations of everyday life, it has been customary to tolerate some degrees of risks in the form of accidents and so forth. This is because it is either not possible to find a way to eliminate accidents or the cost of preventing accidents has been judged to outweigh the gain from the action in question.

There are many ways that mistakes in connection with intraoperative neurophysiological monitoring can be reduced. Following a checklist for setting up equipment, placement of electrodes, which items (including spare ones) to bring to the operating room, and so forth can reduce the risk of forgetting essential elements and setting parameters for stimulation and recording incorrectly. Adhering to specific routines can also help reduce the risk of making mistakes. For example, when many electrodes are to be placed on a patient, mistakes might be made if the electrodes are all applied to the patient and then, after that, all electrodes are connected to the electrode box at one time. The risk of making mistakes in connecting the electrodes is much smaller if each electrode is connected one at a time to the electrode box after it is placed on the patient and before the next electrode is applied to the patient.

The "KISS" Principle of Intraoperative Neurophysiological Monitoring. The risk that something will go wrong is likely to increase with increasing complexity of the equipment and the complexity of the methods used for intraoperative neurophysiological monitoring. A complex computer system that is difficult to set up, with menus with many options, increases the risks of making mistakes. The complex procedure of operating the equipment might also waste time. It is indeed possible to balance your checkbook using a supercomputer, but it is not the most practical option. It

is also possible to use complex equipment for the rather uncomplicated tasks of collecting neurophysiological data. Recording evoked potentials on many channels rarely provides more useful information than what can be obtained by using a few correctly selected recording channels, but it does add to the complexity of recording. This means that also in intraoperative neurophysiological monitoring, it is important to observe the "KISS" principle—Keep It Simple, Stupid. Following the "KISS" principle can save much aggravation and also reduce the risks of minor and major disasters.

Importance of Thinking Ahead. Possible problems to expect should be considered before the operation starts, so that the person who does the intraoperative neurophysiological monitoring is prepared to handle at least the most common problems. Naturally, the highest-quality electronic equipment will provide the most reliable service, but it is important that backup electronic equipment and especially spare electrodes and connectors are available for use within a very short time. Having spare cables and electrodes available in the operating room is important, and it is wise to have redundant electrodes placed on the patient when manipulation during the operation might occur. Attending to every possible detail will be rewarded with fewer problems and better quality of the monitoring. A checklist can help achieve that because it helps keep a person from forgetting important matters.

Advantage of Using a Checklist. The airline industry has been extremely successful in reducing the risks of accidents. One reason for that is meticulously adhering to praxes that are known to involve minimal risks. When boarding a commercial airplane, one will often see the captain (and probably the first officer, who sits on the right side) ticking off a checklist. This is not because the captain does not know how to fly the airplane; the purpose is to avoid forgetting something. This occurs for short trips as well as for long trips; it occurs for large airlines as well as for small airlines and private pilots. The same should be the case for intraoperative neurophysiological monitoring. A checklist helps with remembering all small details, some of which could easily be forgotten even though the person who does the monitoring knows it all. The argument that a person knows how to do a specific job (monitoring or surgery, for that matter) is not an argument against using a checklist.

Unexpected Events. Most problems that occur in connection with intraoperative neurophysiological monitoring happen when not expected. The sudden appearance of electrical interference is a common example of an event that might interrupt monitoring because it obscures the recorded potentials. It will result in the neurophysiologist having to stop the monitoring. If the monitoring is going to be successful, it is necessary to identify the sources and the nature of such suddenly appearing interference within a very short time. The nature of the waveform of interference often tells where it comes from and what has caused the interference. Therefore, it is important that the neurophysiologist observe not only the averaged potentials but also observe the recorded potentials directly and that he/she be able to diagnose the problem and identify its source and distinguish between external electrical interference and interference that is of a biological origin, such as muscle activity.

EQUIPMENT MALFUNCTION. Equipment malfunction is rare now, but if it does happen, it either has to be fixed within a very short time or the operation will continue without the aid of intraoperative neurophysiological monitoring. Thorough knowledge about the equipment and its function is invaluable for troubleshooting and restoration of normal function. Most problems with modern computer equipment are software related and the user needs to know the function (and malfunctions) of the software used in the equipment.

ABSENCE OF RESPONSE. Simple tests can reduce the risk of absence of a response. For example, the risk that no sound being delivered by the earphone when monitoring the auditory system because of failure of the sound generator, or, more likely, a cable, or by earphone malfunction can be reduced by having the sound switched on and having the person who is placing the earphone in the patient's ear listen to the earphone immediately before it is placed in the patient's ear. That will ensure that the earphone is delivering a sound at least in the beginning of the operation. There is often a period where monitoring is not needed. Leaving monitoring running during that time makes it possible to detect malfunctions that might occur during that time. If monitoring is stopped and something happens during that idle time, it might not be possible to resume monitoring when needed and it might be difficult to find out what had happened.

A common cause of absence of evoked responses is that the patient has a disorder that affects evoked responses. Hearing loss or peripheral nerve neuropathy are common causes of inability to get a response. Preoperative tests can avoid such surprises.

Unexpected absence of muscle response to electrical stimulation of a nerve is often caused by the anesthesia team paralyzing the patient. Other causes for a lack of a muscle response include failure to stimulate the nerve adequately; failure to obtain a muscle response in response to cortical stimulation is often caused by too much or inadequate selection of the anesthetics used for anesthetizing the patient (*see* Chap. 16).

Communication Is Important

The neurophysiologist who is responsible for monitoring should communicate frequently with the surgeon, but it is also important to communicate with the anesthesiologist regarding changes in anesthesia and in the patient's vital signs. Such communication is also often beneficial to the anesthesiologist. For instance, an increase in spontaneous muscle activity as a result of a decrease in the level of anesthesia is

often noticeable in electrophysiological record
ings long before the level of anesthesia has
dropped so much that the patient moves. Relaying information about electrophysiological
recorded muscle activity to the anesthesiologist
might avoid the anesthesia becoming so low
that the patient moves spontaneously. Therefore, such information is valuable to the anesthesiologist as well as to the surgeon.

ELECTRICAL AND MAGNETIC INTERFERENCE IN THE OPERATING ROOM

The quality of recorded potentials from the
nervous system and muscles depends on the
level of electrical interference. There are several kinds of interference in the operating room
that can jeopardize intraoperative neurophysiological monitoring. One kind of interference
comes from electrical currents that reach the
amplifiers used in monitoring from other
equipment or from the power line. Another
source of interference in the operating room is
magnetic fields that induce electrical current
that can reach the input of amplifiers used for
monitoring. Biological noise such as that from
muscles and the ongoing EEG can also interfere
with electrophysiological recordings and even
obscure the recorded electrical potentials. Electrical interference from outside and from the
body of the patient can never be totally eliminated, but it can often be reduced and often it
can be reduced to a level where the recorded
potentials can be interpreted directly, or if the
amplitude of the potentials is small, after signal
averaging and appropriate filtering. Thus, it is
essential to successful intraoperative neurophysiological monitoring that interference be
kept at a minimum throughout the entire time
that monitoring is being done. In this section,
we will discuss how to reduce the amount of
interference that reaches the input of the recording amplifiers from nonbiological sources in the
operating room.

The wealth of electrical equipment in the
operating room that operates simultaneously
with the equipment used for intraoperative
neurophysiological monitoring can emit many
kinds of electrical interference. The best known
of these is the signal that originates in the
power line (a frequency of 60 Hz in North
America and 50 Hz in Europe), but many types
of electronic equipment that are in routine use
in the operating room emit many other kinds of
signals that might interfere with recording of
neuroelectrical potentials. Magnetic interference is mainly caused by equipment that contains transformers, which generate a magnetic
field related to the power line frequency.
Deflection coils in old types of video monitors
can emit magnetic field that can generate high-
frequency interference. Several sources of
interference emit electrical signals that are
periodic in nature and that can cause special
problems in connection with the recording of
evoked potentials where signal averaging is
used (*see* p. 313).

Some kinds of interference might not manifest in the beginning of an operation but appear
suddenly. A prerequisite for reducing the emission of such electrical interference signals is to
be able to identify the source of the interference.

Identifying the Sources of Electrical and Magnetic Interference

There are many ways to identify sources of
magnetic and electrical interference. One is
naturally to switch off suspected equipment
and see if the interference disappears. That is
normally not an option during an operation.
However, a closer examination of the operating
room when it is not in use is a more efficient
way to identify sources of interference.

A survey should be performed in all operating rooms to identify possible sources of interference prior to attempting to do intraoperative
neurophysiological monitoring in that location.
Equipment in the operating room that emits
signals that might interfere with the electrophysiological recordings should be identified
and actions taken to eliminate or reduce the
interference. This is best done when the operating room is not in use and when time is not a
limiting factor.

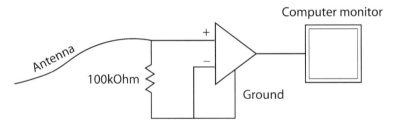

Figure 17.1: Using a standard physiological amplifier to identify sources of electrical interference.

Examining the Operating Room for Sources of Electrical Interference. Identification of sources that generate electric field interference can be done by using the amplifiers and display unit that are normally used for monitoring neuroelectrical potentials intraoperatively. With a piece of wire connected to one of the two differential inputs of an amplifier to act as an antenna (*see* **Fig. 17.1**) the electrical fields of signals that are present near the antenna will appear on the display. The other input to the amplifier should be grounded and a resistor (of about 100 kΩ; *see* **Fig. 17.1**) placed between the ground and the input to which the "antenna" is connected. When the antenna is brought closer to the equipment that is "leaking" an electric signal, the amplitude of the signal that is picked up by the antenna will increase, as can be observed on the computer display of the output from the amplifier.

Most electrical equipment is encased in a metal box that is connected to a ground lead for the purpose of electrical safety. A piece of equipment that is not properly grounded is not only a safety hazard, but improperly grounded equipment is also a source of interference for electrophysiological recordings because the casing no longer acts as an electrical shield. Locating such equipment can easily be done by the methods described above (**Fig. 17.1**). The function of the equipment itself is not usually affected if the ground wire becomes disconnected, and accidental disconnection of the safety ground lead will therefore normally go unnoticed. The only indication of such a loss of grounding might be increased interference in intraoperative electrophysiological recordings.

Another way to identify equipment that emits interference signals is to use a volunteer person placed in the same position on the operating table as the patient who is to be operated upon. With electrodes placed on the volunteer and connected to the input of the physiological amplifiers, no electrical interference should be noted when all other equipment in the operating room is switched off. If interference is present, it must be generated either by the recording equipment itself or by the electrical installation in room such as cables in the floor and walls and the lighting. The frequency of such interference signals is most likely that of the power line and the setup shown in **Fig. 17.1** can be used to find the location of such sources of interference.

Each piece of equipment that will be used by the anesthesia staff and others during the operation can then be switched on one at a time while observing the display of the output of the physiological amplifier for interference. Operating tables that are electrically controlled are frequent sources of interference.

This exercise will not only identify electrical fields, but it will also identify interference that is conducted galvanically to the recording equipment.

The normal operating room situation involves fluid lines that are in contact with the patient and that cannot easily be simulated with such a volunteer patient. There are also other situations in an actual operation that are not easily simulated in an idle operating room. For example, during an operation, changes might be made in the way that the anesthesia equipment is connected to the patient and such

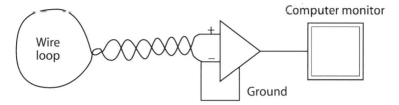

Figure 17.2: Arrangement for identifying a source of magnetic interference.

changes might cause interference with recordings of the neuroelectrical potentials that are to be monitored.

Examining the Operating Room for Magnetic Interference. The sources of magnetic interference can be identified in a way similar to that described for electrical interference, with the difference that a wire in the form of a loop is connected to the two input terminals of the amplifier (**Fig. 17.2**). (One of the inputs should be grounded.) A magnetic field will generate an electrical current in the wire loop. When the loop is moved closer to the source of a strong magnetic field, the amplitude of the pattern on the display of the output of the amplifier will increase. The source of a magnetic field that might generate electrical currents in the electrode leads and thereby act as electrical interference can be identified by searching the area around the operating table with such a loop. The orientation of the loop is important for reception of the magnetic field and the wire loop should therefore be rotated to keep it optimally oriented with regard to the orientation of the magnetic field. If there is doubt about which device is generating the interference, switching off each of the suspected devices one at a time can identify the equipment that is the source of interference.

Transformers such as the power transformers that are a part of most electronic equipment could generate magnetic fields. Powerful light sources in operating microscopes could generate similar magnetic fields and cause interference by the current they might induce in electrode leads. The deflection coils in old types of display monitors can generate strong high-frequency magnetic fields that can act as interference but which can easily be identified by the arrangement in **Fig. 17.2**.

Signature of Different Interference Signals

The waveform of the interference signals often provides important information about the identity of their source and how they have entered the recording system, both factors that are important to the elimination of the interference. The most important signature for identifying the source of interference is its frequency. The frequencies of the signals generated by different equipment are usually different. Interference signals that have the frequency of the power line must be generated by the power line in one or another way. The waveform of the current that the power line delivers is usually nearly sinusoidal, but in electrophysiological recordings, interference from the power line does not always appear as a sinusoidal waveform. Magnetically conducted power-line interference is often rich in higher harmonics, which is a great help in identifying the source of the interference, but, unfortunately, such interference is also often more severe because the harmonics of the power-line frequency might overlap with the spectrum of recorded neuroelectrical potentials.

Interference from the power line can also appear as a sinusoid with a series of sharp spikes superimposed, either with the same frequency as the power-line signal (60 or 50 Hz) or with a frequency twice as high as that of the power-line signal. Such spikes usually originate from equipment that has power regulators that chop the waveform of the power. Inexpensive equipment is the worst offender in this respect. Digital

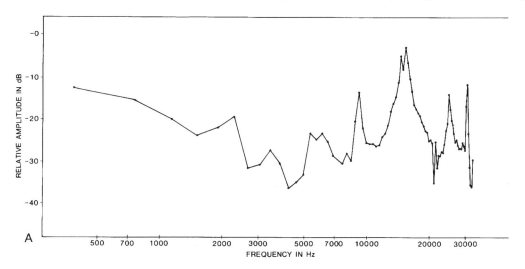

Figure 17.3: The spectrum of typical interference picked up by electrodes placed on the vertex and earlobe for differential recording of the ABR in a patient undergoing an operation to relieve hemifacial spasm. The sampling rate was 100 kHz.

control equipment such as found in blood warmers, infusion pumps, computers, or other digital equipment often radiates electric signals of much higher frequencies than the power line.

Determining the exact frequency of an interference signal might help in identifying the source of the interference. If the waveform (and frequency) of the signal that is picked up by the test loop is the same as that of the interference observed when recording from a patient, then that specific piece of equipment is most likely the source of the observed interference. If the interference waveform is complex, a spectrum analysis of the recorded interference potentials might help in identifying the source of the interference.

*Figure 17.3 shows the spectrum of an interference signal that was picked up by electrodes placed on the vertex and the earlobe for recording the ABR in a patient undergoing an operation where the auditory nerve was at risk. There are sharp peaks with a large amplitude that appear in the spectrum at frequencies of 9.8, 16, 25.7, and 31.6 kHz. The 16-kHz component had an amplitude of approx 10 μV peak to peak at the input of the amplifier. Tests using a wire loop (**Fig. 17.2**) connected to the amplifier showed that the*

*16-kHz signal was generated by a video monitor and it was transmitted to the recording equipment mainly as a magnetic field. The 25-kHz signal seen in the spectrogram in **Fig. 17.3** was generated by the blood pressure monitoring equipment, and it was radiated by the cable to a disposable pressure transducer mainly as a magnetic field. Because equipment that is used in the operating room changes with technological developments, similar signals might not be present in an operating room at a given time. These high-frequency signals have their energy outside the spectrum of the biological signals that are of interest in connection with intraoperative neurophysiological monitoring, but they might exert their effect as interference signals because of aliasing. Aliasing might occur if these high-frequency signals are not sufficiently attenuated by a low-pass filter before being sampled and digitized (see Chap. 18) or because a too low sampling rate is used. Such aliasing can make high-frequency signals appear in the sampled version of the signal with lower frequency than the signals that reach the amplifiers. This means that interference signals that have noticeable energy at frequencies above that of the* *recorded neuroelectrical potentials could interfere with biological signals of much lower frequencies.*

It is important that the neurophysiologist who performs troubleshooting procedures for interference signals has sufficient experience and knowledge to be able to correctly evaluate the nature of the different kinds of electrical and magnetic interference that might be present in the operating room.

How Can Electrical Interference Reach Physiological Recording Equipment

It is important to consider that electrical interference is only a problem when it reaches the recording equipment. Electrical interference can reach the recording equipment in two different ways: as electrical fields that are conducted through capacitance coupling ("through the air") or conducted (galvanically) to the recording equipment through electrically conductive media such as ground leads. Interference signals can also be conducted through the patient or directly to the recording equipment. Therefore, there are two ways to reduce the effect of electrical and magnetic interference, namely to reduce the emission of the interference signal and to reduce the ability of the recording systems to pick up the interference. As a last resort, when these two possibilities have been exhausted, special processing of the recorded electrical potentials from the nervous system is used to reduce the effect of interference on interpretation of the biological signals that are recorded (processing of recorded potentials will be discussed in Chap. 18). Selecting optimal recording parameters, optimal signal processing methods, and optimal stimulus parameters can also reduce the effect of interference (*see* Chap. 18). There are basically five different ways that electrical signals can enter the recording equipment and appear as interference to recorded potentials:

1. Electrical fields can be picked up by unshielded electrode leads (capacitance coupling) from nearby interference sources.

2. Electrical signals can be injected into the recording system by a common path, such as ground loops (galvanic coupling).
3. Electrical current can be galvanically conducted to the patient via other recording or stimulating electrodes that are placed on the patient (such as anesthesia monitoring equipment), by infusion lines or devices that are in galvanic contact with the patient, such as head holders.
4. Electrical interference can be picked up by capacitance coupling to the patient, such as from heating pads or motor-driven operating tables.
5. Interference signals can leak directly into the physiological amplifiers via the power line.

An example of sources of electrical field interference is unshielded equipment or power lines that pass close to recording leads. Perhaps the most common path for electrical interference to reach the input of physiological amplifiers is through the electrode wires. It is also the easiest problem to remedy. Twisting or braiding the wires and keeping them short and placed away from equipment that generate interferences are effective ways of reducing that kind of interference.

Typical examples of galvanically conducted interference is that generated by blood warmers and infusion pumps in which electrical current from the electronic circuits in these devices is conducted to the patient through the fluid that is infused. Devices that are connected electrically to the patient can also cause interference with recorded neuroelectrical potentials. Anesthesia monitoring equipment can cause electrical interference to be "injected" into a patient and picked up from the patient by electrodes that are used for neurophysiological monitoring purposes. There are many other kinds of equipment connected to the patient that can conduct interference signals to the patient. Such equipment might generate a variety of different types of electrical interference signal. For example, electrical stimulation of muscles on the hand for testing the level of paralysis by the anesthesia team can cause sudden electrical interference with recoded neuroelectrical potentials.

Intravenous infusion lines and arterial lines all carry electrically conductive fluids; therefore, electrical signals that these lines might pick up will be conducted to the patient and reach the input of the amplifiers that are used for intraoperative neurophysiological monitoring. Because bags with infusion solutions are often hanging high above the patient, they will act as effective "antennas" that can pick up various types of interference. Infusion lines often pass through electronic devices, such as intravenous pumps or blood warmers, and they can be sources of interference. Intravenous infusion pumps have electronic control circuits that might generate high-frequency electrical signals that might be conducted to the patient via the electrically conducting fluid of these lines. Blood warmers are often powered by the common power line, and this might cause severe interference with electrophysiological recordings because these signals are transferred to the patient via the conductive fluid in the infusion lines. Such interference might not be apparent in the beginning of an operation, but it might "appear suddenly" during the operation as circumstances change and new infusion bags added.

Blood pressure transducers that use intraarterial catheters are electrically connected to the patient, and interference signals can reach the patient from these through arterial lines. Electrical signals might also be conducted to the patient through head holders and other devices that are in direct (galvanic) contact with the patient. The head holder is in contact with the operating table that might be grounded for safety reasons, but the safety ground might provide a ground loop that can cause interference with the frequency of the power line.

Items other than those that are directly connected to the patient, such as heating blankets connected to the power line, might also create electrical interference with intraoperative recordings of neuroelectrical potentials. Electrically controlled operating tables are another frequent source of electrical interference. Although equipment that is connected directly (galvanic

connection) to the patient might be more likely to cause interference, these other devices might radiate enough electrical signals to interfere with recording of neuroelectrical potentials.

The interference from the power line could be caused by equipment, such as anesthesia monitoring equipment, and could become worse if such equipment is connected to power sources (isolation transformers) different than the one used for the equipment used to record evoked potentials. All equipment that is in galvanic contact with the patient should therefore get power from outlets that are supplied by the same isolation transformer.

How Can Magnetic Interference Reach Physiological Recording Equipment?

Alternating magnetic fields can cause interference with the recording of neuroelectrical potentials by inducing electric currents in the electrode leads. Many kinds of equipment in the modern operating room generate such magnetic fields, which can appear as interference in recordings of neuroelectrical potentials.

A magnetic field in itself does not interfere with electrical recordings, and a magnetic field only becomes a source of interference with recording of neuroelectrical potentials when it sets up an electric current in a conductor, such as the electrode leads connected to the recording amplifiers. Magnetic fields might also induce electric currents in cables that connect the "electrode box" to the amplifier, but most modern equipment now have an analog–digital converter located in the "electrode box." The digital signals transmitted to the computer are less sensitive to magnetic interference than analog signals. Many modern recording systems use fiberoptic lines to transmit the digital signals from the electrode box to the amplifiers and these are not affected by magnetic (and electrical) interference.

How to Reduce the Effect of Interference

Electrical or magnetic signals only act as interference when they reach the input of the amplifiers that are used to record neuroelectrical potentials in intraoperative neurophysiological monitoring. To effectively reduce electrical and magnetic interference, it is important to understand how electrical and magnetic fields can reach the input of recording amplifiers and generate an output of these amplifiers that can interfere with the neuroelectrical signals that are recorded for the purpose of intraoperative neurophysiological monitoring. When a source of interference has been identified, its effect on recordings can therefore be minimized in two ways, namely by reducing the emission of the interference signal and by hindering the interference signal from entering the amplifiers.

Electrical Interference. The first action to be taken in efforts to reduce the effect of electrical interference is to reduce the emission of the interference signals and then seek methods to reduce the entrance of the signals into the amplifiers used for recording neuroelectrical potentials. Moving the equipment that emits the interference away from the recording equipment, especially the wires of the recording electrodes, is one option. Twisting or braiding the electrode wires that are connected to the input of a differential amplifier is perhaps the most effective way to reduce interference that is picked up by the electrode wires from electric fields. This method is effective because it will make the two leads that serve as input to a differential amplifiers pick up approximately the same amount of interference. Differential amplifiers are only sensitive to the difference between the potentials that reach the two inputs; therefore, the amount of the interference that appears at the output will be greatly reduced by twisting or braiding electrode wires. If the electrode wires are widely separated, they will pick up different amounts of interference and that will cause a large output of the amplifiers. Using the shortest possible electrode leads is another effective means to reduce the amount of electrical interference that electrode leads can pick up.

The electrode impedance should be kept as low as possible because the leads to electrodes that have high impedance pick up more

interference than leads to low-impedance electrodes. If platinum needle reusable electrodes are used, they must be treated correctly by soaking in a chlorine solution to remove the coating of proteins that otherwise will increase their impedance. (Such treatment [unlike autoclaving] will also remove all kinds of pathogenic organism, including virus and agents that are believed to cause degenerative brain disorders such as Creutzfeldt–Jacobs disease.)

When interference with electrophysiological recordings is caused by unshielded or faulty equipment, the remedy is naturally to repair or replace the equipment. If interference is emitted by intact equipment, the best way to reduce the interference is to move the offending equipment as far away from the patient and the leads of the recording electrodes. If the interference is severe, such equipment should be replaced by equipment that causes less interference. It is usually inexpensive equipment that causes the worst interference and, frequently, the problems are solved by replacing such equipment with equipment of better quality. (Such replacements can often be justified not only by the fact that interference is reduced or eliminated but also because the performance often improves as well.)

The situation is much different, and also more severe, regarding equipment that is in (galvanic) contact with the patient and other methods must be used for reducing the conduction of such interference to the recording equipment or to the patient. Grounding of equipment has often been regarded to be the solution to reducing interference from the power line. Whereas it is true that lack of grounding or faulty grounding of equipment can cause severe electrical interference, it is also true that too many ground connections can increase interference. Multiple groundings can create what is known as "ground loops," a condition in which electric current circulates between the various pieces of equipment and the patient. In many cases, the most effective remedy for reducing electrical interference consists of revising the entire grounding system and connecting all the ground wires from all the equipment to one common point. This, however, is not always possible because most equipment is already grounded internally through the safety grounding through the connection to the power line.

It is also common practice to place a ground connection on the patient, but in fact it is often advantageous to remove ground leads to the patient, because the patient might already be grounded through other equipment, such as the equipment used by the anesthesia team. In summary, it is often better to remove ground connections than add ones for reducing interference.

When recording small-amplitude neuro-electrical potentials (such as evoked potentials) from electrodes placed on the head and interference is reaching the recording electrodes from infusion lines, or from electrodes (e.g., EKG electrodes) placed on different parts of the body, the interference can sometimes be reduced by placing the (only) ground electrode on the patient's neck or on the upper portion of the sternum. This can also often reduce the interference from the electrocoagulator — induced by the return pad usually placed on the patient's thigh. Interference from electrocautery equipment could occur even when it is not in use (but switched on). (Nothing can eliminate the severe interference that always occurs during active use of electrocoagulation.)

Reduction of interference is more difficult when intraoperative neurophysiological monitoring includes recording from parts of the body other than the head. When the two recording electrodes that are connected to a differential amplifier are placed far apart, they will pick up more interference than when placed close together; the placement of the grounding electrode might not be much help in reducing the amount of interference signals.

Modern operating rooms are usually equipped with power regulators and isolation transformers that have leakage detectors. Such devices are useful and they no doubt increase safety in the operating room, but they can also cause the impedance of the power line to increase. If a piece of equipment that draws heavy current in only certain phases of the power waveform is connected to the same isolation transformer as the electrophysiological recording equipment, severe interference might result. The obvious remedy is to connect the particular piece of equipment to a different isolation transformer or, even better, to replace the equipment that is causing the distortion of the waveform of the electrical power with better equipment that does not have such adverse properties.

Magnetic Interference. It is generally more difficult to reduce interference caused by a magnetic field than that caused by electrical fields. Because magnetic fields act as interference by the electric current that the magnetic field induces in the electrode leads, the most effective way of minimizing that kind of interference is to keep electrode leads straight because loops of a wire pick up magnetic fields to a greater extent than a straight wire. Magnetic fields can induce electric currents even in straight wires. The electric current that a magnetic field induces in a straight wire depends on the wire's orientation within the magnetic field and it is therefore worthwhile to change the orientation of electrode wires while observing the interference on the computer display (that shows the output of the recording amplifiers) to find an optimal orientation of the electrode leads. Twisting (or braiding) the electrode leads is helpful in reducing interference from magnetic fields, because it makes the magnetic field induce nearly the same current in each one of the leads that is connected to the input of a differential amplifier.

ELECTRICAL SAFETY IN THE OPERATING ROOM

Exposure to electric current in the operating can place patients and the personnel who works in the operating at risk from electrical shock that can be lethal because it can cause heart arrest and cause injuries in the form of burns of the skin and other tissue or by affecting the nervous system.

Patient Safety

The greatest risk to the personnel in the operating rooms comes from the electric power line. This is also a risk to patients, but there are additional electrical risks to patients. One such risk is related to electrical stimulation of nerves and central nervous system (CNS) structures that are used in intraoperative neurophysiological monitoring. Whenever electric current is used to stimulate peripheral nerves, the spinal cord, or the brain, there is a risk that it can cause neural injury if the stimulus strength exceeds a certain level. Applying excessive electric current to the CNS can have many different effects depending on the location of the application of the current. The only way to avoid that risk is to arrange the electrical stimulation so that it is physically impossible to exceed the stimulus strength that might cause injury. If a current that is higher than the safe limit for stimulation can be selected from the stimulator, then there is always a certain risk that (by operator error) stimuli of an unsafe level might be applied. That risk can be reduced (but not avoided) by appropriate training of those who operate the equipment. A clear display of what stimulus current (or voltage) is in use is important for reducing the risks of mistakes. Anesthetized or unconscious patients do not react to dangerous situations and cannot protect themselves from, for instance, stimulation that might imply a risk of injury. Therefore, appropriate safety precautions must be the responsibility of the people who work in the operating room.

Excessive stimulation of motor nerves can cause extremely strong contractions that can injure muscles. Normally, neural safety mechanisms in the spinal cord prevent that from happening by inhibiting the alpha motoneurons, but these safety mechanisms are not active when stimulating a motor nerve electrically. Passing electric current through the heart can cause ventricular fibrillations or cardiac arrest. Excessive electric current applied to the skin through surface or needle electrodes can cause local irritation or injuries in the form of burns. Stimulation with direct current (DC) is the most dangerous and should never be used for stimulation in anesthetized patients. The injury by electrical current is caused mainly by heat, which is proportional to the product of squared value of the current (I) and tissue resistance (R) through which it flows (I^2R) and the amount of time the current is applied. The surface area of the electrode is important; smaller surface area means a higher risk of burns with the same current. Therefore, needle electrodes involve a greater risk of burns than surface electrodes.

Ineffective return leads (pads) from electrocautery equipment can cause burns at the site of recording electrodes that are placed on the skin and connected to equipment that provide a path to ground. That is probably the most common cause of burns of the skin in anesthetized patients. Amplifiers pose a potential risk of applying electric current to the patient through recording electrodes. Some preamplifiers have optic isolation units that isolate the preamplifiers from the other parts of the amplifiers. The other conceivable safety risk is that the supply voltage of the first stage of the amplifier can be delivered to the patient, which can happen if a short circuit in the preamplifier occurs. That can be prevented by solid-state devices placed at the input of the amplifiers that increase the impedance if the input current should exceed a certain (small) value. The limit of current is usually 5 μA, and such devices cause the currents that exceed that limit to practically disconnect the patient from the amplifier.

The increasing use of transcranial electric stimulation using stimulus strength of as much as 1000 V poses safety questions (7). Transcranial electric stimulation and transcranial magnetic stimulation have been feared to cause seizures, but that fear seems to be unwarranted except in patients with seizure disorders. However, it seems unlikely that excessive stimulation could cause brain damage.

The difference between equipment used in the operating room and that used in the clinic also involves electrical safety features. Equipment used in the clinic is often left in the same room for a long time with permanently installed connecting cables, whereas equipment used in the operating room is often exposed to mechanical stress because it is moved frequently and because parts of it might get wet.

Operating room equipment should not expose the patient to dangerous electric current via recording and stimulating electrodes that are applied for monitoring purposes. This is particularly important when recording directly from surgically exposed portions of the nervous system, which is now done during many types of operation. Thus, equipment used in the operating room must comply with the highest standards of electrical safety.

Safety to Personnel Working in the Operating Room

Isolation transformers that are commonly installed in operating rooms isolate the power supply from the primary hospital power supply circuits and often each operating room has its own isolation transformer making the power supply floating in relation to ground. Line isolation monitors are used to detect the degree of isolation quality and sound an alarm in case the leakage current exceeds a certain amount. Leakage current is the total currents flowing from all equipment in the operating room to ground. In the case of excessive leakage currents these monitors will interrupt the power supply. The amount of accepted leakage current has been established by various safety organizations.[1]

Commonly accepted rules state that accessible conductive parts that are connected together must not have potential difference of more than 100 mV. All accessible conductive parts in operating rooms must be grounded. All electrical power-supply outlets must be tested regularly for loose connections and interruption of the safety ground connection.

The limitation for leakage current is different for different kinds of equipment. Equipment belonging to class I are protected by grounding of accessible conductive parts and enclosures , whereas class II equipment are protected by the use of double or reinforced insulation. Class III equipment comprises devices that have internal power supply (batteries) with voltages not exceeding 60 V DC or 24 V AC.

In the United States, equipment that are to be used in the operating room must be approved by the Food and Drug Administration and routine tests must be performed at regular time intervals to ensure that safety of equipment is maintained during the equipment's lifetime. This interval can be defined by the equipment manufacturer but must not exceed 1 yr. All tested equipment must be labeled with a clearly visible expiration date. These safety standards have the form of recommendations, but some states regulate this matter through the hospital accreditation process.

---

[1]The International Standard IEC 60601-1 edited by the International Electrotechnical Committee sets the European norm (IEC 60601-1   Medical electrical equipment Part 1: General requirement for safety, International Standard, International Electrotechnical Commission, March 1995) and UL 2601 edited by Underwriter Laboratories (UL 2601-1   Medical electrical equipment Part 1: General requirement for safety, Underwriter Laboratories Inc., June 2000) in the United States provides the American norms. These standards also define what equipment states are regarded as being either "Normal condition" or "Single fault condition." In normal condition, all protective means built into the equipment must be operable and function as intended. In single-fault condition, one of the protective means can be faulty, but it is the user's responsibility to determine and correct such conditions promptly.

AAMI Standards and Recommended Practice, Volume 2 Biomedical Equipment. Association for the Advancement of Medical Instrumentation, World Trade Press, Novato, CA *(8).*

The role of cable stray capacitance in causing leakage is defined by $C = S/d$, where d is the dielectric constant and has a fixed value, S is the cable surface ($S = 2rl$, where r is the cable radius and l is the cable length), and d is the cable distance to ground or conductive grounded surfaces. Because cable stray capacitance depends on cable length and its distance from the grounded surfaces, it is important to use cables as short as possible and place it as far as possible from the ground. Because its impedance decreases with increased frequency ($Xc = 1/2fC$, high-frequency current sources cause more leakage than low frequency sources (8).

18

Equipment, Recording Techniques, Data Analysis, and Stimulation

INTRODUCTION

In the early days of intraoperative monitoring, either custom-made equipment or equipment taken from the clinical testing laboratory or the neurophysiological animal laboratories was used in the operating room. Now, there is specialized equipment commercially available for nearly all needs of intraoperative monitoring. This means that the persons who do monitoring do not need to know as much about recording and stimulating equipment as they did earlier. However, knowledge about the basic function of the equipment that is used for intraoperative monitoring is an advantage for optimal use of the equipment and for troubleshooting. The equipment now used for intraoperative monitoring is capable of appropriate signal processing and it has several possibilities for filtering the recorded responses. The user must have sufficient knowledge about the basis for filtering and signal averaging to use these methods in optimal ways. Modern equipment also have many options for display of recorded potentials.

The easy access to advanced digital techniques has increased the number of options for setting parameter for recording and stimulating equipment. Most modern equipment allows both stimulus and recording parameters to be controlled through computer commands. To

From: *Intraoperative Neurophysiological Monitoring: Second Edition*
By A. R. Møller
© Humana Press Inc., Totowa, NJ.

make the best choice of settings, the person who does monitoring must know the optimal settings for, for example, obtaining an interpretable recording of evoked potentials in as short a time as possible.

When evoked potentials are monitored, it is the change in the intraoperatively recorded response from the patient's baseline recording that is important. Because data must be interpreted immediately after being collected, special features are required for the equipment that is used for intraoperative monitoring. Thus, the computer systems should permit instantaneous display of a current recording superimposed on a baseline recording and it should provide online quality control of the recorded potentials.

Breakdowns of good quality equipment used for intraoperative monitoring occur rarely, but a malfunction of monitoring equipment during intraoperative monitoring has serious consequences because it makes it impossible to continue monitoring if the malfunction cannot be corrected within a short time.

EQUIPMENT

Commercially available equipment can perform most tasks required for intraoperative monitoring. Several companies now have equipment available that can record and process many channels of electromyographic (EMGs), and multimodality evoked potentials simultaneously. Most commercial equipment contains everything that is needed in one unit: stimulators, amplifiers, signal averagers, display units, and equipment for storing the results.

Equipment used in the operating room is subjected to rough treatment because it is wheeled in and out of different surgical facilities quite regularly; it is therefore important to buy only high-quality equipment for use in the operating room. The cables that connect the equipment to the patient are now the weakest part of equipment used in the operating room. Cables are subjected to mechanical stress in the operating room and often become wet. Equipment used for intraoperative electrophysiological monitoring (amplifiers, stimulators, and computers)—just as other equipment used in the operating room—should therefore be selected not only on the basis of how well it performs the function for which it was designed but also on the basis of its durability, reliability, and electrical safety features. Because the specifications of equipment do not usually include information about properties that make it fail less often than other equipment, it is tempting to select equipment based on the cost alone. It is unfortunate that many hospitals choose products they buy on the basis of cost alone: The least expensive item that meets the specification is often purchased. It might be necessary for a neurophysiologist to document the need for high-quality equipment thoroughly in order to obtain equipment of high quality, which can suit the use in intraoperative monitoring well.

General Requirements of Equipment for Intraoperative Monitoring

Much of the present commercially available equipment is considerably more complex than necessary and has options that are not used. This complexity complicates its use and might increase the possibility of making mistakes. The availability of inexpensive computing power of modern equipment could be better used to improve signal processing than making fancy displays and unnecessary options. In some equipment, complex displays and many options are accompanied by lack of some important basic functions. For example, the option to continuously observe the output

of the physiological amplifiers used in recording of evoked potentials seems to have disappeared from modern equipment. When using averaging, the raw output from the amplifiers should be displayed continuously for observing interference and the interpretation of what kind of interference has occurred. That function was earlier served by an oscilloscope, but now crowded computer displays often lack the possibility to observe the output of the physiological amplifiers, and only through separate commands can the directly recorded potentials be viewed. That makes it difficult to react properly to suddenly occurring interference.

Optimal techniques for signal averaging and aids in interpreting recorded evoked potentials are features that would be useful as would noise-based averaging (p. 312), and digital filtering (p. 320) could be incorporated to a greater extent in the equipment without decreasing, or sacrificing, its user-friendliness. Commercially available equipment (software) has been slow to incorporate desired features such as the capability to use zero-phase finite-impulse response digital filtering, quality control of the recorded potentials, and practical displays.

Equipment that is designed to meet the need to monitor more than one modality of recorded potentials simultaneously is now widely available. Equipment that is designed especially to assist the person who is doing the monitoring as much as possible by aiding in the interpretation of the recordings will most likely also become more common if monitoring professionals make their needs known. Ideally, such equipment would be more user-friendly and present recorded potentials of all types in the most interpretable form for each type of potentials and it would automate such functions as the detection of changes in the latencies of selected components of the recorded potentials are detected.

Amplifiers

In modern equipment, amplifiers consist of two parts: a preamplifier that is located close to the patient (in what is commonly known as the electrode box) and a main amplifier that is located in the main monitoring equipment.

Many modern preamplifiers contain analog-to-digital converters and some equipment makers provide fiberoptic cables between the preamplifier and the main amplifier, which reduces the electrical noise pick-up.

Manufacturers of intraoperative monitoring equipment provide good quality differential amplifiers for recording a variety of neuroelectrical potentials. The amplifiers have built-in filters to attenuate both low-frequency components (high-pass filters) and high-frequency components (low-pass filters). The filter settings as well as the amplification are usually digitally controlled and should be variable and easy to set within wide ranges. Often, the most commonly used settings are factory set as default options. The possibility for the user to set options as defaults is important.

Common Mode Rejection. A differential amplifier is presumed to sense only the difference in the potentials that appear at its two inputs, so that if identical signals appear at the two inputs of a differential amplifier, there should ideally be no output from the amplifier. However, this cancellation of identical signals that are applied to both inputs is known as the common-mode rejection. Manufacturers now offer amplifiers with common-mode rejection of 90 dB (10^9) times. The common-mode rejection ratio given by manufacturers refers to an ideal situation that is rarely attainable. Thus, the practical obtainable common-mode rejection ratio is lower than that given in the specifications for any amplifier. It is also important to consider that for any amplifier, the common-mode rejection ratio given in the specifications applies only to a certain range of frequencies and common-mode rejection for signals with frequencies outside that range is less. Perhaps even more important is the fact that the common-mode rejection ratio that is given in specifications assumes that the sources of the signal that are applied to each of the two inputs of a differential amplifier have exactly the same internal impedances. Such perfect symmetry can rarely be achieved when amplifiers are used to record biological potentials from electrodes placed on the skin or on neural tissue.

This is another reason why the real common-mode rejection ratio will be less than that specified by the manufacturers.

Earlier, another important feature of amplifiers, namely their input impedance, was a concern. However, modern amplifiers have input impedances of as much as 1000 MΩ and that has eliminated that concern for all practical purposes of work in the operating room.

All of these properties only apply for input signals, the amplitudes of which are below certain values. If these values are exceeded and the amplifiers become overloaded, it affects the input impedances and common-mode rejection.

Maximal Output. All amplifiers have a maximal output voltage, and when that has been exceeded, the amplifier cannot properly amplify the input (which is taken to be the difference in potentials that appear at the two input terminals of a differential amplifier). The maximal output voltage varies among different types of amplifier, but it is usually between 5 and 15 V. When, for instance, the amplification is set at 10,000 times, an input signal (e.g., a sine wave) with an amplitude of 0.5 mV will result in an output signal with an amplitude of 5 V. If the maximal output of the particular amplifier is 5 V, then with that setting of the amplification, any input signal above 0.5 mV will overload the amplifier and the output will be a distorted signal with a maximal amplitude of 5 V. Ideally, the amplifier will resume its normal operation when the amplitude of the input signal again decreases below 0.5 mV; however, this is rarely the case. If an amplifier has been subjected to an input voltage that is much higher than that which gives the amplifier's maximal output (in this case, 0.5 mV), common amplifiers become blocked for a period after being overloaded. During that time, the amplifiers will not amplify the input signal properly and the output signal might be near zero or it might be a slowly varying (noise) signal. Overloading of amplifiers used in intraoperative monitoring can result from stimulus artifacts, interference from electrocoagulators, or other sources of strong intermittent electrical interference.

Overloading of a physiological amplifier is more likely to occur when high amplification is used. One way to minimize the risk of blockage of an amplifier from overloading is to use a lower amplification. When signal averaging is used, the amplification can be reduced considerably from that which has been used traditionally (e.g., from 100,000 times to 5000 times) without noticeable problems because the process of signal averaging in itself increases the dynamic range of signal acquisition (*see* p. 309).

Low-Pass and High-Pass Filters. Two kinds of filters are used in the equipment used for intraoperative monitoring. One type is the electronic filter and the other is the digital filter. All physiological amplifiers have built-in (electronic) filters of two kinds: high-pass and low-pass filters. High-pass filters attenuate low frequencies ("pass" high frequencies). Low-pass filters attenuate high frequencies ("pass" low frequencies). (This terminology, which emanates from electrical engineering, seems slightly illogical and some descriptions of filters and their specifications call low-pass filters "high filters" and high-pass filters are called "low filters." Although this might seem more logical, in this volume we used the engineering terminology for filters.

The frequency band between the cutoff frequencies of the low-pass and the high-pass filters are known as the (band) pass and there are special filters that only pass a band of frequencies (band-pass filters). There are also filters the attenuate a narrow band of frequencies (notch filters).

Filters are usually described by their cutoff frequency, which is usually defined as the frequency at which the attenuation reaches 3 dB, but some manufacturers instead list the frequency at which the attenuation reaches 6 dB[1]. Cut-off frequencies for low and high-pass filters

are usually variable and set by the user, often digitally by computer commands.

For common electronic filters, the attenuation increases gradually as the frequency deviates more and more from the cutoff frequency of the filter. The slope of attenuation, given in dB/octave, is different for different types of filter, and unlike the cutoff frequency, the user usually cannot change the slope because it is related to the type of filter that is used. Thus, the attenuation of a low-pass filter might increase at a rate of 6, 12, 18, or 24 dB/octave above the cutoff frequency, depending on the type of filter (one octave corresponds to an increase, or decrease, in frequency by a factor of 2). The same is true for high-pass filters, the difference being that the attenuation increases as the frequency is lowered at rates of 6, 12, 18, or 24 dB/octave. The specifications for filters in monitoring equipment should give the rate of attenuation not only the cutoff frequency, because it not only determines the efficiency of the filter in attenuating high frequencies or low frequencies but it also determines the amount of phase shift to which the signal is subjected by the filter. Phase shift can cause distortion of the waveform of recorded potentials.

Low-pass filters that are built into amplifiers and attenuate high frequencies before the signal is converted to digital form have their greatest importance in preventing aliasing (*see* p. 315) and should be set according to that task. The main need of filtering for the purpose of obtaining the most interpretable record should be served by digital filters that operate on digital signals (*see* p. 320). High-pass filters placed before analog-to-digital conversion have their greatest importance in removing slow (low-frequency) interference that could otherwise overload the amplifier. High-pass filtering that is done for the purpose of producing an

---

[1]The decibel scale is a logarithmic measure of ratios, such as the ratio between the amplitude of the output and that of the input; thus, it is a measure of attenuation or amplification. For voltage ratios, it is defined as $20 \log_{10}(E_o/E_i)$, where E_i is the input voltage and E_o is the output voltage. An attenuation of 3 dB means that the output is 0.707 times the input, a 6-dB attenuation means that the output voltage is half of the input, a 10-dB attenuation means that the output is 0.3 of the input, a 20-dB attenuation means that the output is 0.1 of the input, and so on.

interpretable record can best be performed by digital filtering (*see* p. 320).

Most electronic filters will shift components of recorded potentials, such a peaks and valleys, in time by an amount that depends on the spectrum of the individual peaks in relation to the filter's cutoff frequency and the type of filter that is used. This severely limits the use of electronic filters for aggressive filtering of recordings of evoked potentials where interpretation depends on the ability to determine the absolute values of the latencies of different peaks, such as is the case in the clinic. The reason that ordinary electronic filters shift the different components of a signal differently is that the phase shift that they introduces is not a linear function of frequency *(9,10)*.

The errors introduced by phase shifts are largest when electronic high-pass filters are used, and these errors become greater when these filters have a steep slope of attenuation, but also low-pass filters have phase shift that can cause peaks of a response to shift in time. Common electronic high-pass filters can also cause severe distortion of the waveform and even cause peaks to appear inverted *(11)*. If the phase shift was a linear function of frequency, the shift in time would be the same for all components of a signal, such as the auditory brainstem response (ABR) or the somatosensory evoked potential (SSEP), and the shift in time could therefore be easily compensated for by adding a certain value to the observed latency time of the various peaks. However, filters such as the Bessel filter are more difficult to design than conventional electronic filters *(12)*.

It is a fact that the adverse effects of the phase shift and distortion of the waveform by electronic filters with less steep slope of attenuation has led many manufacturers of amplifiers for physiological signals to use filters with slopes of attenuation of only 6 or 12 dB/octave for both high-pass and low-pass filters, but low-pass filters with slopes of 6 dB/octave often provide insufficient attenuation of the high-frequency interference signals to avoid aliasing (*see* p. 315). High-frequency interference signals are often present in operating rooms as more and more digital equipment and other equipment that "radiate" high-frequency signals has been added to the operating room apparatus. Thus, it is not uncommon for high-frequency components of such interference signals to be folded down into the frequency range of evoked potentials by aliasing (*see* p. 316) if these components are insufficiently attenuated before sampling and digitizing. This occurs often because the rate of attenuation of the electronic low-pass filters that are built into common physiological amplifiers is too low. Therefore, it is advantageous to use low-pass filters that have slope of 24 dB/octave. (The use of a too low sampling rate also contributes to that problem.)

Because high-pass filters are more likely to cause distortion of recorded potentials than low-pass filters, it is preferable to use high-pass filters with 6-dB/octave slopes of attenuation, but filters with 12-dB/octave slopes are acceptable. Low-pass filters should have slopes of at least 18 dB/octave and preferably 24 dB/octave because of the need of attenuating high-frequency interference signals (*see* p. 317).

Notch Filters (Line Frequency Rejection Filters). Many amplifiers have notch filters that are intended for reducing interference from the power line (60 or 50 Hz). However, the use of notch filters is strongly discouraged when recording evoked potentials because notch filters can cause a sharp stimulus artifact to appear as a damped oscillation that can interfere with the biologic potentials that follow and that could be interpreted as part of the recorded bioelectric potentials because the waveform is reproducible. Thus, as a general rule, notch filters should never be used in intraoperative neurophysiological monitoring where stimulus artifacts are present or when the recorded potentials contains sharp waves.

Electrical Stimulators

The electric stimulators used to stimulate neural tissue in connection with neurophysiological recordings usually deliver rectangular impulses, the amplitudes (voltage or current) and durations of which are variable within a wide range as is the repetition rate. A stimulator should be able to generate impulses at a rate in the range of 0.5 and 250 pps. It should be possible to control the stimulus rate continuously or in small steps in order to reduce interference from periodic signals when signal averaging is employed (*see* p. 310). Many computer-controlled stimulators have the option to make the repetition rate vary randomly within a small range and that can reduce the effects of periodic interference signals for recording of evoked potentials when used as stimuli in connection with signal averaging. The repetition rate should be varied in a random fashion by 5–10% of the selected mean repetition rate. The (mean) stimulus rate should be chosen so that it is not a submultiple of the frequency of a periodic interference signal, such as the power-line frequency.

Stimulators used in connection with intraoperative neurophysiological monitoring should have the capability to deliver double pulses with variable intervals. The duration of the delivered impulses should also be variable, from approx 0.05 to 2 ms, and it should be easy to invert the stimulus polarity.

It should be possible to choose between constant-voltage output and constant-current output of the stimulator (*see* Chap. 11) and the stimulus level (voltage or current) should be clearly displayed to reduce the risk of mistakenly setting the stimulus at a level that might cause injury.

There should also be a way to (physically) limit the possibility of a stimulator delivering a current that is in excess of what is regarded to be safe. Stimulators that can deliver a continuous direct current (or voltage) should be avoided entirely in the operating room for reasons of safety. Inexpensive disposable stimulators, some of which deliver a direct electric current, might be effective in stimulating a nerve, but such stimulation might also injure the nerve. Such stimulators should not be used in intraoperative assessment of the function of nerves and central nervous system (CNS) structures.

Stimulators that are used in intraoperative monitoring must have a stimulation isolation unit that causes the output current to be delivered between the two output leads without producing any appreciable current flow between the output leads and the ground. Such isolation units are absolutely essential, for both reducing stimulus artifacts and for patient safety.

Many manufacturers of equipment for intraoperative monitoring now also offer special and separate stimulators for transcranial electrical stimulation as part of equipment for intraoperative monitoring. Magnetic stimulators are offered by some companies as separate equipment.

Constant-Current Versus Constant-Voltage Stimulation. Stimulators can either deliver a constant (or nearly constant) voltage or a (nearly) constant current. Which one of these two options is optimal for use depends on the individual circumstances. Because it is the amount of electric current that flows through the neural tissue that determines the degree of stimulation, it would be ideal that the stimulator delivers a current to the neural tissue that is independent of changes in external circumstances, such as electrode impedance and shunting of current around the neural tissue by fluid and other tissues.

Constant-current stimulators are suitable when the source of variability in the current that is delivered to a nerve is changes in the electrode impedance. Using a constant-current stimulator will prevent changes in the electrode impedance from causing a change in the delivered stimulus current and thus reduce the effect of changes in the electrode impedance on the current delivered to the nerve in question, thus reducing changes in the efficacy of the stimulation. When electrodes placed on the skin are used to deliver electrical stimulation to a peripheral nerve, the electrode impedance will often change spontaneously; thus, a constant-current stimulator would be the best choice. Therefore, it is common in clinical studies where peripheral nerves are stimulated to use a stimulator that delivers a constant current. Some of the stimulus current flows through non-neural tissue located adjacent to the nerve that is to be stimulated, therefore shunting current around the nerve. That shunting of current does not vary very much when stimulating peripheral nerves either with surface electrodes or needle electrodes and, therefore, shunting of stimulus current is not a major concern when stimulating peripheral nerves using electrodes placed on the skin.

In the brain and the spinal cord, however, the situation is different because some fraction of the current applied will be shunted away by the fluid that surrounds the nerve that is to be stimulated *(13,14)*. The amount of current that is shunted away from the nerve will vary from time to time. At one moment, the field might be flooded by cerebrospinal fluid (CSF) and later the fluid will move away and make the area relatively dry. Such change in the degree of wetness causes a varying degree of shunting of stimulus current that is applied for the purpose of stimulating a nerve or other nervous tissue. Stimulation with constant current would therefore result in much of the stimulus current being shunted away when the area is wet, but much less current is lost to shunting when the area is dry, making the current that passes through the tissue that is to be stimulated vary *(13,15,16)* (**Fig. 18.1**). If, for example, a constant voltage is applied to the stimulating electrode in the cerebella pontine angle (CPA), then the change in the shunting of current as a result of the change in condition of the area from wet to dry will not affect the current delivered to a certain volume of tissue and will provide a rather stable delivery of a stimulation of a nerve that is located in such an environment. If the electrode impedance is negligible, the current that flows through a nerve that is located between the stimulating electrodes would be determined only by the electrical resistance of the nerve.

However, because constant-current stimulators have been used so frequently in clinical studies, it was controversial to suggest that the use of stimulators of the constant-voltage type might be more suited for monitoring the facial nerve in operations in the CPA *(13,14)*. It was later suggested that a stimulating electrode insulated except at its tip ("flush-tip" stimulating electrode) *(17)* would reduce the effect of current shunting if a constant-current stimulator is used. Although this is true, it seems more logical to use stimulators that deliver a constant voltage for stimulating in a surgical field where

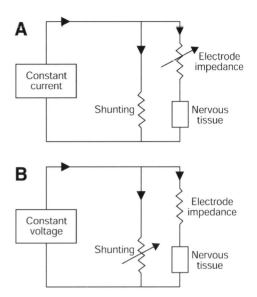

Figure 18.1: Illustration of how a change in electrode impedance and shunting can affect the stimulus current that is delivered to a nerve: (**A**) using a constant-current stimulator; (**B**) using a constant-voltage stimulator.

the degree of wetness and, thus, shunting of stimulus current varies over time. Many modern stimulators can be set to deliver either a constant voltage or a constant current.

A stimulator that delivers a semiconstant voltage with an inner impedance of 1 kΩ together with an electrode impedance of about 3 kΩ, which makes the total inner impedance about 4 kΩ, is suitable for stimulating nerves where the shunting of current varies. With such a stimulator, the current that passes through any part of the tissue is relatively independent of changes in the electrical shunting of the stimulus current caused by changes in the amount of fluid covering the operative field, and the same setting of the output of the stimulator can be used when the operative field is very wet as well as when it is relatively dry.

Thus, choice of the type of stimulator—constant voltage or constant current—that is most suitable depends on whether it is the electrode impedance or the shunting of the stimulus current that is likely to vary most. (These matters are also discussed in connection with monitoring cranial motor nerves and pedicle screws; *see* Chaps. 10 and 11.)

Output Limitations. Electrical stimulators of the constant-current type have limitations as to the load under which they can deliver a certain current. Again, recalling Ohm's law, it becomes evident that if a stimulator is set to deliver 1 mA of current and the electrode impedance is 10 kΩ, the required voltage will be 10 V, which is within the limits of most stimulators. Many stimulators can also deliver 10 mA at that impedance (10 kΩ), which will require a voltage of 100 V. However, if a current of 20 mA is required and the electrode impedance is 10 kΩ, most stimulators will fail because it would require a voltage of 200 V to drive 20 mA through such a load.

Constant-voltage stimulators have similar limitations regarding the current they can deliver into low-impedance loads. Thus, if a constant-voltage stimulator is set to deliver 5 V to an impedance (electrode and tissue impedance) of 5 kΩ, it would only require a current of 1 mA, which is well within the range of all stimulators. Many stimulators set to deliver 50 V with an electrode impedance of 1 kΩ can also provide the required current (50 mA). However, if the voltage were set at 100 V with the same electrode impedance, it would require 100 mA to be delivered, which might be outside the limit of many stimulators. (This amount of voltage is only needed for transcranial electrical stimulation of the motor cortex; *see* Chapter 10.)

Stimulating Electrodes. Needle or surface electrodes are suitable for stimulating peripheral nerves. The same type of needle electrode as used for recording potentials can also be used for stimulation (e.g., subdermal platinum or stainless-steel needle electrodes), but surface electrodes such as EKG pads of the size used in children can also be used for stimulating peripheral nerves and dermatomes. The use of large-surface electrodes stimulates structures other than those anticipated being stimulated and surface electrodes might cause pressure injury when used for extended periods of time. Needle electrodes do not have these disadvantages and they can be placed very close to a peripheral nerve, thus effectively stimulating a specific nerve without stimulating other structures. When stimulating electrodes are placed on motor nerves (or mixed nerves), it is helpful to have the stimulation switched on at the time the electrodes are applied, and observing muscle contractions caused by the stimulation can help position stimulating electrodes close to the respective nerve (naturally, this is provided that the patient is not paralyzed when the electrodes are being placed).

Probing the surgical field to find the location of a motor nerve such as the facial nerve can be done by application of electrical stimulation by the use of a monopolar handheld stimulating electrode *(13)*. An all-metal hypodermic needle is used as a return electrode.

> *Some investigators have described surgical dissection instruments that also could function as stimulating electrodes* (18) *when connected to a stimulator. The purpose of designing such instruments was to be able to warn the surgeon when dissection is being done near a motor nerve.*

The stimulating electrode should be connected to a stimulator via an appropriate interface (stimulus isolation unit) placed outside the sterile field in a way similar to that described for the electrode box used for recording electrodes. Similar arrangements should be made when electrical stimulation of the spinal cord, spinal nerves, or surgically exposed peripheral nerves is done.

Magnetic Stimulation

Magnetic stimulation is used to stimulate peripheral nerves and CNS structures. Magnetic stimulation involves applying an impulse or a train of impulses of a strong magnetic field to the structure in question. The magnetic field is generated by a coil through which a strong electric current is passed. It is not the magnetic field that causes the activation of neural tissue but, rather, the induced electric current. Magnetic stimulation has advantages over electrical stimulation in that it can activate nerves and brain tissue noninvasively (extracranial) without causing any pain. However, the equipment used for magnetic stimulation is bulky and there are limitations regarding how close in time magnetic impulses can be generated. Magnetic stimulation has some use in stimulation of the motor cortex for monitoring motor systems (*see* p. 183).

Sound Generators

Sound generators used in connection with recording ABR (and compound action potentials [CAP] from the auditory nerve and the auditory nervous system) in the operating room should be able to deliver rectangular impulses to an earphone to produce click sounds. The duration of these impulses are usually fixed at 100 μs, which is the standard duration used for most intraoperative monitoring as well as for clinical ABR testing (but not the optimal duration *[19]*). The polarity of the clicks should be easily reversible to produce rarefaction or condensation clicks.

The rate at which stimuli are presented should be variable from 5 to 80 pps, with the most important range being 30–50 pps. It should be possible to modulate the rate of the impulses delivered to the earphone so that the rate varies from 5 to 10% randomly. This will reduce the effect of interference signals that are periodic in nature. If this option is not available, the repetition rates should be variable in small steps so that a repetition rate can be selected that is not a submultiple of the periodicity of electrical interference that might be present. The output of an audio-stimulator should be variable in 5-dB steps, to make it possible to stimulate at different sound intensities. The sound delivered should be calibrated in hearing level (dB HL).

Most audio-stimulators are designed to be used in connection with a specific type of earphone, but they should be sufficiently versatile so that other types of earphones can also be used. However, if earphones are chosen that are different than those supplied with the specific audio-stimulator being used, then it is necessary to calibrate the sound (*see* Chap. 6).

Most manufacturers that supply auditory test equipment offer earphones. Most common are insert earphones that connect to the patient's ear through a (plastic) tube with a length of 20–30 cm. Insert earphones that use a plastic tube for connecting the sound from the transducer to the ear canal are commonly supplied together with intraoperative monitoring equipment. The sound that reaches the ears is delayed from the time the electrical signal is applied to the earphone because of the travel time of the sound in the tube (by approx 1 ms for a tube of 34 cm length). That delay increases the separation of stimulus artifact and response.

Some manufacturers still offer the old TDH39 earphone, which should not be used in the operating room or in the clinic for obtaining ABRs. The inexpensive "Walkman" type of earphone (Chap. 6, **Fig 6.2**), which has been in use for many years, still offers an alternative to the much more expensive insert earphones and it in fact provides a better quality of acoustic signal.

Light Stimulators

Most commercially available visual stimulators are goggles fitted with light-emitting diodes. These are supposed to stimulate the eye through a closed eyelid. Light stimulators have been described that make use of light-emitting diodes bonded to contact lenses *(20),* but this type of device is not commercially available. The light-emitting diodes that are either bonded to contact lenses or placed in goggles can be driven by a common electrical stimulator that can deliver pulses of approx 100 mA. If a constant-voltage stimulator is used, a suitable resistor (of about 1000 Ω) must be placed in series with the light-emitting diodes to limit the current. The duration of the current pulse should be variable between 1 and 50 ms at a repetition rate of 1–5 pps, thus well within the range of most electrical stimulators.

The goggles commonly used in the clinic are usually too bulky for use in the operating room, especially when operating near the eyes. More recently, fiberoptic cables have been used to conduct white light of high intensity to the eye in anesthetized patients. High-intensity light stimulators for use in the operating room have been described (21).

Audio-Amplifiers and Loudspeakers

As mentioned in Chap. 11 in connection with recording muscle potentials (EMG), it is often of great value to have the recorded potentials made audible so that the surgeon can "hear" the potentials (13,22,23). Commercially available EMG amplifiers have built in audio-amplifiers and loudspeakers that have a circuit that suppresses the sound during the time the stimulus is being delivered.

Computer Systems

Currently, computer systems are often based on personal computers using one of Microsoft's operating systems (XP or 2000). Because the hardware of personal computers has sufficient computational and storage capacity for intraoperative monitoring tasks, the focus should be on the available software when selecting a computer system for use in intraoperative neurophysiological monitoring. Often manufacturers are tempted to include many more options than suitable or necessary for use in intraoperative monitoring. Software should include the possibility of setting defaults for types of monitoring so that it is not necessary to (manually) set the parameters for different kinds of monitoring such as the most common modalities of evoked potentials (ABR and SSEP). The computer system should allow digital filtering, artifact rejection, quality control, and so forth in connection with signal averaging. It should be possible to easily review the current settings (amplification, filter cutoff frequencies, stimulus parameters, etc.).

Display Units. The display is an important part of a monitoring system. It should be easy to change and have the ability to show several forms of recorded potential. It is important that the display unit be sufficiently large and the resolution enable fine clarity. The display unit should be able to display at least 8 channels (most modern equipment can display 16 channels) simultaneously. The averaged waveform of sensory evoked potentials, as well as other types of potentials, and a baseline should be

displayed simultaneously. Most manufacturers provide different modes of display such as single traces of, for example, averaged potentials, "water fall" displays (stack), and various forms of trend displays. However, the most practical use in connection with recording of evoked potentials is a simple display of the current recording superimposed on the baseline recording. That provides immediate information about changes in the recorded potentials. The "water fall" displays are suitable for record keeping, showing the history of changes in recorded potentials.

The possibility of displaying different modalities of recorded potentials is important, but there is also a risk of overloading the person who does monitoring by overcrowded displays. Many equipment makers also offer displays of the surgeon's view through a microscope, which is useful for keeping the person who does monitoring aware of what happens in the surgical field. A separate display unit for that purpose is perhaps more suitable than having it together with traces of recorded potentials.

It is important to display the recorded signals directly. This is true even when the recorded potentials are not of sufficient amplitude to be discerned without signal averaging. A direct display of the recorded potentials makes it possible to detect and examine interference signals that might appear in the beginning of a recording as well as at any time (unexpected) during intraoperative monitoring. A display of the raw output of the amplifiers is important for diagnosing the interference that might occur at any time during monitoring and identify the source of electrical interference or other kinds of interference. Switching between displaying averaged responses and the direct output of the physiological amplifiers should be simple, requiring only a minimal number of keystrokes, or, even better, the directly recorded potentials should be shown in a separate window. When displaying only the averaged potentials, the only indication of interference is that all responses are rejected and that is not useful information for identification of the source of the interference.

RECORDING TECHNIQUES

Recording of electrical potentials from nerves, the CNS, and muscles are basic parts of intraoperative neurophysiological monitoring. Three main kinds of potential are recorded in the operating room, namely responses from muscles (EMG potentials) and near-field and far-field potentials from the nervous system. Recordings of these potentials have both commonalities and differences. A fourth kind of neuroelectrical potential are action potentials recorded from single nerve fibers or cell bodies (unit potentials) and from clusters of nerve cells (multiunit recordings); they have become of importance recently for guidance of lesions in the CNS and for implantation of electrodes for deep brain stimulation (DBS).

Recording of Far-Field Evoked Potentials

Far-field sensory evoked potentials such as ABR, SSEP, and visual evoked potential (VEP) are recorded from electrodes placed on the body surface (the scalp). The electrodes used for such recordings can be needle electrodes or surface electrodes. The recording electrodes can be arranged so that both of the electrodes that are connected to a differential amplifier record the same kind of potentials or so that one electrode does not record the evoked potentials in question (using a noncephalic reference electrode).

The amplitude of far-field sensory evoked potentials is mostly less than 1 μV. Even under the best possible recording conditions with a minimal amount of electrical interference, the amplitude of these potentials is lower than the background spontaneous activity from the brain (EEG). Therefore, it is necessary to use signal averaging techniques to obtain records that are interpretable (*see* p. 310).

Recording of Near-Field Evoked Potentials From Peripheral Nerves and the CNS

Near-field sensory evoked potentials are obtained with recording electrodes placed directly on the surgically exposed neural structures. For the purpose of intraoperative monitoring, near-field recordings are done from the

auditory nerve, cochlear nucleus, spinal cord, and the cerebral cortex. Recording of electrical potentials from muscles (EMG) and compound action potentials (CAPs) from peripheral nerves are other examples of near-field responses that are used in intraoperative monitoring. Such potentials can be recorded by placing needle electrodes percutaneously in the structures from which recording is to be made, thus not always requiring surgical exposure. (Unit potentials recorded by microelectrodes from nerve fibers or cell bodies might also be regarded as near-field potentials.)

Near-field potentials can be recorded using equipment similar to that used to record far-field sensory evoked potentials. Because EMG potentials, CAP from nerves, and EMG potentials have much larger amplitudes than far-field evoked potentials, recordings of such potentials do not require signal averaging to make the responses interpretable. Therefore, such recordings can be interpreted immediately after they are acquired and they can usually be observed directly on a computer screen after being amplified or only a few responses might need to be averaged.

Using EMG recordings to detect muscle contractions is far superior to visual observation of muscle contractions. Although several devices that have been described to detect facial muscle contractions using mechano-transducers *(24,25)*, recording EMG potentials is now the most common method for detecting contractions of specific muscles *(13,16,20,26)*.

Bipolar or Monopolar Recordings. Near-field potentials can be recorded either by monopolar recording electrodes or bipolar recording electrodes. Monopolar recording electrodes are easier to place on the structure from which recording is to be made but have less spatial specificity than bipolar recording electrodes.

SIGNAL PROCESSING AND DATA ANALYSIS

Even under the most favorable conditions, the amplitudes of far-field sensory evoked potentials are too small to be discernable in the background noise consisting of ongoing brain activity (EEG) and residual interference from sources outside the patient. Filtering and signal averaging are the two ways used to enhance the responses so that they become interpretable.

Signal Averaging of Evoked Potentials

The use of signal averaging to enhance evoked potentials that appear in a background of noise is based on three assumptions:

1. That the potentials evoked by individual stimuli have the same waveform.
2. That the individual components of the response appear with the same time delay (latency) after the stimulus is delivered.
3. That the waveform of the interfering noise does not have a fixed-time relationship to the presentation of the individual stimuli.

When the signal fulfills the above three criteria and the background noise consists of random noise, then the ratio between the response and the background noise (signal-to-noise ratio [SNR]) is improved by a factor that is the square root of the number of responses that are added together. Adding four responses thus results in a twofold improvement in the SNR. In the same way, it is necessary to increase the number of responses that are added from 1000 to 4000 in order to achieve a twofold increase in the SNR obtained by averaging 1000 responses. if the purpose is to increase the SNR by a factor of 2 when 4000 responses have been averaged, then 16,000 responses must be added instead of 4000. Thus, if the amplitude of the signal is only slightly smaller than that of the noise, a relatively small number of responses need to be added in order to achieve a considerable improvement of the SNR, but when the amplitude of the signal is small compared with the noise, it will take many added responses to obtain the same degree of improvement in the SNR. Thus, when the amplitude of the signal is small compared with that of the noise, signal averaging becomes a slow process to improve the SNR.

The improvement of the SNR by a factor that is the square root of the number of responses that are added is only achieved when the background noise is random noise and when all responses are identical. However, because none of the above-mentioned three criteria is fulfilled under practical circumstances, the improvement in the SNR through signal averaging of neuroelectric potentials is always less than optimal. Management of background noise that is not random (periodic or semiperiodic signals that are buried) is discussed.

All signal averagers in current use employ digital summation of the responses to many identical stimuli. Therefore, the responses are sampled and converted to digital form before they are summed. The interval at which the sampling is performed determines the highest-frequency component that can be handled correctly. Thus, if a sampling interval of 40 μs is chosen (25 kHz sampling rate), only signals with frequencies below 12.5 kHz will be faithfully reproduced in the digitized waveform. In practice, the sampling rate has to be kept somewhat higher than twice the upper frequency limit of interest and the input signal must be properly filtered, to sufficiently reduce the amplitudes of the signals that occur at frequencies higher than half the sampling rate (see p. 315).

Effect of Periodic Interference Signals. Background noise seen in intraoperative recordings is a mixture of biological signals, such as muscle potentials, EEG potentials, and electrical interference potentials, some of which might be more or less periodic. The effects on the averaged responses of the interference that is periodic or semiperiodic in nature can be completely different from those seen when the noise has a random or nearly random character. Although the effects of random noise can be reduced by the signal averaging technique, as described earlier, a similar reduction in the interference from periodic signals can only be realized if certain conditions are fulfilled. Thus, if the repetition rate of the stimulus happens to be a submultiple of the frequency of one such interference signal, the interference signals will add in very much the same way as the stimulus-related responses when the responses are averaged; this means that periodic interference signals might appear in the averaged response with an amplitude that is not much less than it was before averaging. This, in turn, means that periodic interference signals can totally obscure the response. Because signal averaging does not enhance the responses in the noise in such a case, it does not help to add more responses.

When recordings are made from the scalp, spontaneous brain activity (EEG) is a substantial source of background noise, which can be regarded as quasiperiodic in nature, but it is electrical signals generated by various pieces of electrical equipment that constitutes the most severe problems in intraoperative monitoring, because these signals are often periodic in nature.

Naturally, the best way to handle a situation in which interference from periodic signals is present is the same as for nonperiodic signals, namely to reduce the amount of interference that reaches the recording system as much as possible (as discussed in Chap. 17). However, because it is usually not possible to totally eliminate interference in recordings made in the operating room, there is a need to reduce the effects of interference signals on evoked potentials.

An effective way to reduce the effect of periodic interference signals is to set the stimulus repetition rate so that it is not a submultiple of the frequency of the interference, a process that might necessitate the ability to change the repetition rate in small steps. Probably the best way to reduce the effects of periodic interference signals is to modulate the stimulus repetition rate with a random signal. About 5–15% random variation in the stimulus repetition rate is likely to reduce this problem substantially, without having any significant influence on the response. This technique has been used for many years, but it has not yet come into general widespread use and it has not been incorporated into commercial equipment.

Artifact Rejection. When signal averaging is used in connection with recording of evoked potentials, the effect of intermittent interference, the amplitude of which is much larger than those of the recorded potentials, can be eliminated using artifact rejection. Artifact rejection works by excluding recordings in which the amplitude exceeds a certain value. This means that the potential that follows a stimulus is first examined with regard to the amplitude of any component that occurs within the recording time window before it is added to form the averaged response. Commercially available signal averaging equipment for recording sensory evoked potentials has the capabilities for artifact rejection. Some equipment allow the user to set the signal amplitude that triggers artifact rejection and it should be set so that all responses that contain intermittent interference are rejected, whereas all other responses are included in the average. If the threshold for the artifact rejection is set too low, then too many responses will be rejected, and the time it takes to obtain an interpretable recording will be unnecessarily prolonged. If the threshold for rejection is set too high, interference could be included in the averaged response.

Some equipment does not allow the user to set the artifact rejection level; instead, that is set at the maximal output (or slightly less) of the amplifier. That means that the level at which artifact rejection occurs cannot be set independently. If the artifact reject is fixed at a value near the maximal output of the amplifier, artifacts will overload the amplifier and that might affect the following responses because it takes some time for the amplifier to recover. Therefore, artifact rejection level should be set at a faction of the maximal output of the amplifier.

If the artifact rejection is activated by periodic interference signals, it will enhance the appearance of the periodic interference in the averaged response. Continuous interference, such as from the power-line frequency (60 Hz in North America and 50 Hz in Europe), should never be allowed to activate artifact rejection. If the observation window is shorter than one period of the interference, artifact rejection of such interference might result in part of the interference wave to add, generating an odd-looking artifact in the averaged response.

When the background noise contains low-frequency components or slow baseline changes and artifact rejection is based on the amplitude of the recorded signal, these low-frequency components might lead to the activation of artifact rejection. Because this elimination of records occurs in synchrony with the low-frequency components, it might result in the averaged recording appearing as a slanted line on which the response is superimposed. However, a simple computer program (or high-pass digital filtering) can restore the response to a straight horizontal line. If the recorded potential appears on a curved line, as might happen when the interference is a low-frequency signal, the best remedy is to use a zero-phase finite-impulse response digital high-pass filter to remove such a baseline shift.

Some (most) equipment examines the entire record for artifacts; however, it would be advantageous to be able to exclude the earliest part of a record that contains the stimulus artifact from examination for artifacts. This possibility is useful in connection with recordings of responses to electrical stimulation where a large stimulus artifact occurs before the response appears. The equipment should permit the user to select a fraction of the total analysis time window in which the artifact rejection routine checks the amplitude and in which a signal with high amplitude will result in rejection.

Reducing Effects of Amplifier Blockage. The technique for eliminating transient interference from averages of evoked potentials by artifact rejection works well as long as the amplification that is used is low enough so that the amplifier does not become blocked by these transients. However, if the transients are strong enough to block the amplifiers, the amplifiers might fail to work properly when the interference stops and averaging is resumed. Interference resulting from electrocoagulation is an example of interference that often causes blockage of the amplifiers that are being used to record the evoked potentials. Such blocking can last for several seconds after cessation of the electrocoagulation. This means that the output of the amplifiers can be nearly

zero or that the amplification might be lower than normal for several seconds after cessation of electrocoagulation. Many amplifiers generate different types of noise signals as a result of such overloading, and most amplifiers will not operate properly for some time after they begin to recover from overloading. If the output is zero (no amplification), the recording will not be rejected if rejection is based on the amplitude of the signal exceeding a certain value. Because the averaged response is the sum of all recordings that are not rejected divided by the number of recordings, accepting "empty" recordings will result in a lowering of the amplitude of the averaged response. During the recovery period of the amplifiers, the signal might be amplified, but it is often distorted and the amplification is not optimal.

These adverse effects of amplifier blockage can be remedied by having the computer that performs the averaging continue to reject responses for a certain time (a few seconds) while the amplifier is recovering following cessation of electrocoagulation. This means that the computer program must be able to identify when amplifiers have been blocked for a certain time compared with what is caused by a single transient. In fact, more sophisticated computer programs can recognize exactly when the amplifiers have fully recovered after being overloaded because they are able to identify normal noise background. Such computer programs will allow only the recordings that have normal noise background to be added.

Ways to Optimize Signal Averaging. Artifact rejection, as just described, totally eliminates responses that contain too much noise from the average. Other and more sophisticated methods than artifact rejection have been designed to improve the efficiency of signal averaging. One methods, known as weighted averaging *(27,28)* increases the efficiency of signal averaging. Other methods of enhanced signal averaging have been described *(29)*. Such routines are, however, not implemented in equipment that is generally commercially available, despite the fact that the necessary computer capability is now widely available.

Noise that interferes with recording evoked potentials often vary over time. For example, interference from muscle activity often appears in bursts. If all responses with such varying background noise are added together in the conventional way using an ordinary averaging technique, adding more responses might in fact decrease the quality of the averaged response. This paradox might occur because the responses that are added later contain more noise than those that were added earlier. This problem can be reduced by assigning weighting factors to the individual responses, with the values of these weighting factors being dependent on the amount of background noise. Thus, recordings that contain more noise will add less to the resulting average than recordings that contain less noise. Responses that contain a great deal of noise (but less than that needed to trigger the artifact rejection routine) are given less weight than recordings that contain less noise [Bayesian statistics, see ref. 30; sorted averages, see ref. 31)]. Such assigning of different weights to each response, depending on the noise content before the responses are added, can increase the efficiency of signal averaging when the level of the background noise varies over time (30,32). In this way, relatively noise-free recordings will contribute more to the averaged response than noisier responses. Weighted recordings are obtained by first multiplying each recording by a factor that depends on the noise content before the recordings are added together.

Averaging Slowly Varying Evoked Potentials. When signal averaging is used to enhance signals that are buried in noise, it must be remembered that the validity of this technique is based on the assumptions that the waveform of the signals does not change during the period over which averaging is being done and that the time relationship to the stimulus is unchanged during the period over which the averaging is being done. If the waveform of the recorded evoked potentials changes, the averaged response will be the average of the different waveforms of the signal, which means that the waveform of the averaged response will be different from the waveforms of the individual potentials that were averaged; further, the amplitude of the averaged response is likely to be smaller than the amplitude of the responses. This is particularly important to bear in mind when many responses are averaged over long times. The error that could be introduced by averaging many responses is particularly noticeable when ABRs are recorded under unfavorable conditions (low amplitude and a large amount of interference).

Reducing the time over which the responses are averaged can reduce this problem. Filtering of the recorded signal can reduce the number of recordings that must be summed in order to obtain an interpretable record, and when proper filtering is done, the time required to obtain interpretable records in many cases is decreased considerably. It is therefore important to use optimal filtering in addition to the averaging technique to enhance the evoked potentials in intraoperative monitoring and, of course, reduce interference as much as possible.

Quality Control of Evoked Potentials. When signal averaging is used to recover signals buried in noise, the neurophysiologist must ascertain that the averaged waveform is the signal (evoked potential) and not just filtered noise. Repeating the recording is the standard way of verifying this when averaged responses are used clinically. Because the time it takes to obtain an interpretable recording is important in intraoperative monitoring, this method is disadvantageous because it increases the time it takes to obtain an interpretable record. When aggressive filtering is performed after signal averaging, the waveform of filtered noise might resemble evoked potentials, making it even more important to have the means to ensure that the displayed potentials are an evoked response rather than just filtered noise.

One method to obtain a measure of the reliability of an averaged response (illustrated in **Fig 18.2**) compares an averaged response with a similar average in which every other recording is inverted (± average) *(30,33,34)*. Adding and

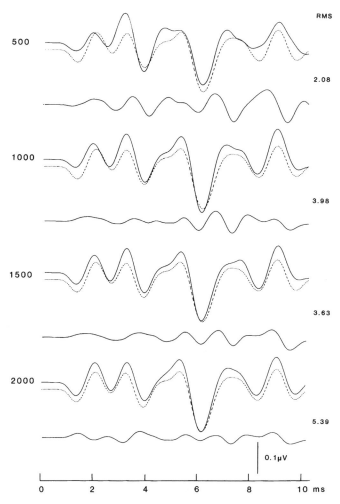

Figure 18.2: Illustration of the use of the ± average for quality control of ABR recordings during intraoperative monitoring. The ABR was recorded in the operating room showing the results of including a different number of responses (given by legend numbers) in the averaged response. The dashed lines show the average of 2500 responses (baseline), whereas the solid lines that nearly follow the dashed lines show the average of a few number of responses (number of responses are shown to the left of each curve). The single solid lines are the ± average of the same number of responses as shown on the curve above it. The vertical scale is the same. The numbers to the right show the ratio between the RMS value of the ordinary average and that of the ± average. Both types of averages were filtered with the W50 zero-phase digital filter described earlier in this volume.

subtracting every other response cancels any signal that is identical, and thus any evoked potential will be canceled by this procedure. This method provides quantitative measures of the validity of recorded potentials such as far-field evoked potentials without requiring replication of the record. It makes use of the assumption that recorded evoked potentials to every stimulus are identical, whereas the superimposed noise varies from time to time. The averaged responses will appear clearer and more consistent as more responses are added, whereas the amplitude of the ± average will remain irregular even when more responses are included. The ratio between the root mean square (RMS) value of the ordinary average and that of the ± average becomes a measure of the amount of noise that the averaged response contains (**Fig 18.2**). If the response is real (different from noise), this ratio will increase as more and more responses are added.

Thus, this method for quality control does not prolong the time it takes to obtain an interpretable recording because the ± average can be obtained simultaneously with ordinary averaging. Examples of ABR recorded in an anesthetized patient undergoing a neurosurgical operation to remove a skull base tumor (**Fig. 18.2**) shows how the ± average decreases in amplitude as more responses are added, and the ratio of the RMS values of the ordinary average and the ± average increases. (Other investigators Wong and Bickford, 1980 *[34]* have used the ratio of variance; the RMS value is the square root of the variance; hence, the RMS values are equivalent to the square root of the values used by Wong and Bickford).

If the response contains a stimulus artifact, as it usually does, it is important not to include this part of the recording in these calculations. For ABR and SSEP recordings, computation of the RMS value should begin 2–3 ms after the stimulus is delivered when recording SSEP, and computation of the RMS value should not include parts of the average that are beyond the region of the response. Before the computation of the RMS value, the mean value of the recorded potentials should be subtracted from the recording. (Such "demeaning" can be done by computing the mean value of all the samples of the signal [not including the earliest period in which the artifact occurs] and then subtracting the mean value from all samples.)

Other methods for quality control of evoked potentials have been described and some of these are implemented in some of the commercially available equipment for use in the operating room.

How to Avoid Aliasing

Aliasing is the term used to describe what happens when a signal that contains energy at frequencies higher than one-half the sampling rate is digitized. The problem of aliasing is probably greatest in connection with averaging of evoked potentials, but it can be a problem in connection with any recorded potentials because practically all modern equipment for intraoperative monitoring digitize recorded potentials before they are displayed or processed. The Nyquist theorem tells us that we can sample and digitize frequency components up to one-half the sampling frequency and preserve the signal faithfully as a digital record. Signals with frequencies higher than half the sampling rate (known as the Nyquist frequency) will be "folded" around the Nyquist frequency after sampling and thus appear as components with a lower frequency in the digitized record. Therefore, high-frequency components must be attenuated by suitable (electronic) low-pass filtering before they are sampled and digitized. Therefore, signals that are to be converted into digital form must not contain (noticeable) energy at frequencies above the Nyquist frequency. This is avoided by using a sufficiently high sampling frequency and by low-pass filtering the signal that is to be sampled and digitized so that components of the signal that have energy above the Nyquist frequency are sufficiently attenuated. Unfortunately, modern equipment for intraoperative monitoring rarely let the user select the sampling frequency.

It has been mentioned elsewhere in this volume that digital filters have advantages over electronic filters for filtering of neuroelectrical potentials. However, electronic filters cannot be entirely substituted by digital filters because only electronic filters that operate on the signal before it is sampled can limit the energy above the Nyquist frequency and thus avoid aliasing. The purpose of low-pass filtering the signal from the amplifiers before it is digitized is to avoid aliasing in connection with sampling of the input signal before analog-to-digital conversion and averaging. The effect of using different sampling frequencies is illustrated in **Fig. 18.3**, which

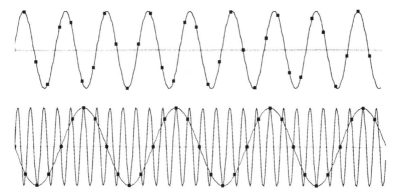

Figure 18.3: A sinusoidal signal at different frequencies that is sampled at 8kHz (125-µs interval) (Nyquist frequency of 4kHz). **(A)** A 2.2-kHz sine wave, sampled at 8 kHz. The sampling points are indicated by squares. **(B)** A 7-kHz sine wave, sampled at 8 kHz. The superimposed sine wave shows the 1 kHz wave that results from aliasing. (From Applet demonstration.)

shows how a correct sampling of a sinusoidal signal can reproduce the signal correctly (**Fig. 18.3A**) and how sampling at too few points (**Fig. 18.3B**) can distort the signal and create signals with frequencies that do not exist in the original signal before sampling has been performed. In the example in **Fig. 18.3B**, a signal with a frequency of 1 kHz is created by sampling a sinusoidal signal of 7 kHz at a sampling rate of 8 kHz.

Sampling a 7-kHz sine wave at a 8-kHz sampling rate violates the sampling theorem and results in an erroneous signal of 1 kHz. That means that the 7-kHz signal that was sampled does not appear as a 7-kHz signal in the digitized form but as a 1-kHz signal (8–7 kHz = 1 kHz).

However, it is rare that biological potentials from the nervous system contain energy at so high frequencies. It is much more likely that such high frequency components are interference signals (Chap. 17, **Fig. 17.3**). Consequently, if such signals exist at the output of the recording amplifiers, they will result in low-frequency interference in the averaged records. Therefore, it is the user's task to make sure that the signals that are sampled and converted to digital form do not contain noticeable energy at frequencies below the Nyquist frequency. In fact, because the slope of attenuation of low-pass filters is finite, it is important to select a cutoff frequency of the low-pass filter in the amplifier that is sufficiently lower than the

Nyquist frequency in order to attenuate the energy of interference signals appropriately; how much lower depends on the slope of attenuation of the filter used and the intensity of the high-frequency interference. If the output of the amplifiers is not attenuated sufficiently, such high-frequency signals might appear as low-frequency interference because of aliasing.

The signal displayed in **Fig. 17.3**, was sampled at 100 kHz, thus a Nyquist frequency of 50 kHz. When that interference signal was sampled at a rate of 25 kHz (**Fig. 18.4A**), low-frequency components that were not seen when the signal was sampled at 100 kHz appear. The strong component at approx 30 kHz (**Fig. 17.3**) now appears as a peak in the spectrum at approx 8 kHz and other high-frequency components of the original signal have been transposed to much lower frequencies.

One of the reasons for that was that the low-pass filter that was set to a cutoff frequency of 3.4 kHz only had a slope of attenuation of 6 dB/octave and that provided insufficient attenuation to suppress these high-frequency components that were present in the signal before it was sampled and digitized. Aliasing of the high-frequency components has occurred because of the lower sampling rate (25 kHz with a Nyquist frequency of 12.5 kHz) causing the spectrum above 12.5 kHz to be transposed to lower frequencies. The component in the original signal that has large energy at approx 25 kHz give rise

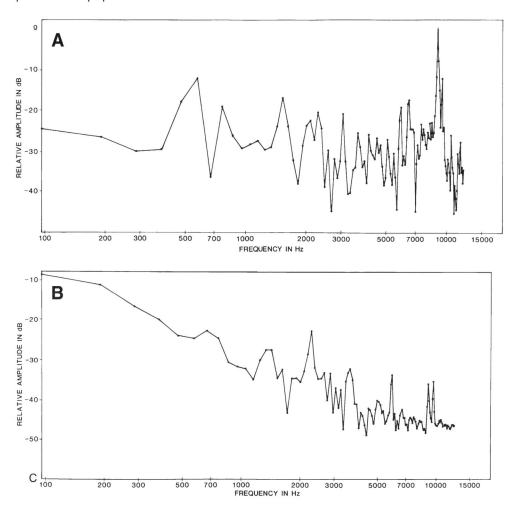

Figure 18.4: The effect of aliasing of a complex interference signal with considerable energy at several high frequencies (spectrum of the signal using a sampling rate of 100 kHz is shown in **Fig. 17.3**, Chap. 17). (**A**) The signal the spectrum of which is shown in **Fig. 17.3** (Chap. 17) but sampled at a rate of 25 kHz. The signal was low-pass filtered before sampling with a filter set to a cut-off of 3.4 kHz and it had a slope of 6 dB/octave. (**B**) Same as in (**A**), but after the low-pass filter was changed to 18 dB/octave.

to a component of approx 500 Hz in the signal after sampling at 25 kHz.

The waveform of the interference signals is altered when the sampling rate is changed from 100 kHz (**Fig. 18.5A**) to 25 kHz (**Fig. 18.5B**), and it is seen that increasing the slope of the low-pass filter that attenuates these high-frequency components in fact reduces the low-frequency components in the sampled and digitized waveform (**Fig. 18.4C**). The change of the low-pass filter that reduced the amplitude of

the high-frequency interference thus reduced low-frequency components in the digitized signal to acceptable levels.

If a sampling rate of 25 kHz is maintained, the remedy to reduce the low-frequency components seen in **Fig. 18.5B** is to attenuate components above the Nyquist frequency (12.5 kHz). That can be done by increasing the slope of attenuation of the low-pass filter that is used to filter signals before analog-to-digital conversion. A change from 6 dB/octave to 18 dB/octave

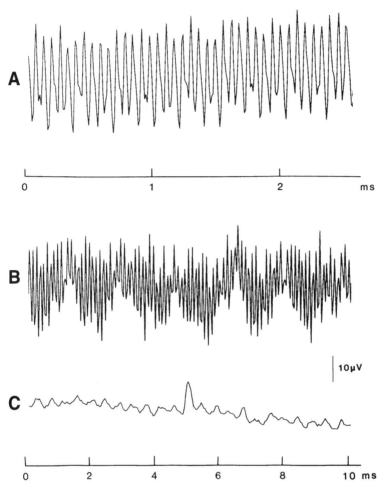

Figure 18.5: The waveform of the digitized signals, the spectra of which are seen in Fig. 17.3 and 18.4. The effect of different sampling rates and different filter settings. (**A**) Sampling rate of 100 kHz and low-pass filter with an attenuation slope of 6 dB/octave and a cutoff frequency of 3.4 kHz (from **Fig. 17.3**). (**B**) Sampling rate of 50 kHz and a low-pass filter with a cutoff frequency of 3.4 kHz and an attenuation slope of 6 dB/octave. (**C**) Same as in (**B**), but the low-pass filter has a slope 18 dB/octave.

seen in **Fig. 18.5C** reduced these components. The low-frequency components in the sampled and digitized signal decreased considerably, despite the fact that it was the high-frequency components of the analog signal that were attenuated.

Thus, it is obvious from the illustrations in **Figs. 18.4** and **18.5** that low-frequency components can arise from aliasing of high-frequency interference components that are not sufficiently

attenuated by the electronic filters before the signal is sampled and converted to digital form. The low-pass filtering that is usually built into physiological amplifiers, such as those commonly used to record evoked potentials, often has a slope of only 12 or 6 dB/octave. A low-pass filter with a slope of 6 dB/octave and set at a cutoff frequency of 3 kHz will only have an attenuation of 20 dB at 30 kHz and 14 dB at 15 kHz, which means an attenuation of only five times. This degree of attenuation is often insufficient to attenuate the high-frequency interference signals that can occur in the operating room to a degree that the aliased components do not interfere with recording of neuroelectrical potentials.

The presence of high-frequency interference components prompted a change in the slope of the attenuation of the low-pass filters in the amplifiers that are used in the operating rooms to amplify evoked potentials from 6 dB/octave to 24 dB/octave. With a cutoff frequency of 3 kHz, the attenuation of a filter with a 24-dB/octave slope is about 40 dB at 13.6 kHz, which means that a 13.6-kHz signal is attenuated by a factor of about 100.

The same results as those obtained by this extra filtering could have been achieved by using a sampling rate of 100 kHz and 1024 data points instead of 256 and then using digital filtering of the averaged response to remove the high-frequency components. This, however, increases the size of the file of the recorded data and requires more computer power for processing of the data, because it generates a larger number of samples in each recording.

In summary, the effect of aliasing on high-frequency interference can be reduced either by adequate filtering of the signal before it is sampled or by increasing the sampling rate. When a high sampling rate is used, high-frequency interference will appear as a high-frequency interference signal, but that can be removed by digital filtering. The choice of which one of these two options to use depends on the availability of suitable electronic filters and on the computer power that is available. If faster computers are available, increasing the sampling rate for solving the problems associated with interference from high-frequency signals might be preferred over analog filtering. However, it is not always a user option to change the sampling rate of modern equipment for intraoperative monitoring.

Filtering

Above, we discussed the need of (electronic) filters of a signal before it is sampled and digitized. In the following, we will discuss the use of filters to enhance recorded neuroelectrical potentials to facilitate interpretation of recorded responses. Filters can enhance the appearance of recorded potentials by attenuating components of the recorded potentials that do belong to the response (noise), making the signal appear cleaner. Filters can also attenuate components of the response that are not important for its interpretation. By increasing the ratio between the response (signal) and the interference (noise) (the SNR), adequate filtering decreases the number of responses that require averaging before an interpretable response can be obtained. In addition, proper selection of filtering techniques can enhance particular features of the response that are of interest, such as the peaks in the ABR or SSEP, thereby making it easier to interpret the recordings. Adequate filtering can extract the most useful information in the responses and enhance the information by displaying it in a more readable way. This is important when evoked potentials are used as a diagnostic aid in the clinic, but it might be even more important for obtaining an interpretable recording in the operating room, where interference might be greater and where it is important to be able to interpret the recording with fewer averaged responses because of the necessity to obtain an interpretable record in as short a time as possible.

When evoked potentials are filtered to suppress noise (improve the SNR), the goal is usually to avoid, as much as possible, attenuating the spectrum of the response while attenuating the energy that is outside the spectrum of the signal as much as possible. However, the assumption that the entire spectrum of evoked potentials must be preserved in order to obtain an interpretable record is not always valid: often only parts of the spectrum of the evoked responses are important for interpreting potentials such as ABR, SSEP, and VEP. For instance, it is easy to show that the low-frequency components of the ABR do not contribute to the identification of the peaks of the response. Because it is the peaks and particularly their latencies that are the most important features of the ABR (as is the case for many other sensory evoked potentials), it is advantageous to enhance these peaks. Evoked potentials such as the ABRs are often rich in low-frequency components, and reducing the low-frequency components of the recorded responses makes it easier to identify the peaks. Filtering might affect the recorded response unfavorably. For example, the use of electronic filters can shift components in time and thereby affect the measurement of latency of individual components of the responses and electronic filters can prolong a sharp initial stimulus artifact so that it covers parts of the response.

The functions of electronic filters can be done by digital filters and digital filters have advantages. Whereas electronic filters that operate on the recorded signal before it is converted to digital form are necessary to avoid aliasing (see p. 315) filtering using computer programs (digital filters) has many advantages over electronic filters for the purpose of improving the appearance of recorded neuro-electric potentials. Many of the disadvantages of electronic filtering can be overcome by the use of zero-phase digital filters that have a finite-impulse response.

Electronic filters were discussed earlier in connection with discussions of equipment. In this part of the chapter, we will discuss digital filters.

Digital Filters. The development of digital computers made it possible to design filters that operate on digitized signals using arithmetic operations implemented by computer programs. Such filters are much more flexible than electronic filters and the filtering process does not need to be physically realizable as is the case for electronic filters. Thus, whereas electronic filters must always operate on the past history of a signal, a digital filter can operate just as well on the future of a signal because the signal that is to be filtered is stored in the computer as a digital file. Therefore, digital filters can be designed to have no phase shift and have a finite-impulse response. Such "zero-phase finite-impulse" digital filters can perform the same attenuation of spectral components as electronic filters, but without causing any shift in the location of the components of recorded potentials (9,35). Digital filters with finite-impulse response that are implemented in the

time domain also have the advantage that they do not cause any spread of energy beyond the duration of their impulse response independent of how large the amplitudes of the signals that are being filtered are. Electronic filters will always cause spread of energy in time, which is important when the recorded potentials have large stimulus artifacts.

When digital filters are used along with signal averaging, it is practical to filter the averaged response rather than to filter the signal before it is averaged, as is done when conventional electronic filters are used. Because the averaging process is a linear process that consists of a summation of responses, filtering after averaging is equivalent to filtering before averaging, except that the artifact rejection will not be affected by the filtering and might therefore work differently, depending on whether the filtering is performed before or after averaging.

Digital filters that are used in commercially available equipment for intraoperative monitoring are often designed to emulate ordinary electronic filters, such as Butterworth filters having low-pass, high-pass, or band-pass characteristics. Zero-phase digital filters can be designed so that they have exactly the same attenuation of signals above or below a certain frequency as ordinary electronic filters, but without a phase shift. Digital filters can also be designed to enhance specific components of the waveform of a signal.

Digital filtering can be performed either in the time domain or in the frequency domain. When digital filtering is done in the frequency domain, the signal that is to be filtered is first Fourier-transformed to obtain its frequency spectrum. The filtering is then done by arithmetic operations on the spectrum of the signal, after which an inverse Fourier transform is made to return the signal to the time domain. When digital filtering is done in the time domain, the sampled and digitized signal is processed directly, and the filtering is done by convolving the signal with a weighting function, which is equivalent to the impulse response of the filter.

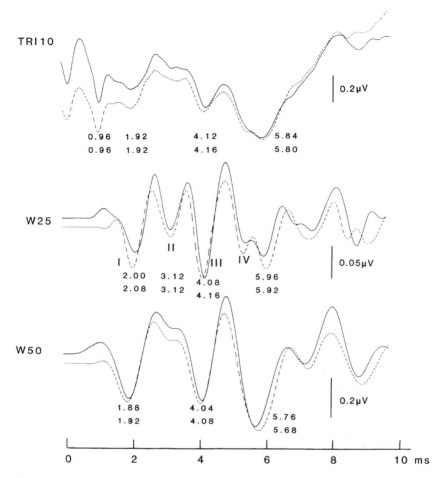

Figure 18.6: ABR recorded in the traditional way (differentially between vertex and mastoid). Each curve is the average of 8192 responses. The responses were sampled at 40-μs intervals. Solid lines: response to rarefaction click; dashed lines: response to condensation clicks. Top curves: filtered only by electronic filters (10–3400 Hz). Tri 10: additional low-pass digital filtering with a filter that has a triangular weighting function (*see* **Fig. 18.7**); W25: digital filtering with a weighting function that provided band-pass characteristics (W25 in **Fig. 18.7**); W50: digital filtering with a filter that has a wider weighting function than the W25 filter (*see* **Fig. 18.7**).

There are several advantages to doing the filtering in the time domain and having the filter function described by its weighting function rather than by its frequency transfer function *(35)*. The arithmetic operation of filtering that consists of convolving the signal with a weighting function might use more computing power than filtering in the frequency domain, but the abundance of computing power in modern equipment makes that difference irrelevant.

Several different kinds of digital filter have been described for use in connection with evoked potentials *(9,10,35)*. The efficiency of zero-phase finite-impulse response digital filters in enhancing the peaks of ABR recordings is demonstrated in **Fig. 18.6**.

A filter that has a triangular weighting function only smoothes the ABR curve (**Fig. 18.7**, TRI10), as would be done by a low-pass filter. The two other filters have characteristics that

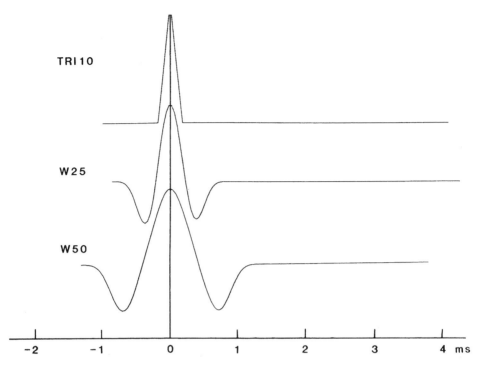

TRI 10

W 25

W 50

−2   −1   0   1   2   3   4 ms

Figure 18.7: Weighting functions of three zero-phase digital filters with finite-impulse response. The time scale assumes a sampling interval of 40 µs.

allow the peaks of the ABR to appear more clearly. One of these filters reproduces peaks I, III, and V of the ABR but does not usually reproduce peaks II and IV. The filter that is suitable for use in clinical testing (**Fig. 18.6, W25**) *(36)* has a narrower weighting function than the W50 filter and it reproduces all of the peaks in the ABR (**Fig. 18.7**, W25). (The W25 and W50 weighting functions resembles truncated $\sin(x)/x$ functions.) The greater noise suppression by the W50 filter makes that filter more suitable for use in intraoperative monitoring than the W25 filter illustrated in **Fig. 18.6** (W25). The fact that W50 filter in **Fig. 18.6** only reproduces peaks I, III, and V of the ABR is not a great disadvantage in intraoperative monitoring (**Fig. 18.8**).

The shape of the frequency transfer function of the three filters, the weighting functions of which are shown in **Figs. 18.6** and **18.8**, is different from that of common electronic band-pass filters. The filter with the triangular weighting function (**Fig. 18.9A**) has a transfer function that is similar to an electronic low-pass filter reproducing signals with no attenuation up to a certain frequency, above which it attenuates the signal to a degree that increases with increasing frequency. The filters in **Fig. 18.9B,C** attenuate both low- and high-frequency spectral components of the signal, but they do not have a part that is flat as commonly used electronic filters. The shapes of the frequency transfer functions of these two filters (**Fig. 18.9B,C**) thus differ from those of the electronic band-pass filters (or a combination of low-pass and high-pass filters) that are commonly used in physiological recording.

The previously discussed digital filters have no phase shift; the peaks in a record that is filtered by these filters appear precisely at the same location as before filtering. However, if similar band-pass filtering had been done using analog (electronic) filters, the latencies of the peaks would have been shifted in time and with a different amount for different

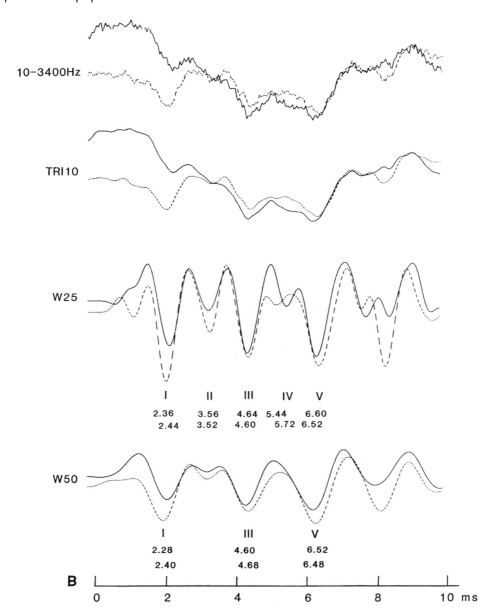

Figure 18.8: Similar recordings as in **Fig. 18.6**, but obtained in the operating room from a patient undergoing an microvascular decompression operation of CN VIII. This graph also shows latency values obtained using computer programs that automatically identify the peaks. Reprinted from: Møller AR. *Evoked Potentials in Intraoperative Monitoring.* Baltimore; MD: Williams and Wilkins; 1988, with permission.

settings of the cutoff frequencies of the electronic filters.

Because the background noise also becomes attenuated by the same filtering process, two advantages have been gained: (1) a clearer recording, thus making more accu-

rate interpretation possible, and (2) a reduction in noise, with the obvious consequence that fewer responses need to be averaged in order to obtain an interpretable recording and, consequently, an interpretable record can be obtained in a shorter time. This is illustrated

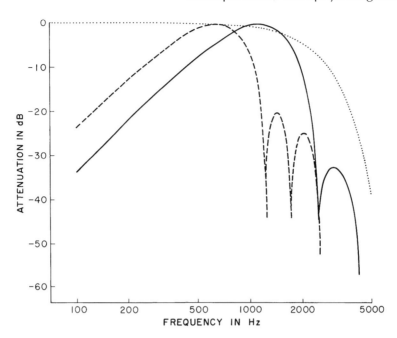

Figure 18.9: Frequency transfer functions of the three digital filters, the weighting functions of which are seen in **Fig. 18.7**. TRI10, Dotted lines; W25, solid lines; W50, dashed lines. The frequency scale corresponds to a sampling rate of 25 kHz.

in the examples ABRs obtained during a neurosurgical operation shown in **Figs. 18.10** and **18.11**. Although the unfiltered averaged responses are noisy to an extent that makes it impossible to identify any of the peaks, peaks I, II, and III appear clearly after filtering with the W50 digital filter.

It would be difficult to determine the latencies of any of the peaks of the ABR in **Fig. 18.11** from examining the raw recordings. Low-pass filtering using the triangular weighting function improves the recording to a point where it might be possible to identify peak V, but not without some difficulty. However, after filtering with the W50 digital filter (**Fig. 18.11**), the record shows a clearly identifiable and reproducible peak V and possibly also a peak III. This shows that digital filtering can thus improve the quality of the averaged responses of ABR of low amplitude with strong interference.

Similar filtering is also beneficial when monitoring other evoked potentials, such as SSEPs. Traditionally, it is the long-latency

components of SSEP that are used for monitoring these responses, but if short-latency components of the upper limb SSEP are to be evaluated, such monitoring can be used even when the patient is under inhalation anesthesia (*see* Chap. 7). Because the amplitude of such potentials is much smaller than the later cortical responses, suitable filtering is valuable for extracting important information. Filters similar to those described to record ABR are just as suitable for this application, provided that the filter functions are chosen appropriately.

Such filtering can enhance the early peaks in a recording of SSEP to median nerve stimulation and thus reduce the number of responses that need to be averaged to obtain an interpretable response (**Fig. 18.12**). Generally, short-latency components of SSEP recorded in response to lower limb stimulation are variable and more difficult to identify.

It is important to emphasize that the weighting functions of zero-phase digital filters, such as those just described, do not have time as

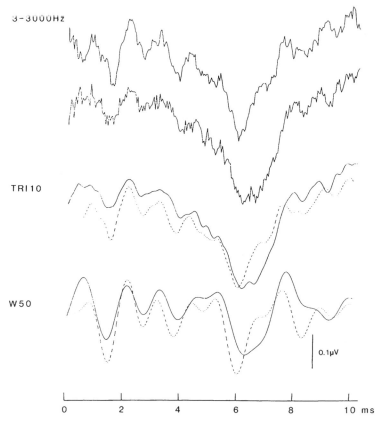

Figure 18.10: Recording of ABR from an electrode placed on the vertex using a noncephalic reference obtained from a patient during an operation to relieve hemifacial spasm. The two upper curves are repetitions of summations of 2048 responses using a filter setting of 3–3000 Hz (6 dB/octave). The middle curves are the same recordings (the repetition is shown by the dashed line), but after low-pass filtering with the TRI10 filter. The lower curves show the same recording, but after digital band-pass filtering with the W50 filter (the weighting function is shown in **Fig. 18.7**). The sampling rate was 25 kHz and each record consists of 256 data points.

their horizontal axis, as does the impulse response of an analog (electronic) filter. Rather, the weighting functions of digital filters have the number of samples as the horizontal axis. Thus, the time axis depends on the sampling interval that is used: the triangular filter shown in **Fig. 18.7** is eight samples wide, which means that it is 0.8 ms wide when a 100-μs sampling interval is used, but it is 0.32 ms wide when a 40-μs sampling interval is used, as in the recordings of the ABR in **Figs. 18.8–18.11**.

More Complex Filtering. Many "intelligent" ways to filter evoked potentials and extract

information from potentials obscured by noise that is not stationary random noise have been proposed and tested (28,38,39). When the spectra of the signal (for instance, evoked potentials) and of the unwanted background noise are known, it is possible to design a filter that will separate the signal from the noise in an optimal way and to define the filter so that it provides an optimal reduction in the mean square difference (error) between the response and the true response. The mathematical basis for this is known as "Wiener filtering" (39,40) and it presumes that the signal (evoked potential) does not vary during the

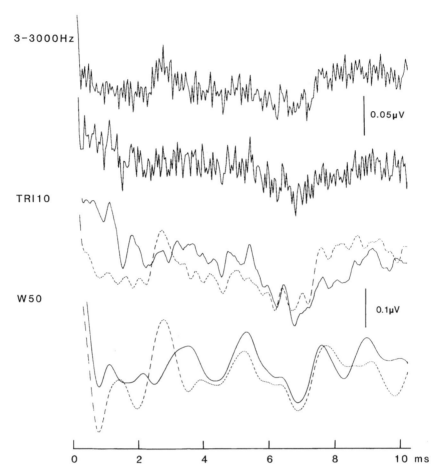

Figure 18.11: Similar recordings of ABR as in **Fig. 18.10**, but recorded in a situation of low amplitude of the response and severe interference. The two top curves are consecutive recording showing the average of 2048 responses each. These two recordings appear as solid and dashed lines in the digitally filtered responses (TRI 10 and W50 filters) in the two lower pairs of curves. The sampling rate was 25 kHz and each record consists of 256 data points.

observation time and that the noise is a stationary broad-band noise. The method further requires that the spectrum of the signal (such as an evoked potential without noise) and that of the background noise are known. However, this kind of complex processing of evoked potentials is not commonly incorporated in commercially available equipment for intraoperative monitoring.

Other more sophisticated systems for filtering evoked potentials makes use of two-dimensional filtering based on Fourier

analysis of the raw responses computed along the time axis as well as along the cross-trial sequence axis. Such filtering has been proven effective in processing of evoked potentials (28) by a method similar to that used for image processing (41). One of the great advantages of these systems is that they can be used when the evoked potentials are expected to change during the recording period. Although there has been little practical experience in the use of such signal processing, it seems to be powerful and could represent one

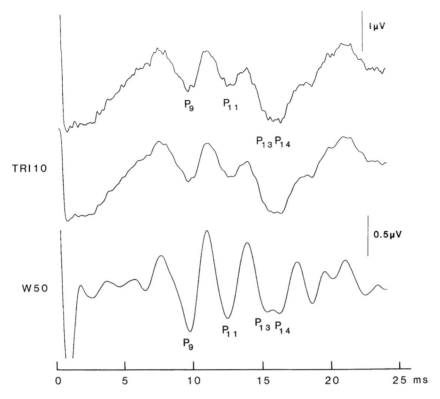

Figure 18.12: SSEP recorded in response to median nerve stimulation in a patient undergoing a neurosurgical operation. Each recording consists of 256 data points. The effects of the same type of filtering as shown in **Figs 18.10** and **18.11** are shown. In this case, the sampling interval was 100 μs and, thus, the base of the triangular weighting function was 0.8 ms, compared to 0.320 ms when used to filter the ABR. The base of the W50 filter was similarly prolonged.

very efficient way to quickly obtain interpretable responses. It has been claimed earlier that the required computing power is large. The feasibility of such processing was demonstrated many years ago by using an array processor connected to a minicomputer of the 1980s (LSI 11/73) (28), which then provided processing in sufficiently short time to make it useful in intraoperative monitoring. With the present state of computers, such analyses could be done using much less complex equipment. However, these techniques have, unfortunately, not found their way to commercially available equipment. The lack of commercially available equipment has also had the result that little experience in their practical use has been acquired.

Reducing Stimulus Artifacts

When an electrical stimulus is used to elicit the response that is to be monitored, some of the stimulus current might spread to the sites of the recording electrodes and thereby be amplified in a way similar to that of the response. This type of interference is known as the stimulus artifact. The electrical signals that are used to drive an earphone to generate an acoustic stimulus can act in a similar way and cause stimulus artifacts to appear in the recorded signal. Magnetic types of acoustic transducer (such as earphones of older design) generate a magnetic field that might also give rise to a stimulus artifact because the magnetic field can create electric currents in the electrode leads. Unshielded earphone leads might cause interference from the electrical signal used to drive the earphone if the leads are unshielded and placed close to the recording electrode leads. Modern earphones produce less stimulus artifacts than older ones. The electrical signal used to drive other transducers, such as light-emitting diodes used to generate flash stimuli in connection with recording VEPs, can cause stimulus artifacts.

Stimulus Artifacts From Electrical Stimulation. The largest and most troublesome stimulus artifacts usually appear in connection with electrical stimulation. Because electrical stimulation of nerves uses electrical impulses of durations between 50 and 200 µs (0.05 and 0.2 ms), the stimulus would not overlap in time with the response and the stimulus artifact itself should therefore not interfere with the response. The stimulus artifact from electrical stimulation only become a problem when it gets smeared out in time (prolonged) by the action of the amplifiers and filters so that it interferes with the recorded potentials. In some instances, the interference from the stimulus artifact might be so severe that it totally obscures the response. Amplifiers might prolong the stimulus artifact if the stimulus artifact overloads the amplifiers. Therefore, one way to reduce the effect of a stimulus artifact is to prevent the stimulus artifact from overloading the amplifier.

Reducing the amplitude of the stimulus, in fact, is the most effective way of reducing the effect of stimulus artifacts. The worst situation usually occurs when recordings are done close to the site of the electrical stimulation. Recording the response from a peripheral nerve to electrical stimulation of the nerve itself at a short distance from the recording site is probably one of the worst situations with regard to stimulus artifacts interfering with the response. In this situation, the response appears with a short latency time after cessation of the stimulus impulse.

When recording is to be made close to the site of stimulation, as, is the case when measuring the nerve conduction time of an exposed nerve, the bipolar recording technique and bipolar stimulation should be used. Even more effective in reducing the stimulus artifact is the use of a tripolar electrode *(42,43)* (Chap. 15, **Fig. 15.2**). The use of a tripolar stimulating electrode eliminates the current path away from the stimulating electrode because the stimulating current has two electrodes through which it can return to the stimulator. Choosing optimal electrode position for electrical stimulation, using correct (low) amplification, selecting the proper type of filtering (digital), and removing the stimulus artifact using computer programs before the averaged signal is subjected to digital filtering are measures that normally can reduce the appearance of stimulus artifacts to acceptable levels.

When signal averaging is used, alternating the polarity of the stimulus can sometimes be of help in reducing the stimulus artifact. This is widely used when recording auditory evoked potentials (alternating rarefaction and condensation clicks); however, this technique should be used cautiously because the stimulus of one polarity might elicit responses that are different from the responses elicited with the inverted polarity. This difference is particularly pronounced in patients with high-frequency hearing loss, such as that commonly seen in elderly patients. Electrically evoked responses from nerves are also dependent on the polarity of the stimulation; therefore, alternating the polarity of the stimuli is not advisable.

Stimulus artifacts can be removed digitally from a digitized record. This method of eliminating stimulus artifacts was used in **Figs. 18.8–18.11**. Used in connection with digital filters that have finite-impulse responses and implemented in the time domain rather than in the frequency domain has made it unnecessary to use shielded earphones when recording ABR intraoperatively and it has considerably reduced the effects of the stimulus artifact on responses that are elicited by electrical stimulation. However, such techniques have not gained acceptance by manufacturers of equipment for intraoperative monitoring. Leakage (spreading of energy) can be eliminated in the time domain *(35)*, but that cannot be done when the filtering is done in the frequency domain.

19

Evaluating the Benefits of Intraoperative Neurophysiological Monitoring

Introduction
Reduction of Postoperative Deficits from Intraoperative Monitoring
Which Operations Should be Monitored?
Efficacy of Intraoperative Monitoring
Consequences of False-Positive and False-Negative Responses
Evaluation of Benefits From Electrophysiological Guidance of the Surgeon
     in an Operation
Benefits From Research in the Operating Room

Guidelines for intraoperative monitoring have been issued by various bodies. The Therapeutics and Technology Subcommittee of the American Academy of Neurology has concluded that the following are useful and noninvestigational: (1) EEG, compressed spectral array, and somatosensory evoked potential (SSEP) in CEA and brain surgeries that potentially compromise cerebral blood flow, (2) auditory brainstem response (ABR) and cranial nerve monitoring in surgeries performed in the region of the brainstem or inner ear, and (3) SSEP monitoring performed for surgical procedures potentially involving ischemia or mechanical trauma of the spinal cord *(44)*. Earlier, the National Institutes of Health Consensus Development Conference (held December 11–13, 1991) stated in a "Consensus Statement" that

There is a consensus that intraoperative real-time neurologic monitoring improves the surgical management of vestibular schwannoma, including the preservation of facial nerve function and possibly improves hearing preservation by the use of intraoperative auditory brainstem response monitoring.

From: *Intraoperative Neurophysiological Monitoring: Second Edition*
By A. R. Møller
© Humana Press Inc., Totowa, NJ.

Intraoperative monitoring of cranial nerves V, VI, IX, X, and XI also has been described, but the full benefits of this monitoring remains to be determined.

In the "Conclusion and Recommendation" of this report it is stated: "The benefit of routine intraoperative monitoring of the facial nerve has been clearly established. This technique should be included in surgical therapy of vestibular schwannoma. Routine monitoring of other cranial nerves should be considered" (Consensus Statement 1991, p. 19).

INTRODUCTION

The benefits from monitoring that is aimed at reducing postoperative neurological deficits should be evaluated both regarding their ability to reduce the risk of iatrogenic injuries to the nervous system in patients who are operated upon and regarding its ability to improve the quality of medical care in general, including providing economic savings. Investigators have concluded that published studies provide sufficient evidence to make recommendation of mandatory use of intraoperative monitoring in many kinds of operations *(45)*. On the basis of studies of literature on outcome and complications, these authors recommend that monitoring be performed in operations on supratentorial central nervous system (CNS) structures (tumors, aneurysms, etc.), brainstem tumors, intramedullary spinal cord tumors, conus–cauda equina tumors; rhizotomy for relief of spasticity, and spina bifida with tethered cord.

Monitoring of SSEP is generally regarded as beneficial in intraoperative assessment of the functional integrity of sensory pathways including peripheral nerves, the dorsal column, and the sensory cortex. Because SSEP cannot provide reliable information on the functional integrity of the motor system, these authors (45) also conclude that monitoring of motor evoked potentials is an important part to assess the functional integrity of descending motor pathways in the brain, the brainstem, and especially the spinal cord.

Although monitoring of ABR is the standard technique for monitoring in operations in the cerebellopontine angle and the posterior fossa, it is also valuable in monitoring general functions of the brainstem (46). It is regarded by many surgeons that mapping techniques such as of the surface of the cortex for determining the location of the central sulcus important and that of the motor nuclei of the VIIth, IXth–Xth, and XIIth cranial nerves on the floor of the fourth ventricle is of great value in identification of "safe entry zones" into the brainstem. However, other techniques, although safe and feasible, have not gained similar acceptance.

The advantage of many of these techniques that are regarded of value in improving outcome and/or decrease the risk of complications have not been confirmed using established quantitative statistical methods of study. The success and the feasibility of the use of spinal motor evoked potentials have been studied in a survey (47) recommending the use of SSEP and motor evoked potentials together in operations where there were risk of spinal cord injury. Auditory evoked potentials (auditory brainstem response [ABR] and compound action potential [CAP] from CN VIII and the

cochlear nucleus) have been found to reduce the occurrence of postoperative hearing loss in studies using historical data (48). The use of motor evoked potentials has been studied in retrospective reviews by several authors who found that SSEP and motor evoked potentials were effective in detecting changes in functions during operations (49,50). However, little quantitative data are available regarding the efficacy of motor evoked potentials in reducing the risk of postoperative complications.

The advantage of using neurophysiological methods for intraoperative guidance and diagnosis has been established for operations to repair peripheral nerve injuries (42). Some studies have shown that neurophysiological recordings improve the outcome for microvascular decompression operations for hemifacial spasm (51,52), but some surgeons have questioned the value of this method of electrophysiological guidance in such operations (53). Some surgeons feel that operations involving placement of electrodes for deep brain stimulation (DBS) should only be carried out with neurophysiological guidance, whereas studies have not been able to find noticeable advantages regarding accuracy in placement (and thus better outcome) or in reduced complications or side effects (54).

There is also a need for evaluating the use of electrophysiological methods in the operating room from an economic point of view because a reduction of potential complications reduces associated cost of medical care. The benefits from the use of neurophysiological monitoring in the operating room also has an economic impact for surgeons and the hospital in that it makes procedures feasible that otherwise were not regarded as safe or feasible. The ability of intraoperative monitoring to reduce the stress on the surgeon should also be regarded as a noteworthy benefit. Few of these benefits from intraoperative monitoring have been verified in statistical studies, but they have been regarded to be of sufficient value that intraoperative monitoring is requested systematically by surgeons. Quantitative information about the intrinsic benefit of intraoperative monitoring is also important for the purpose of deciding which kinds of operation should be monitored.

REDUCTION OF POSTOPERATIVE DEFICITS FROM INTRAOPERATIVE MONITORING

The benefit from reduction of the risk of postoperative neurological deficits has importance in two ways: benefit to the patient (improvement of medical care) and economic benefits for the health care provider. Justification of the use of intraoperative neurophysiological monitoring should rely on quantitative evaluation of the reduction of the risk of postoperative neurological deficits. Therefore, it is an important task for those who do intraoperative monitoring to document the advantages of monitoring. Evaluation of these benefits depends on reliable information about the efficacy of intraoperative monitoring in reducing such risks.

It is not possible to evaluate the benefit of intraoperative neurophysiological monitoring using the conventional double-blind technique. Instead, comparison with historical data has been done, but that method has several kinds of error. One noticeable source of error is the lack of reliable data regarding postoperative deficits in general. Surgeons are usually reluctant to publish their statistics regarding postoperative neurological deficits that can be related to surgical operations. The other uncertainty is related to improved surgical techniques that also have reduced the occurrences of postoperative deficits.

Perhaps the best known benefits are from operations to correct spinal deformities (55,56) and other operations affecting the spinal cord using SSEP and motor evoked potential monitoring (57–63). Such operations had a low rate of severe postoperative neurological deficits, but the deficits in question (paraplegia) were devastating. This means that a reduction from, for example, 1% of severe deficits to 0.5% would be an important improvement regarding human suffering. It would also mean an enormous cost saving even if only cost of care was counted and that saving could justify intraoperative monitoring on a pure economic basis. The reduction in human suffering, not only regarding the individual patients but also for their relatives, is naturally far more important than the bare economic aspects. Benefits from monitoring auditory evoked potentials in operations where the auditory nerve has been at risk have been reported by many investigators (48,64,65), but some investigators have questioned the benefits from such monitoring in specific operations (66). Another use of monitoring of sensory evoked potentials has been reported regarding operations such as carotid surgery (endarterectomy) (67,68).

Studies of the use of facial nerve monitoring in middle ear surgery, both primary and revision surgery, has shown a significant reduction of iatrogenic facial nerve injuries in such operations (69). Similar studies regarding facial nerve monitoring in parotid gland surgery were less convincing regarding benefits from monitoring (70). Likewise, the use of intraoperative monitoring has been found to reduce iatrogenic injuries in connection with insertion of pedicle screws. It has been shown that intraoperative SSEP recording has a good predictive value regarding postoperative absence of deficits in skull base operations (100%) but less effective regarding prediction of postoperative deficits (90%) (71). Other studies agree that intraoperative monitoring of SSEP and ABR can reduce the risk of iatrogenic injuries (72,73), whereas monitoring of VEP seems less efficient in reducing iatrogenic injuries (74), although new techniques might have made such monitoring more effective (21). Intraoperative guidance of the surgeon has been demonstrated to increase the outcome of specific operations such as MVD for HFS (52), and repair of peripheral nerves (42,43). More recently, the use of electrophysiological methods for guidance of implantation of electrodes for DBS or lesions in the basal ganglia and thalamus has gained use and it has been regarded to increase the precision of such procedures (75), although some investigators have failed to find such advantages (54).

The fact that it has not been possible to study the efficacy of intraoperative monitoring with regard to reducing postoperative neurological deficits by using the methods commonly utilized is an obstacle in evaluating the benefits of intraoperative neurophysiological monitoring. It has been difficult to use methods such as double-blind studies that are commonly used to assess the efficacy of medical treatments. Surgeons who have been acquainted with the use of intraoperative neurophysiological monitoring are often reluctant to deprive their patients of intraoperative monitoring because they believe such monitoring to be beneficial to their patients and that excludes the use of studies where patients are randomly assigned for monitoring.

The use of historical data in assessing the frequency of postoperative deficits before and after the introduction of intraoperative monitoring has been cited *(48,76–78)* but such studies have been criticized as providing an overestimation of the role of intraoperative monitoring in reducing postoperative neurological deficits because other developments and improvements in surgical techniques have also contributed to the observed improvement regarding the occurrence of postoperative neurological deficits.

Evaluation of Postoperative Neurological Deficits

A prerequisite for being able to evaluate the neurological deficits that might have been acquired during an operation is that adequate preoperative and postoperative testing are done of the parts of the nervous system that are relevant. For example, complete hearing tests, which should include pure tone audiograms and determination of speech discrimination scores using recorded test words (not "live voice"), should be performed both before and after operations in which there is a risk of injury to the auditory nerve. Evaluations of facial function have improved with the development of a standard grading scale *(3,79)*, but such evaluations still rely on a physician's examination of the patient and can never be totally objective. More objective tests of facial

function have been described *(80,81)* utilizing measurements of the excursions (movements) of selected points on the face using computer programs that display the outlined face of the patient and measure the excursions as the patient performs voluntary face movements. The results derived from both sides of the patient's face are then compared to information obtained before the operation. Such objective methods of evaluating neurological deficits are only available for a few kinds of operations.

Assessment of many other kinds of neurological function still relies on subjective evaluation. For example, evaluation of the function of eye muscles even when evaluated by specialists in this area to a great extent relies on subjective judgments.

Even the most thorough examination and evaluation of postoperative deficits rarely reflect the handicap to which the person is subjected. For example, hearing tests rarely involve evaluation of tinnitus and many times do not include speech discrimination tests. The results of commonly used vestibular tests poorly correlate with the patient's handicap. Examination of motor deficits that are done after an operation involving the spinal cord is mostly concerned with distal limbs thus involving the corticospinal system (lateral system; *see* Chap. 9), whereas much less attention is paid to the medial system that controls the proximal limb muscles and trunk muscles. The reason is that the patients are observed postoperatively while in bed and the focus is on deficits in the use of hands and feet. The implication for a patient with chronic postoperative pain cannot be assessed by a physician's examination of the patient. Postoperative evaluations should be done by persons who are trained to perform the evaluations, and the surgeon who operated on the patient or any member of the surgical team should not do the examination and evaluation of postoperative deficits.

Loss of quality of life is almost never assessed in studies of complications in surgical procedures although it has been shown that decreased quality of life is a rather common complication to operations that involves the

CNS even in cases where there are no objective signs of complications *(82,83)*.

Cost/Benefit Analysis of Reduction in Iatrogenic Injuries Through Monitoring

Only a few kinds of operation have been analyzed regarding the economic feasibility of intraoperative monitoring. Difficulties in estimating the reduction in the likelihood of acquiring a postoperative neurological deficit through the use of intraoperative monitoring and difficulties in estimating the economic implications of neurological deficits *(77)* are two factors that hamper cost/benefit analysis of intraoperative monitoring *(72,73)*. In a few kinds of operation, the cost/benefit ratio has been evaluated. In operations on the middle ear, studies have shown that facial nerve monitoring, for primary and revision surgery is economically beneficial *(69)*. Similar results were obtained regarding monitoring in association with insertion of pedicle screws *(77,78)*. Estimates regarding operations in the cerebellopontine angle also show evidence that intraoperative monitoring is cost-effective *(84)*.

The most extensive cost/benefit analysis of intraoperative neurophysiological monitoring has been presented in connection with operations that might affect the spinal cord. Scoliosis and other back operations have a low rate of occurrence of complications even without monitoring, but the complications of such operations, which are in the form of paraplegia or quadriplegia, are so severe and often affect young people who can be expected to live for a long time that the consequences of even a very few occurrences of such complications are enormous (*see* Chap. 10). Even very conservative estimates of the advantages of intraoperative monitoring show substantial economic benefit from monitoring (Chap. 10).

Although it is relatively easy to accurately determine the costs of implementing intraoperative neurophysiological monitoring, it is much more difficult to estimate the costs involved when postoperative neurological deficits occur and that is one reason why it is difficult to estimate the economic benefit from intraoperative

neurophysiologicalal monitoring. Estimates of the economic costs of postoperative neurological deficits are usually restricted to estimates of cost of care, but such estimates should include an estimate of the economic value of human suffering and loss of quality of life—not only the actual cost of care, for an individual. The value of human suffering has been conspicuously neglected in past discussions of the cost/benefit ratio of implementing any new addition to health care, including intraoperative neurophysiologicalal monitoring.

It is not possible to place a monetary value on every specific type of neurological deficit, and even if this was possible, the monetary values on specific deficits would vary from person to person. The courts of law in the United States grant monetary compensations to patients who have lost neural function resulting from injuries that were regarded as caused by malpractice. Compensation for suffering are often granted when losses of body functions are considered by the courts of law, making the compensation far in excess of the cost of care. If the amounts granted in malpractice suits were used as guidelines for estimating the value of loss of neural functions, the economic costs of iatrogenic injuries would be enormous and would dwarf the costs of the intraoperative monitoring that could reduce the incidence of postoperative neurological deficits. This would be a strong argument to justify the use of intraoperative monitoring in many operations.

Toleikis (77) has reported that his service had monitored more than 1000 patients during placement of more than 5000 pedicle screws. Postoperative assessment showed that only one patient had acquired postoperative neurological deficits caused by a misplaced pedicle screw. This patient had a threshold for stimulation of the pedicle screw that exceeded the established "warning threshold," but the surgeon elected to leave the screw in place. The patient's problems were resolved after removal of the screws and no permanent deficits remained.

Without monitoring, it has been reported that from 2 to 10% of operations have complications in connection with placement of pedicle screws (77). This means that 20–100 patients of every 1000 would have some problems that were related to placement of pedicle screws. The use of monitoring has substantially decreased the risks in connection with placement of pedicle screws and, therefore, reduced complications. Such monitoring is also cost-effective. The estimated cost of monitoring 1000 patients is $1,000,000. If monitoring was implemented, it would have prevented complication in 20 patients (using the lowest estimate of 2%). The direct cost of such complications was estimated to be $50,000 for each patient, but this figure is conservative and the costs of medical treatment for complications from nerve root injuries and rehabilitation can easily exceed $50,000. This means that the direct economic saving from monitoring would be at least $50,000 × 20 = $1,000,000 for each 1000 patients who are operated upon, which means that monitoring is economically sound. Everybody would agree that complications from pedicle screw misplacement means a substantial decrease in quality of life, which cannot be measured in money. Also, consider that the estimates of direct costs are conservative and that the lowest reported rate of complications (2%) without monitoring was used in these calculations. If the highest reported rate of complications is used (10%) the economic savings become substantially greater.

Operations in the cerebellopontine angle, such as those to remove acoustic tumors, carry a large risk of the patient losing facial function postoperatively. Loss of facial function is not only a cosmetic handicap, but it also causes impairment of the eye and makes it difficult for the patient to eat and it definitely implies great loss of quality of life. It is encouraging that the NIH Consensus Conference of Acoustic Tumors (1991) found intraoperative monitoring of value in preventing the loss of facial function following removal of acoustic tumors in the cerebellopontine angle.

However, to date, there have been no estimations published on the economic implications of losing facial function and, consequently, it has not been possible to estimate the benefits of preventing the loss of facial function in economic terms. If loss of facial function would be compensated economically in a similar way as the court of law often compensate loss of function in malpractice lawsuits, the use of intraoperative monitoring of facial function would appear as a highly cost-effective preventative method. Similar reasoning would apply to intraoperatively monitoring of auditory function.

In evaluating human suffering in monetary terms, what are the implications of an elderly person losing facial function compared to a person who could be expected to live for many years? What are the implications of a young musician suffering hearing loss compared with a person who does not have to communicate verbally in a noisy environment?

Several cranial nerves are at risk of injury in skull base operations and the use of intraoperative monitoring can reduce the risk of losing function of cranial motor nerves postoperatively. Loss of function of either CN III or CN XII causes perhaps the most severe handicaps, the risks of which can be reduced by intraoperative neurophysiological monitoring. Cost/benefit analysis has not been applied to such aspects of intraoperative injuries.

Other Benefits From Neurophysiology in the Operating Room

The value of intraoperative neurophysiological monitoring is not limited to reducing the risk of postoperative deficits. For example, intraoperative neurophysiological monitoring have the following benefits:

- Promote the development of better operating methods.
- Improve the outcome of an operation by helping the surgeon reach the therapeutic goal of the operation.
- Shorten the time required to carry out an operation.
- Give the surgeon a feeling of security.

These advantages of monitoring are difficult to evaluate quantitatively (and impossible to assign monetary values), but they contribute noticeably to reducing the risk of postoperative neurological deficits and thereby increasing the quality of medical care in general, and those aspects of the use of monitoring no doubt in many cases reduces the cost of medical care.

WHICH OPERATIONS SHOULD BE MONITORED?

It is important to know the benefits that intraoperative neurophysiological monitoring offers to both the patient and the surgeon when deciding which patients and/or operations should be monitored. Current pressure to increase control over the costs involved in medical care places great demands on health care providers to produce evidence that intraoperative monitoring is indeed cost-effective. Thus, decisions relating to which patients should be monitored intraoperatively are not only based on the benefits to the patient that can be expected from such intraoperative monitoring but also on the immediate cost of intraoperative neurophysiological monitoring in relation to the savings in costs that such monitoring represents regarding postoperative care.

Traditionally, additions to medical care have been introduced and used because of their improvement of the quality of medical care rather than for saving costs. For instance, when intraoperative monitoring of blood pressure was first introduced to the operating room regimen, the (only) question at the time was whether or not it contributed significantly to the promotion of good health care. Naturally, the goal of modern medicine should be to reduce the risks related to the occurrence of any postoperative deficit as much as possible and utilizing all possible means for that goal. Unfortunately, this goal is unrealistic because of present economical constraints on health care, limited availability of skilled personnel, and other resources that cause the quality of medical care to depend on factors other than

scientific and technical capabilities. Because pure economic factors play important roles for decisions regarding the use of new additions to health care, economically based arguments for the implementation of intraoperative neurophysiological monitoring are important in each individual operation.

The question about which patients could (possibly) benefit from intraoperative neurophysiological monitoring depends on many factors that are not always easy to define. One such factor is the patient's preoperative condition. There is no reason to monitor hearing in a patient who is already deaf from the disease for which he or she is being treated or from other causes. Patients with total facial palsy cannot possibly benefit from intraoperative facial monitoring nor can patients with peripheral neuropathies that prevent obtaining preoperative SSEPs. Therefore, decisions on whether a certain type of monitoring should be used in a certain patient must rely on the assessment of the patient's preoperative situation.

Naturally, systems that cannot be affected by the operation should not be monitored. Thus, it would seem unjustified to monitor ABR during an operation to remove a tumor in the frontal portion of the brain. However, it must be considered that ABR is a good indicator of general brainstem function and, therefore, patients who are in poor general condition might benefit from monitoring ABR even if the operations are performed far from the anatomical location of the neural territory covered by ABR monitoring. Thus, a decision on whether to do intraoperative neurophysiological monitoring must be made on the basis of each individual patient as is the case in medical treatment in general.

There might be legal ramifications pertaining to when intraoperative neurophysiological monitoring is employed. A patient who acquires a postoperative deficit following an operation in which monitoring was not done could claim that the likelihood of he or she acquiring the deficit might have been lessened if intraoperative monitoring had been done. An interesting question arises as to whether a surgeon's choice to not use intraoperative monitoring can result in a law suit against (and subsequent conviction of) the surgeon for negligence because known techniques to achieve the best possible outcome of an operation were not utilized.

EFFICACY OF INTRAOPERATIVE MONITORING

The decrease in the risk of postoperative neurological deficits through the use of intraoperative monitoring depends on the quality of monitoring and the expertise of the individuals who are doing the monitoring. If a change in neural function is not detected for one reason or another, then the monitoring is not useful. This is known as a false-negative result. There are many reasons why that might occur. For example, the wrong system might be monitored or the person who is responsible for monitoring might not understand what the changes in the recorded electrical potentials means, or the changes could be obscured in one way or another. If the surgeon does not take action in response to detected changes in function, monitoring has no value. Alarming the surgeon when there is actually no surgically induced change in neural function (false-positive responses) might jeopardize the credibility of the monitoring team and cause the surgeon not to respond when real changes occur.

CONSEQUENCES OF FALSE-POSITIVE AND FALSE-NEGATIVE RESPONSES

In medical diagnostics or in screening for specific diseases, a false-negative response to a test might result in a disease condition being overlooked because the test (mistakenly) indicated an absence of disease. This might result in delay of treatment or no treatment at all. A false-positive response to a test (indicating the presence of a disease when in fact there is no disease present) is less harmful because the results only cause unnecessary additional tests

and examinations and could possibly result in treating a disease that does not exist.

False-negative results in intraoperative neurophysiological monitoring might result in a patient acquiring a postoperative neurological deficit because the occurrence of neural injury was not detected intraoperatively. False-negative results in intraoperative monitoring are therefore serious.

Some investigators have defined false-positive responses in intraoperative monitoring to include all changes in the recorded potentials that do not result in neurological deficits. That definition is unfortunate and reminds one of Russian Roulette. The fact that changes can occur with a minimal risk of neurological deficits is the basis of intraoperative monitoring that makes it possible to detect changes in function before these changes are associated with injuries that cause permanent deficits. This makes it possible to use intraoperative neurophysiological monitoring not as a warning of an eminent disaster but, rather, to provide information that indicates when a particular portion of the nervous system has been affected in a way that might eventually result in a postoperative neurological deficit.

Whereas a false-negative response might result in a serious postoperative neurological deficit, a false-positive response essentially causes only an increase in surgical time; however, if false-positives occur often, they might diminish the surgeon's confidence in intraoperative monitoring. Unexpected dramatic events in the recorded potentials, such as total loss of the recorded potentials, are often signs of a serious condition in the patient's status that must be addressed immediately to avoid the risk of a catastrophic operative outcome. Therefore, a delay in reporting such a change to the surgeon to check equipment or some other possible technical difficulty will most likely reduce the surgeon's chances to reverse the manipulation that caused the change and thereby increase the risk of the patient's acquiring a permanent postoperative neurological deficit. Therefore, such unusual events should be promptly reported to the surgeon. If, in fact, the change in the recorded neuroelectrical potentials had been caused by a technical problem, the cost of alerting the surgeon unnecessarily would be small—simply resulting in a few minutes of lost operating time.

There might be another type of false-positive response in connection with intraoperative monitoring that deserves attention, namely the situation in which the results of intraoperative monitoring show a change in the function of a specific part of the nervous system while, in fact, the observed change in function was caused by harmless events such as irrigation with a cool solution.

Therefore, the number of false-negative responses should be kept to an absolute minimum by all available means, whereas, conversely, false-positive responses (according to the strict definition mentioned above) should be tolerated and in fact might be used to respond to changes in neural function before the likelihood of postoperative permanent deficits become noticeable.

EVALUATION OF BENEFITS FROM ELECTROPHYSIOLOGICAL GUIDANCE OF THE SURGEON IN AN OPERATION

The advantages of guidance of the surgeon in operations are more difficult to evaluate than the benefit from reducing the risk of postoperative deficits. Neurophysiologicalal guidance has made repair of peripheral nerves and treatment for some disorders of cranial nerves more efficient. Additionally, it is the impression that neurophysiologicalal guidance has increased the precision with which therapeutical lesions in specific structures of the CNS can be made and it has made precise implantations of electrodes for permanent stimulation possible. This has increased the efficacy of treatments of many forms of movement disorder and pain, the value

of which is difficult to quantify. However, reviews of articles published regarding a specific operation, pallidotomy, and implantation of electrodes for DBS has not shown advantages of neurophysiologicalal guidance regarding precision or in regard to complication (54). These studies examined published reports. The results of such studies of the literature might not be representative because it is seems more likely that surgeons who use complex procedures will publish their results than surgeons who use less sophisticated methods. This means that studies of published reports on the results of lesioning and implantation of electrodes in the thalamus and the basal ganglia might be biased toward studies using neurophysiologicalal guidance.

BENEFITS FROM RESEARCH IN THE OPERATING ROOM

Even more difficult to evaluate are the advantages from basic and applied research that are done in connection with the use of electrophysiological techniques in the operating room. However, research in the operating room has contributed to development of better treatment, better operating methods with less risk of postoperative deficits, and better understanding of the function of the normal nervous system and the pathological nervous system. Some of these benefits have immediate impact, whereas others have long-term benefit. Converting these benefits into monetary values is impossible and it is even difficult to estimate the extent of the contribution to better care from research. Most people will agree that this aspect of bringing electrophysiology to the operating room can produce enormous progress in the treatment of disorders of the nervous system. In fact, this kind of research has been responsible for much progress in surgical and medical treatment of many different disorders.

References to Section VI

1. Cottrell J, Smith DH. *Anesthesia and Neurosurgery*. Philadelphia, PA: Mosby; 2001.
2. Albin M. *A Textbook of Neuroanesthesia with Neurosurgical and Neuroscience Perspectives*. New York, NY: McGraw-Hill; 1997.
3. Sloan T. Anesthesia and motor evoked potential monitoring. In: Deletis V, Shils JL, eds. *Neurophysiology in Neurosurgery*. Amsterdam: Elsevier Science; 2002.
4. Samra SK. Effect of isoflurane on human nerve evoked potentials. In: Ducker TB, Brown RH, eds. *Neurophysiology and Standards of Spinal Cord Monitoring*. New York, NY: Springer-Verlag; 1988:147–156.
5. McPherson RW, Bell S, Traystman RJ. Effects of thiopental, fentanyl, and etomidate on upper extremity somatosensory evoked potentials in humans. *Anesthesiology* 1986;65:584–589.
6. Harper CM, Nelson KR. Intraoperative electrophysiological monitoring in children. *J. Clin. Neurophysiol.* 1992;9:342–356.
7. MacDonald DB. Safety of intraoperative transcranial electrical stimulation motor evoked potential monitoring. *J. Clin. Neurophysiol.* 2002;19:416–429.
8. Išgum V, Deletis V. Electrical safety in the operating theatre. In: Deletis V, Shils JL, eds. *Intraoperative Neurophysiologicalal Monitoring in Neurosurgery*. New York; 2004.
9. Doyle DJ, Hyde ML. Analogue and digital filtering of auditory brainstem responses. *Scand. Audiol. (Stockh.)* 1981;10:81–89.
10. Boston JR, Ainslie PJ. Effects of analog and digital filtering on brain stem auditory evoked potentials. *Electroenceph. Clin. Neurophysiol.* 1980;48:361–364.
11. Janssen R, Benignus VA, Grimes LM, Dyer RS. Unrecognized errors due to analog filtering of brain-stem auditory evoked responses. *Electroenceph. Clin. Neurophysiol.* 1986;65:203–211.
12. Doyle DJ, Hyde ML. Bessel filtering of brain stem auditory evoked potentials. *Electroenceph. Clin. Neurophysiol.* 1981;51:446–448.
13. Møller AR, Jannetta PJ. Preservation of facial function during removal of acoustic neuromas: Use of monopolar constant voltage stimulation and EMG. *J. Neurosurg.* 1984;61: 757–760.
14. Yingling C. Intraoperative monitoring in skull base surgery. In: Jackler RK, Brackmann DE, eds. *Neurotology*. St. Louis, MO: Mosby; 1994:967–1002.
15. Stecker MM. Nerve stimulation with an electrode of finite size: differences between constant current and constant voltage stimulation. *Comput. Biol. Med.* 2004;34:51–94.
16. Yingling C, Gardi J. Intraoperative monitoring of facial and cochlear nerves during acoustic neuroma surgery. *Otolaryngol. Clin. North Am.* 1992;25:413–448.
17. Prass R, Lueders H. Constant-current versus constant-voltage stimulation. *J. Neurosurg.* 1985;62:622–623.
18. Kartush J, Bouchard K. Intraoperative facial monitoring. Otology, neurotology, and skull base surgery. In: Kartush J, Bouchard K, eds. *Neuromonitoring in Otology and Head and Neck Surgery*. New York: Raven; 1992: 99–120.
19. Møller AR. *Hearing: Its Physiology and Pathophysiology*. San Diego: Academic; 2000.
20. Møller AR. Electrophysiological monitoring of cranial nerves in operations in the skull base. In: Sekhar LN, Schramm Jr VL, eds. *Tumors of the Cranial Base: Diagnosis and Treatment*. Mt. Kisco, NY: Futura;1987:123–132.
21. Pratt H, Martin WH, Bleich N, Zaaroor M, Schacham SE. A high-intensity, goggle-mounted flash stimulator for short-latency visual evoked potentials. *Electroenceph. Clin. Neurophysiol.* 1994;92:469–472.
22. Prass RL, Kinney SE, Hardy RW, Hahn JR, Lueders H. Acoustic (loudspeaker) facial electromyographic monitoring: Part II. Use of evoked EMG activity during acoustic neuroma resection. *Otolaryngol. Head Neck Surg.* 1987;97:541–551.
23. Prass RL, Lueders H. Acoustic (loudspeaker) facial electromyographic monitoring. Part I. *Neurosurgery* 1986;19:392–400.
24. Jako G. Facial nerve monitor. *Trans. Am. Acad. Ophthalmol. Otolaryngol.* 1965;69:340–342.
25. Sugita K, Kobayashi S. Technical and instrumental improvements in the surgical treatment of acoustic neurinomas. *J. Neurosurg.* 1982;57: 747–752.
26. Lanser M, Jackler R, Yingling C. Regional monitoring of the lower (ninth through twelfth) cranial nerves. In: Kartush J, Bouchard K, eds. *Intraoperative Monitoring in Otology and Head and Neck Surgery*. New York, NY: Raven; 1992:131–150.

27. Hoke M, Ross B, Wickesberg R, Luetken-hoener B. Weighted averaging. Theory and application to electrical response audiometry. *Electroenceph. Clin. Neurophysiol.* 1984;57: 484–489.

28. Sgro J, Emerson R, Pedley T. Methods for steadily updating the averaged responses during neuromonitoring. In: Desmedt J, ed. *Neuromonitoring in Surgery.* Amsterdam: Elsevier Science; 1989:49–60.

29. Lam BS, Hu Y, Lu WW, Luk KD. Validation of an adaptive signal enhancer in intraoperative somatosensory evoked potentials monitoring. *J. Clin. Neurophysiol.* 2004;21:409–417.

30. Elberling C. Quality estimation of averaged auditory brainstem responses. *Scand. Audiol. (Stockh.)* 1984;13:187–197.

31. Muhler R, von Specht H. Sorted averaging: principle and application to auditory brainstem responses. *Scand. Audiol. (Stockh.)* 1999;28: 145–149.

32. Hoke M, Ross B, Wickesberg R, Luetkenhoener B. Weighted averaging: theory and application to electrical response audiometry. *Electroenceph. Clin. Neurophysiol.* 1984;57:484–489.

33. Schimmel H. The (+/-) reference: accuracy of estimated mean components in average response studies. *Science* 1967;157:92–94.

34. Wong PKH, Bickford RG. Brain stem auditory potentials: the use of noise estimate. *Electroenceph. Clin. Neurophysiol.* 1980;50:25–34.

35. Møller AR. Use of zero-phase digital filters to enhance brainstem auditory evoked potentials (BAEPs). *Electroenceph. Clin. Neurophysiol.* 1988;71:226–232.

36. Møller MB, Møller AR. Brainstem auditory evoked potentials in patients with cerebellopontine angle tumors. *Ann. Otol. Rhinol. Laryngol.* 1983;92:645–650.

37. Møller AR. *Evoked Potentials in Intraoperative Monitoring.* Baltimore; MD: Williams and Wilkins; 1988.

38. Boston JR, Møller AR. Brainstem auditory evoked potentials. *Crit. Rev. Biomed. Eng.* 1985;13(2):97–123.

39. Walter DO. A posterior "Wiener filtering" of average evoked responses. *Electroenceph. Clin. Neurophysiol.* 1969;27:61–70.

40. Doyle DJ. Some comments on the use of Wiener filtering for the estimation of evoked potentials. *Electroenceph. Clin. Neurophysiol.* 1975;38:533 534.

41. Gonzalez RC. *Digital Image Processing.* Boston, MA: Addison-Wesley; 1977.

42. Happel L, Kline D. Intraoperative neurophysiology of the peripheral nervous system. In: Deletis V, Shils JL, eds. *Neurophysiology in Neurosurgery.* Amsterdam: Academic; 2002:169–195.

43. Happel L, Kline D. Nerve lesions in continuity. In: Gelberman RH, ed. *Operative Nerve Repair and Reconstruction, Volume 1.* Philadelphia, PA: J.B. Lippincott; 1991:601–616.

44. Lopez JR. The use of evoked potentials in intraoperative neurophysiological monitoring. *Phys. Med. Rehabil. Clin. North Am.* 2004;15: 63–84.

45. Sala F, Krzan MJ, Deletis V. Intraoperative neurophysiological monitoring in pediatric neurosurgery: why, when, how? *Childs Nerv. Syst.* 2002;18:264–287.

46. Angelo R, Møller AR. Contralateral evoked brainstem auditory potentials as an indicator of intraoperative brainstem manipulation in cerebellopontine angle tumors. *Neurol. Res.* 1996; 18:528–540.

47. Legatt AD. Current practice of motor evoked potential monitoring: results of a survey. *J. Clin. Neurophysiol.* 2002;19:454–460.

48. Møller AR, Møller MB. Does intraoperative monitoring of auditory evoked potentials reduce incidence of hearing loss as a complication of microvascular decompression of cranial nerves? *Neurosurgery* 1989;24:257–263.

49. Bose B, Sestokas AK, Schwartz DM. Neurophysiologicalal monitoring of spinal cord function during instrumented anterior cervical fusion. *Spine* 2004;4:202–207.

50. Langeloo DD, Lelivelt A, Louis Journee H, Slappendel R, de Kleuver M. Transcranial electrical motor-evoked potential monitoring during surgery for spinal deformity: a study of 145 patients. *Spine* 2003;28:1043–1050.

51. Haines SJ, Torres F. Intraoperative monitoring of the facial nerve during decompressive surgery for hemifacial spasm. *J. Neurosurg.* 1991;74:254–257.

52. Møller AR, Jannetta PJ. Monitoring facial EMG during microvascular decompression operations for hemifacial spasm. *J. Neurosurg.* 1987;66:681–685.

53. Hatem J, Sindou M, Vial C. Intraoperative monitoring of facial EMG responses during microvascular decompression for hemifacial spasm. Prognostic value for long-term outcome:

a study in a 33-patient series. *Br. J. Neurosurg.* 2001:496–499.

54. Hariz MI, Fodstad H. Do microelectrode techniques increase accuracy or decrease risks in pallidotomy and deep brain stimulation? A critical review of the literature. *Stereotact. Funct. Neurosurg.* 1999;72:157–169.

55. Nash CL, Lorig RA, Schatzinger LA, Brown RH. Spinal cord monitoring during operative treatment of the spine. *Clin. Orthop.* 1977;126:100–105.

56. Brown RH, Nash CL. Current status of spinal cord monitoring. *Spine* 1979;4:466–478.

57. Deletis V. Intraoperative neurophysiology and methodologies used to monitor the functional integrity of the motor system. In: Deletis V, Shils JL, eds. *Neurophysiology in Neurosurgery*. Amsterdam: Academic; 2002:25–51.

58. Langeloo DD, Lelivelt A, Journee JH, Slappendel R, de Kleuver M. Transcranial electrical motor-evoked potential monitoring during surgery for spinal deformity: a study of 145 patients. *Spine* 2003;28(10):1043–1053.

59. Nuwer MR, Dawson EG, Carlson LG, Kanim LE, Sherman JE. Somatosensory evoked potential spinal cord monitoring reduces neurologic deficits after scoliosis surgery: Results of a large multicenter study. *Electroenceph. Clin. Neurophys.* 1995;96:6–11.

60. Kothbauer KF. Motor evoked potential monitoring for intramedullary spinal cord tumor surgery. In: Deletis V, Shils JL, eds. *Neurophysiology in Neurosurgery*. Amsterdam: Academic; 2002: 73–92.

61. Nuwer MR. Use of somatosensory evoked potentials for intraoperative monitoring of cerebral and spinal cord function. *Neurol. Clin.* 1988;6:881–897.

62. Nuwer MR, Daube J, Fischer C, Schramm J, Yingling CD. Neuromonitroing during surgery. Report of an IFCN committee. *Electroenceph. Clin. Neurophysiol.* 1993;87:263–276.

63. Tsirikos AI, Aderinto J, Tucker SK, Noordeen HH. Spinal cord monitoring using intraoperative somatosensory evoked potentials for spinal trauma. *J. Spinal Disord. Tech.* 2004;17:385–394.

64. Linden R, Tator C, Benedict C, Mraz C, Bell I. Electro-physiological monitoring during acoutic neuroma and other posterior fossa surgery. *J. Sci. Neurol.* 1988;15:73–81.

65. Polo G, Fischer C, Sindou MP, Marneffe V. Brainstem auditory evoked potential monitoring during microvascular decompression for hemifacial spasm: intraoperative brainstem auditory evoked potential changes and warning values to prevent hearing loss:prospective study in a consecutive series of 84 patients. *Neurosurgery* 2004;54:104–106.

66. Kveton JF. The efficacy of brainstem auditory evoked potentials in acoustic tumor surgery. *Laryngoscope* 1990;100:1171–1173.

67. Haupt WF, Horsch S. Evoked potential monitoring in carotid surgery: a review of 994 cases. *Neurology* 1992;42(4):835–838.

68. Dinkel M, Schweiger H, Goerlitz P. Monitoring during carotid surgery: somatosensory evoked potentials vs. carotid stump pressure. *J. Neurosurg. Anesthesiol.* 1992;4:167–175.

69. Wilson L, Lin E, Lalwani A. Cost-effectiveness of intraoperative facial nerve monitoring in middle ear or mastoid surgery. *Laryngoscope* 2003;113:1736–1745

70. Terrell JE, Kileny PR, Yian C, et al. Clinical outcome of continuous facial nerve monitoring during primary parotidectomy. *Arch. Otolaryngol. Head Neck Surg.* 1997;123:1081–1087.

71. Bejjani GK, Nora PC, Vera PL, Broemling L, Sekhar LN. The predictive value of intraoperative somatosensory evoked potential monitoring: review of 244 procedures. *Neurosurgery* 1998;43:498–500.

72. Fisher RS, Raudzens P, Nunemacher M. Efficacy of intraoperative neurophysiologicalal monitoring. *J. Clin. Neurophysiol.* 1995;12: 97–109.

73. Møller AR. Intraoperative neurophysiological monitoring in neurosurgery: benefits, efficacy, and cost-effectiveness. In: *Clinical Neurosurgery, Proceedings of the Congress of Neurological Surgeons' 1994 Meeting*. Baltimore; MD: Williams and Wilkins; 1995: 171–179.

74. Cedzich C, Schramm J, Mengedoht CF, Fahlbusch R. Factors that limit the use of flash visual evoked potentials for surgical monitoring. *Electroenceph. Clin. Neurophysiol.* 1988; 71:142–145.

75. Starr PA, Turner RS, Rau G, et al. Microelectrode-guided implantation of deep brain stimulators into the globus pallidus internus for dystonia: techniques, electrode locations, and outcomes. *Neurosurg. Focus* 2004;17:20–31.

76. Radtke R, Erwin W, Wilkins R. Intraoperative brainstem auditory evoked potentials: signifi-

cant decrease in post-operative morbidity. *Neurology* 1989:187–191.

77. Toleikis JR. Neurophysiologicalal monitoring during pedicle screw placement. In: Deletis V, Shils JL, eds. *Neurophysiology in Neurosurgey.* Amsterdam: Elsevier; 2002:231–264.

78. Toleikis JR, Skelly JP, Carlvin AO, et al. The usefulness of electrical stimulation for assessing pedicle screw placements. *J. Spinal Disord.* 2000;13:283–289.

79. House J, Brackmann D. Facial nerve grading system. *Otolaryngol. Head Neck Surg.* 1985;93: 146–167.

80. Brach JS, Van Swearingen JM, Lenert J, Johnson PC. Facial Neuromuscular Retraining for Oral Synkinesis. *Plastic Reconstr. Surg.* 1997;99: 1922–1931.

81. Johnson PC, Brown H, Kuzon WM, Balliet R, Garrison JL, Campbel J. Simultaneous quantitation of facial movements: the maximal static response assay of facial nerve function. *Ann. Plastic Surg.* 1994;32:171–179.

82. Kato BM, LaRouere MJ, Bojrab DI, Michaelides EM. Evaluating quality of life after endolymphatic sac surgery: the Ménière's Disease Outcomes Questionnaire. *Otol. Neurotol.* 2004;25: 339–344.

83. Nikolopoulos TP, Johnson I, O'Donoghue GM. Quality of life after acoustic neuroma surgery. *Laryngoscope* 1998;108:1382–1385.

84. Kombos T, Suess O, Brock M. Cost analysis of intraoperative neurophysiologicalal monitoring (IOM). *Zentralbl. Neurochir.* 2002;63: 141–145.

APPENDIX
Cranial Nerves: Anatomy and Physiology

We have 12 cranial nerves; some are sensory nerves, some are motor nerves, and some are part of the autonomic nervous system.

I.	Olfactory	Sensory:	Smell
II.	Optic	Sensory:	Vision
III.	Oculomotor	Motor:	Eye Movements: Innervates all extraocular muscles, except the superior oblique and lateral rectus muscles. Innervates the striated muscle of the eyelid.
		Autonomic:	Mediates pupillary constriction and accommodation for near vision.
IV.	Trochlear	Motor:	Eye Movements: Innervates superior oblique muscle.
V.	Trigeminal	Sensory:	Mediates cutaneous and proprioceptive sensations from skin, muscles, and joints in the face and mouth, including the teeth and the anterior two-thirds of the tongue.
		Motor:	Innervates muscles of mastication.
VI.	Abducens	Motor:	Eye Movements: Innervates lateral rectus muscle.
VII.	Facial	Motor:	Innervates muscles of facial expression.
		Autonomic:	Lacrimal and salivary glands.
		Sensory:	Mediates taste and possible sensation from part of the face (behind the ear).
		Nervous intermedius:	Pain around the ear; possibly taste.
VIII.	Vestibulocochlear	Sensory:	Hearing
			Equilibrium, postural reflexes, orientation of the head in space.
IX.	Glossopharyngeal	Sensory:	Taste
			Innervates taste buds in the posterior third of tongue.
		Sensory:	Mediates visceral sensation from palate and posterior third of the tongue.
			Innervates the carotid body.
		Motor:	Muscles in posterior throat (stylopharyngeal muscle).
		Autonomic:	Parotid gland.
X.	Vagus	Sensory:	Mediates visceral sensation from the pharynx, larynx, thorax, and abdomen.
			Innervates the skin in the ear canal and taste buds in the epiglottis.
		Autonomic:	Contains autonomic fibers that innervate smooth muscle in heart, blood vessels, trachea, bronchi, esophagus, stomach, and intestine.
		Motor:	Innervates striated muscles in the soft palate, pharynx, and the larynx.
XI.	Spinal accessory	Motor:	Innervates the trapezius and sternocleidomastoid muscles.
XII.	Hypoglossal	Motor:	Innervates intrinsic muscles of the tongue.

FUNCTIONS OF THE CRANIAL NERVES

CN I. Olfactory nerve: Communicates chemical airborne messages to the brain.

CN II. Optic nerve: Communicates optic information. Variations in contrast are the most powerful stimulations of the visual system.

CN III. Oculomotor nerve: Controls all of the extraocular eye muscles, except the trochlearis and the lateral rectus muscles; thus, it innervates the superior, the inferior, the medial rectus, and the inferior oblique muscles. This muscle moves the eye in all directions; therefore lesions to CN III affect essentially all eye movements and cause the eye to be deviated downward and outward. It also innervates the eyelid and makes it possible to close the eye when lying down. Lesions to CN III cause ptosis (partial closure of the eyelid). CN III contains autonomic fibers that control the size of the pupil and stretches the lens to achieve accommodation. Lesions to the CN III essentially make the eye useless.

CN IV. Trochlearis nerve: Controls the trochlear muscle, and contraction of this muscle causes the eye to move downward when it is in a position medial to the midline. Lesions of CN IV affect downward and inward movements of the eye.

CN V. Trigeminal nerve: This nerve's sensory portion — the portio major — innervates the skin of the face and the cornea. This portion of CN V thereby communicates sensory information about touch and pain from the face and the mouth. CN V is the nerve that causes toothache and the severe pain of trigeminal neuralgia. Lesions to the sensory portion of CN V cause a loss of sensation of the face. Loss of corneal sensation could result in corneal bruises.

The motor potion of CN V — the portio minor — controls the muscles of mastication. Lesions to the motor portion of CN V cause atrophy of the mastication muscles.

CN VI. Abducens nerve: Controls eye movements from the midline toward the side. Lesion to CN VI prevents movements of the eye from the midline and outward.

CN VII. Facial nerve: Controls the face. CN VII is often monitored intraoperatively because it is at risk in all operations to remove acoustic tumors and it is involved in diseases such as hemifacial spasm. The autonomic fibers of CN VII control both tear glands and salivary glands. A loss of facial function is cosmetically important and makes it difficult to eat, and the lack of tears and the inability to close the eye might result in injures to the cornea.

Nervus intermedius: Perhaps taste. Deep ear pain (geniculate neuralgia).

CN VIII. Vestibulocochlear nerve: The two parts of this nerve communicate auditory information and information about head movements. Whereas the covering of the nerve fibers of most of the brainstem cranial nerves changes from peripheral myelin to central myelin a few millimeters from the brainstem, the transitional zone for CN VIII is in the internal auditory meatus, which means that CN VIII throughout its entire intracranial course is covered with central myelin and it has no epineurium. This means that CN VIII has mechanical properties similar to those of the brain, making it more fragile than other cranial nerves.

The vestibular portion of CN VIII communicates to the brain information gathered by the inner ear about the position of the head. In fact, we can do quite well without the vestibular portion of CN VIII, but if it is injured on one side only, severe balance disturbances can result; however, one can adapt to such dysequilibrium depending on one's age (better when younger than when older).

CN IX. Glossopharyngeal nerve: Communicates sensory information from the throat to the brain and information about blood pressure to the cardiovascular centers. The motor portion of CN IX controls the stylopharyngeal muscle. Lesions of CN IX will cause a loss of gag reflex on the affected side and a risk of choking on food. Lesions on one side will likely have little effect on cardiovascular function, but a loss of CN IX on both sides is fatal.

CN X. Vagus nerve: This nerve's name means the "vagabondering" nerve, descriptive in that it travels around in a large portion of the body. This nerve conveys parasympathetic input to the entire chest and abdomen. The vagus nerve also controls the vocal cords, the heart, and the diaphragm. The most noticeable effect of unilateral lesions to CN X is hoarseness, because the vocal cord on the affected side cannot close. Although CN X carries information to and from the heart, unilateral lesions to CN X have little effect on the cardiovascular system, but the effect of bilateral severance of the vagal nerve is severe. The vagus nerve might carry more complex sensory information from the lower body.

CN XI. Spinal accessory nerve: Controls muscles in the neck and shoulder (sternocleidomastoid and trapezoid muscles). Lesions of CN XI cause atrophy of the muscles that are innervated by that nerve.

CN XII. Hypoglossal nerve: Controls movements of the tongue. Unilateral lesions to CN XII cause deviation of the tongue and atrophy of the tongue on the affected side. Bilateral lesions make it almost impossible to speak and swallowing is impaired.

Abbreviations

μS:	Microseconds	ICC:	Central nucleus of the inferior colliculus
AAF:	Anterior auditory field	IPL:	Interpeak latency
ABI:	Auditory brainstem implants	ISI:	Inter stimulus interval
ABR:	Auditory brainstem response	kHz:	Kilohertz
AI:	Primary auditory cortex	kOhm:	Kiloohm
AICA:	Anterior inferior cerebellar artery	LED:	Light-emitting diodes
AII:	Secondary cortex	LGN:	Lateral geniculate nucleus
AP:	Action potentials	LL:	Lateral lemniscus
AVCN:	Anterior ventral cochlear nucleus	mA:	Milliampere
CAP:	Compound action potentials	ma:	Milliampere
CCT:	Central conduction time	MAC:	Minimal end-alveolar concentration
cm:	Centimeter	MCA:	Middle cerebral artery
CM:	Cochlear microphonics	MEP:	Motor evoked potentials
CMAP:	Compound muscle action potential	MGB:	Medial geniculate body
CMN:	Centromedian nucleus	MGP:	Medial segment of globus pallidus
CN I-XII:	Cranial nerves I-XII	MI:	Primary motor cortex
CN:	Cochlear nucleus	mm:	Millimeter
CNAP:	Compound nerve action potentials	MOhm:	Megaohm
CNS:	Central nervous system	ms:	Millisecond
CPA:	Cerebellopontine angle	MSO:	Medial superior olivary nucleus
CPG:	Central pattern generator	mv:	Millivolts
CSF:	Cerebrospinal fluid	MVD:	Microvascular decompression (operations)
CT:	Corticospinal tract		
DAS:	Dorsal acoustic stria	NF2:	Neurofibromatosis type 2
dB:	Decibel	NIHL:	Noise induced hearing loss
DBS:	Deep brain stimulation	NMEP:	Neurogenic motor evoked potentials
DC:	Direct electric current	NTB:	Nucleus of the trapezoidal body
DCN:	Dorsal cochlear nucleus	PAF:	Posterior auditory field
DPV:	Disabling positional vertigo	PD:	Parkinson's disease
DRG:	Dorsal root ganglia	PeSPL:	Peak equivalent sound pressure level
ECoG:	Electrocochleographic	PICA:	Posterior inferior cerebellar artery
EEG:	Electroencephalographic (potentials)	PMC:	Premotor cortical (areas)
EKG:	Electrocardiogram (or electrocardiographic)	pps:	Pulses per second
		PVCN:	Posterior ventral cochlear nucleus
EMG:	Electromyographic (potentials)	REZ:	Root exit zone (or root entry zone)
EPSP:	Excitatory postsynaptic potential	RMS:	Root mean square
GPe:	Globus pallidus external part	SI:	Primary somatosensory cortex
CPG:	Central pattern generator	SMA:	Supplementary motor area
GPi:	Globus pallidus internal part	SNc:	Substantia nigra pars compacta
GPN:	Glosso-pharyngeal neuralgia	SNR:	Signal-to-noise ratio
HD:	Huntington's disease	SNr:	Substantia nigra is the pars reticulata
HFS:	Hemifacial spasm	SOC:	Superior olivary complex
HL:	Hearing level	SP:	Summating potential
Hz:	Hertz, cycles per second	SSEP:	Somatosensory evoked potentials

STN:	Subthalamic nucleus		V:	Volts
TC-MEPs:	Transcranial motor evoked potentials		VAS:	Ventral acoustic stria
			VEP:	Visual evoked potentials
TES:	Transcranial electrical stimulation		Vim:	Intermediary nucleus of the thalamus
TGN:	Trigeminal neuralgia		μS:	Microsecond
TIVA:	Total intravenous anesthesia		μV:	Microvolt
TN:	Trigeminal neuralgia		μA:	Microamps

Index

A

Abducens nerve (CN VI), 177, 207, 343

Abnormal muscle response, 256

Acoustic tumor operations, *see* vestibular schwannoma

Action potentials, nerve fibers, 22, 230, 268

Aliasing, how to avoid, 315

Alpha motoneurons, 157,168, 185, 187, 193

Amplifiers,
common mode rejection, 301
filters, 302
maximal output, 301

Anatomy,
auditory pathways, 61
basal ganglia, 155, 158, 159
cerebellum, 162
cerebral cortex, 62, 65, 71, 81, 82, 157, 160, 173
ear, 55
motor pathways, 157
somatosensory system, 70
spinal cord, 70, 157, 164, 167
visual pathways, 82

Anatomical location of nerve injuries, assessment, 230

Anesthesia requirements,
ABR, 124
cortical evoked somatosensory potentials, 142
guidance for implantation of electrodes for deep brain stimulation, 271
identification of central sulcus, 249
monitoring motor systems, 189, 279
monitoring sensory systems, 279
recording of EMG, 191
recording of EMG potentials, 282
visual evoked potentials, 147

Anesthesia,
basic principles, 279
effect on neuroelectric potentials, 281
inhalation, 279
intravenous, 280

muscle relaxants, 281
total intravenous (TIVA), 280

Anteriorlateral (somatosensory) system, 72

Artifacts, stimulus,
nature, 301, 303, 312, 315, 328
reducing, 304, 307, 320, 327, 328

Ascending auditory pathways,
classical, 61
electrical potentials, 65
non-classical, 62

Ascending somatosensory pathways,
anteriorlateral system, 72
dorsal column system, 70

Ascending visual pathways, 82

Audio amplifiers and loudspeakers, 308

Auditory brainstem implants (ABI),
monitoring placement of electrodes, 267

Auditory brainstem responses (ABR),
as indicator of brainstem manipulations, 118
display, 93
electrode placement, 90
farfield potentials (ABR), 86
interpretation, 105
monitoring, 85
neural generators, 68
optimal filtering, 300
optimal stimulation, 87
processing, 67, 303, 308, 313
stimulus artifact, 301, 303
wave form, 66

Auditory evoked potentials (near field),
interpretation, 105
recording from auditory nerve, 93
recording from cochlear nucleus, 94

Auditory nerve,
as generator of peak I and II of ABR, 69
conduction block, 106
conduction velocity, 69
recording compound action potentials from, 93, 103